Neuroscience: Psychopathology and Diseases

Neuroscience: Psychopathology and Diseases

Edited by Trevor Cornfield

hayle
medical

New York

Hayle Medical,
750 Third Avenue, 9th Floor,
New York, NY 10017, USA

Visit us on the World Wide Web at:
www.haylemedical.com

ISBN: 978-1-63241-889-0

Cataloging-in-Publication Data

Neuroscience : psychopathology and diseases / edited by Trevor Cornfield.
    p. cm.
Includes bibliographical references and index.
ISBN 978-1-63241-889-0
1. Neurosciences. 2. Psychology, Pathological. 3. Nervous system--Diseases. I. Cornfield, Trevor.
RC343 .N48 2020
616.8--dc23

Table of Contents

Permissions

List of Contributors

Index

Preface

The field of medicine that deals with the disorders of the nervous system is referred to as neurology or neurological medicine. It encompasses the diagnosis and treatment of the conditions of the central and peripheral nervous system, and associated tissues, blood vessels, muscles and coverings. Some of the subspecialties of this field include clinical neurophysiology, brain injury medicine, neuromuscular medicine, sleep medicine, pain medicine and neurocritical care, among others. A neurological examination is required if the patient is suspected of having a neurological disorder. It is generally focused on determining if there exist lesions in the central and peripheral nervous systems. Neuroimaging and other neurological tests show correlations between observed and reported mental difficulties as well as provide insights into neural function and differences in brain structure. This book covers in detail some existing theories and innovative concepts revolving around neurological medicine. Different approaches, evaluations, methodologies and advanced studies on neurology have been included herein. A number of latest researches have been included to keep the readers up-to-date with the global concepts in this field.

This book is a comprehensive compilation of works of different researchers from varied parts of the world. It includes valuable experiences of the researchers with the sole objective of providing the readers (learners) with a proper knowledge of the concerned field. This book will be beneficial in evoking inspiration and enhancing the knowledge of the interested readers.

In the end, I would like to extend my heartiest thanks to the authors who worked with great determination on their chapters. I also appreciate the publisher's support in the course of the book. I would also like to deeply acknowledge my family who stood by me as a source of inspiration during the project.

Editor

Improvement and Neuroplasticity after Combined Rehabilitation to Forced Grasping

Michiko Arima, Atsuko Ogata, Kazumi Kawahira, and Megumi Shimodozono

Department of Rehabilitation and Physical Medicine, Kagoshima University Graduate School of Medical and Dental Sciences, Kagoshima, Japan

Correspondence should be addressed to Michiko Arima; michiko@m3.kufm.kagoshima-u.ac.jp

Academic Editor: Pablo Mir

The grasp reflex is a distressing symptom but the need to treat or suppress it has rarely been discussed in the literature. We report the case of a 17-year-old man who had suffered cerebral infarction of the right putamen and temporal lobe 10 years previously. Forced grasping of the hemiparetic left upper limb was improved after a unique combined treatment. Botulinum toxin type A (BTX-A) was first injected into the left biceps, wrist flexor muscles, and finger flexor muscles. Forced grasping was reduced along with spasticity of the upper limb. In addition, repetitive facilitative exercise and object-related training were performed under low-amplitude continuous neuromuscular electrical stimulation. Since this 2-week treatment improved upper limb function, we compared brain activities, as measured by near-infrared spectroscopy during finger pinching, before and after the combined treatment. Brain activities in the ipsilesional sensorimotor cortex (SMC) and medial frontal cortex (MFC) during pinching under electrical stimulation after treatment were greater than those before. The results suggest that training under electrical stimulation after BTX-A treatment may modulate the activities of the ipsilesional SMC and MFC and lead to functional improvement of the affected upper limb with forced grasping.

1. Introduction

The grasp reflex is a primitive reflex that may reappear in the presence of lesions in the frontal lobe. Involuntary movements and dystonia are well-known features of neurodegenerative diseases in the basal nucleus. They are both distressing symptoms and have specific impacts on the quality of life of patients. There are several effective drugs for involuntary movements, such as L-DOPA, trihexyphenidyl hydrochloride, clonazepam, and botulinum toxin type A (BTX-A) [1, 2]. However, the need to treat or suppress the grasp reflex has rarely been discussed in the literature.

BTX-A is a very effective treatment for spasticity and dystonia in patients with stroke, cerebral palsy (CP), or spinal cord injury (SCI) [3]. To our knowledge, there has been no report on treatment with BTX-A for the grasp reflex.

The objective of this case report is to describe the use of BTX-A treatment accompanied by both repetitive facilitative exercises (RFE) and object-related training under low-amplitude continuous neuromuscular electrical stimulation (NMES) for a patient with the grasp reflex after infarction

of the right putamen and temporal lobe. The patient showed functional improvement after BTX-A treatment. The change in brain activity was examined using near-infrared spectroscopy (NIRS).

2. Methods/Case Report

2.1. Design and Subject. This was a single-patient case study. A 7-year-old boy with right cerebral infarction suffered from left hemiplegia, forced grasping, and unilateral spatial neglect. Brain CT scan revealed cerebral infarction of the right putamen and temporal lobe (Figure 1). Two months later, he was admitted to our hospital for rehabilitation for his hemiplegia. The severity of hemiplegia of the left extremities according to the Brunnstrom stage (BRS) was 2 in the upper limb, 1 in the hand, and 4 in the lower limb. He underwent physical and occupational therapy, including RFE [4, 5] and vibratory stimulation of his palm to reduce forced grasping [6]. After his forced grasping improved, he could grasp and release objects voluntarily. After the three-month admission, he could walk independently and returned to usual school

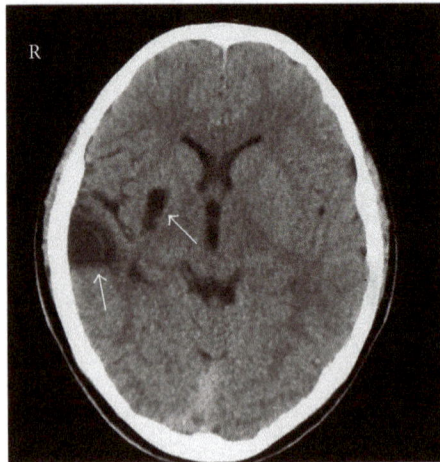

FIGURE 1: Brain lesion in computed tomography (CT). Low-density areas (arrows) in the right putamen and temporal lobe are observed.

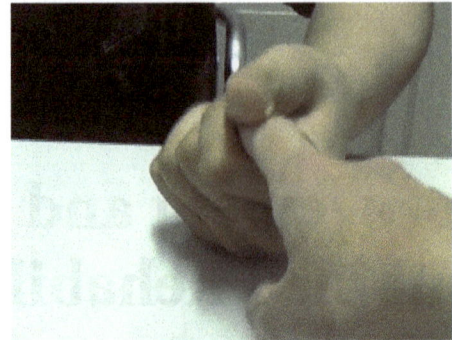

(a)

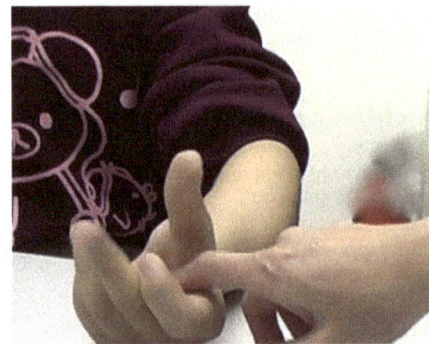

(b)

FIGURE 2: Improvement of the patient's grasp reflex. (a) The patient could not open his hand when the examiner inserted his index finger into the patient's palm before BTX-A treatment. (b) The patient could open his hand when the examiner elicited the grasp reflex after BTX-A treatment.

life. The severity of hemiparesis of the left extremities (BRS) was 6 in the upper limb, 4 in the hand, and 6 in the lower limb. One year after discharge, he developed muscular spasticity and rigidity, and these symptoms gradually deteriorated as he grew older. The effect of vibratory stimulation on his forced grasping weakened. About 2 years later he fell and broke his left upper arm, and his left upper limb developed involuntary movement. This involuntary movement consisted of flexing at the elbow, pronate, and he held his left upper limb behind his body because it would rise up suddenly when he walked. Therapeutic trials with amantadine (100 mg/day) and trihexyphenidyl hydrochloride (2 mg/day) showed a slight benefit. He was treated with botulinum toxin for his upper limb when he was 17 years old. With the improvement of spasticity of the upper arm, the grasp reflex and involuntary movement of the upper limb almost completely disappeared. However, the spasticity of the upper limb and improvement of the grasp reflex deteriorated 2 to 3 months later.

He was admitted again for BTX-A treatment at 4 months after his discharge. The severity of left hemiparesis BRS was 5 in the upper limb, 3 in the hand, and 5 in the lower limb. Forced grasping and involuntary movement of the upper limb were so remarkable that he could not use tools with his left hand. The Simple Test for Evaluating Hand Function (STEF) score on admission was only 8 points. The STEF was designed to evaluate the speed of manipulation (catching or pinching objects and carrying them) of objects (10 different shapes and sizes) using an upper limb [7]. The maximum number of points is 100. The Modified Ashworth Scale (MAS) of his hemiparetic upper limb was 2~3 in the upper limb and 3 in the fingers. The MAS is an established and reliable tool which uses a 6-point scale (0, 1, 1+, 2, 3, 4) to score the average resistance to passive movement for each joint [8]. MAS 0 indicates "no increase in muscle tonus." MAS 4 indicates "affected part(s) rigid in flexion or extension."

2.2. Interventions. The patient was treated by the injection of 200 units (U) of BTX-A (Botox; Allergan, Irvine, CA, USA)

under electromyography (EMG) guidance soon after admission. BTX-A was injected into the following muscles: left biceps (50 U), flexor carpi radialis (25 U), flexor carpi ulnaris (25 U), flexor digitorum superficialis (35 U), flexor digitorum profundus (25 U), flexor pollicis longus (20 U), flexor pollicis brevis (10 U), and adductor pollicis (10 U), respectively. One week after the BTX-A injections, the spasticity of the left upper limb and the fingers improved and the grasp reflex and involuntary movement nearly disappeared (Figure 2). He could grasp and release objects, but the muscle was still weak. The MAS of the upper limb was 1~2, and those of the fingers were 2.

RFE were applied after the BTX-A injections. RFE were designed to elicit and maintain movements isolated from synergy, including the movement of each isolated finger using a stretch reflex, skin-muscle reflex, and alpha-gamma linkage. The hypothesized mechanism of the newly designed facilitation exercises for the fingers is shown in Figure 3 [9]. In patients with hemiparesis, descending motor tracts involved in movements intended by the patient do not discharge because of a low excitation level. If the excitation level in these neural circuits is adjusted and excitation is timed to discharge by the facilitation techniques, upon neuronal excitation of the patient's intention which originates in the prefrontal/premotor cortex, these neural circuits would discharge and realize movement intended by the patient.

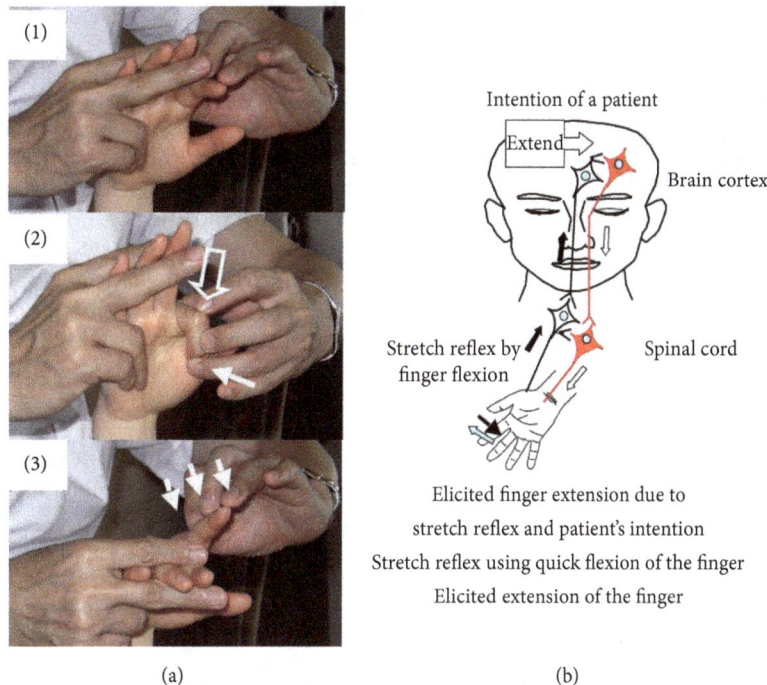

FIGURE 3: Hypothesized mechanism of a newly designed facilitation exercise for the hemiplegic upper limb and fingers. (a) Facilitation for extension of the isolated finger is performed as follows: (1) the finger is quickly flexed by the therapist; this elicits the stretch reflex; (2) the therapist instructs, "Extend" and pushes the proximal phalanx to flex the metacarpophalangeal (MP); and (3) the therapist applies slight resistance against finger extension to maintain extension of the finger. The thick arrow and thin arrow indicate manipulation to induce the stretch reflex and light touch (resistance) to maintain the α-γ linkage, respectively. (b) Descending motor tracts related to the patient's intention to move will respond to excitation of the patient's intention when these neural tracts are excited to a sufficient excitation level by facilitation techniques and result in the realization of movements by the patient's intention. Modified from Figure 1 in Kawahira et al. (2010).

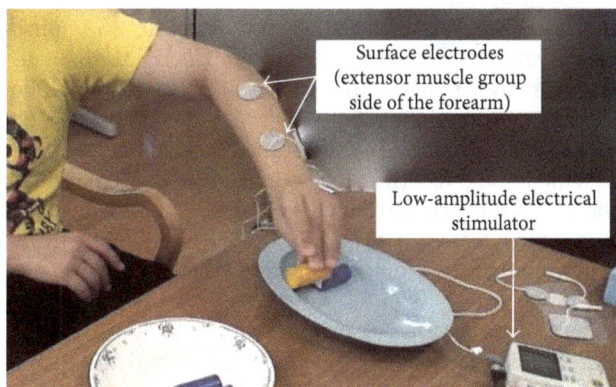

FIGURE 4: Effect of continuous electrical stimulation on the patient's ability to carry 5 pegs. The electrodes were attached to the extensor side of the forearm. The patient was instructed to carry each peg from one dish to another dish. The length of time required to carry the 5 pegs improved from 19.4 s without continuous electrical stimulation to 14.5 s with continuous electrical stimulation.

When low-amplitude continuous NMES was applied to the left wrist and finger extensor muscles with surface electrodes, he could grasp and release objects easily (Figure 4). The stimulation pulse was a symmetrical biphasic waveform, with a pulse width of 250 μs and frequency of 20 Hz. The intensity of the electrical current was adjusted to produce slight contraction of the target muscle without inducing obvious limb/joint movement while the patient remained at rest and was subjectively comfortable. He repeated the training to grasp and release the object under NMES. RFE were applied under NMES [10] for about two weeks.

The function of the hand and upper limb improved over two weeks from a STEF score of 8 to 31 points. The severity of hemiparesis of the hand improved from BRS 3 to 5 when he was discharged.

2.3. Functional NIRS (fNIRS). The effect of BTX-A treatment combined with both RFE and object-related training under low-amplitude continuous NMES (BTX-A treatment combined with NMES) was examined by using NIRS. NIRS was performed before and after BTX-A treatment combined with NMES.

Thirty-four channels of a 52-multi-channel NIRS device (OMM-3000/16, Shimadzu Co., Kyoto, Japan) were placed in 2 reticular patterns on both sides around the sensorimotor cortex (SMC) of the patient. The bottom row of channels was set parallel to the T3-F7 (left) and T4-F8 (right) line, since C3 and C4 should be covered by a total of 3 or 4 channels. T3, T4, F7, F8, C3, and C4 are defined in the International 10–20 system of electroencephalography. Each channel measures the fluctuation of the concentration of oxygenated hemoglobin ([oxy-Hb]) and the concentration of

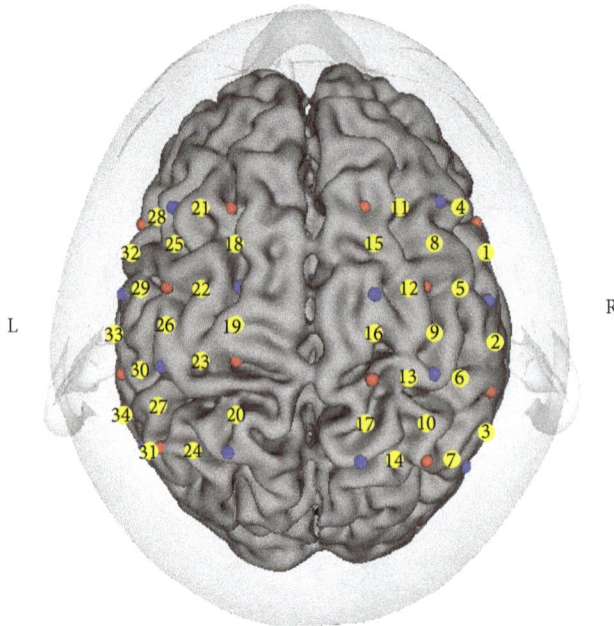

FIGURE 5: Projection of the probes and the channels onto the brain surface, using MRI data and a 3D position detector. Red: source, blue: detector, and yellow: channel.

deoxygenated hemoglobin ([deoxy-Hb]) using 3 wavelengths (780 nm, 805 nm, and 830 nm) according to the Beer-Lambert law. These [oxy-Hb] values reflect not only the hemoglobin density but also the path length of light. Each channel is configured by a pair of source/detector probes, which are separated by a distance of 30 mm. The channel is supposed to be set at the midpoint between the two probes 20~30 mm under the scalp (see Figure 5).

The source probe emitted light sequentially to avoid cross-talk noise, and the sampling time was adjusted to 0.1 s which was sufficiently fast to measure the fluctuation.

The time course data were acquired at each channel during the pinching test. The patient sat on a chair during the experiment. The patient was instructed to relax for 10 s, and then the operator ordered the patient to start pinching with the left thumb and index finger every 2 s at the operator's command. After 20 s of pinching, the patient was instructed to relax for 10 s; 5 cycles of this 10 s rest, 20 s pinching task, and 10 s rest were performed for averaging (Figure 6). Two conditions were investigated: (1) voluntary finger pinching and (2) voluntary finger pinching with continuous electrical stimulation of the wrist extensor muscles.

The statistical significance of differences in hemodynamic responses was assessed by a general linear model (GLM); the time course of Δ oxy-Hb was correlated with the design matrix using a boxcar function. The statistical significance of differences in all GLM analyses was based on an adjusted alpha level of less than 0.05, which corresponded to T values greater than 2.3 [11].

3. Results

The effect of BTX-A treatment combined with NMES on brain activity was examined by NIRS.

There was an increase in activation (increase in [oxy-Hb]) in the ipsilesional SMC after BTX-A treatment combined with NMES compared with that before BTX-A treatment (Figures 7(a) and 7(b)).

When continuous NMES was applied to the extensor side of the forearm during pinching, there was activation in both SMC and ipsilesional prefrontal cortex (PFC) before BTX-A treatment combined with NMES (Figure 8(a)). The activation area was more localized at the ipsilesional SMC after BTX-A treatment (Figure 8(b)).

In a comparison of the activation area after BTX-A treatment combined with NMES, the activation area with continuous electrical stimulation of the extensor side of the forearm (Figure 8(b)) was smaller than that without continuous electrical stimulation (Figure 7(b)).

4. Discussion

The grasp reflex and involuntary movement after cerebral infarction improved with a decrease in spasticity by BTX-A treatment combined with both RFE and object-related training under continuous NMES. NIRS detected an increase in blood flow in the right cerebral motor cortex during left hand pinching after BTX-A treatment combined with NMES. More regional activity of the right motor cortex was detected during continuous electric muscle stimulation of the extensor side of the forearm.

The grasp reflex can be elicited in neonates and early infants as a result of insufficient control of the spinal mechanism by the immature brain, but the reflex gradually disappears as the infant grows, due to increased inhibition accompanying brain maturation [12]. Adult patients with lesions in the frontal lobes sometimes exhibit a grasp reflex of the hands and feet [12]. The reappearance of each of these reflexes in adults is attributed to the release of the spinal reflex center from the disturbed higher brain mechanism, suggesting that these reflexes are only inhibited and not lost after infancy [13].

In a study by De Renzi and Barbieri [14], the palmar grasp reflex was elicited in 21 (66%) of 32 patients with a medial frontal lesion and in 8 (26%) of 30 patients with a lateral frontal lesion. On the other hand, a small percentage of patients with a deep lesion including the basal ganglia without frontal cortical damage were reported to exhibit a positive palmar grasp reflex [14], and the extension of a supplementary motor area (SMA) lesion into more lateral regions of area 6 may increase the strength of the grasp reflex [15].

In our patient, it seems that inhibitory stimuli from upper brain structures were obstructed by lesion of the right putamen to release the spinal grasp reflex center.

A major role of the basal ganglia could be to achieve a balance between excitatory and inhibitory thalamocortical influences. The basal ganglia appear to "gate" sensory input at various levels [16]. There is some indirect evidence that

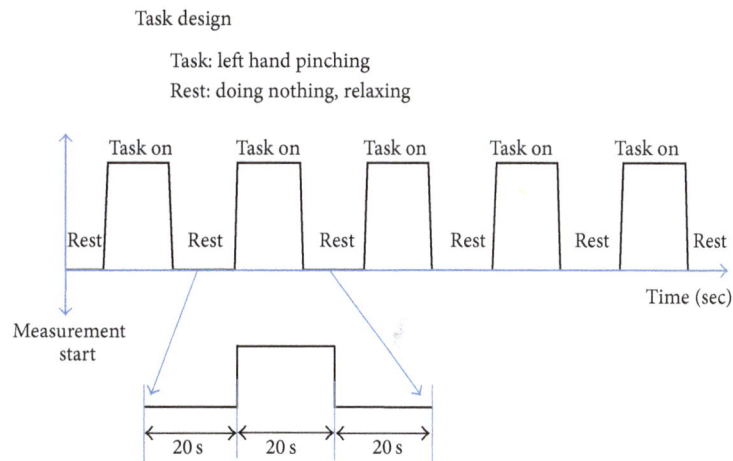

FIGURE 6: The procedure of the pinching task. The patient was instructed to relax for 10 s, and then the operator ordered the patient to start pinching with the left thumb and index finger every 2 s at the operator's command. After 20 s of pinching, the patient was instructed to relax for another 10 s: 5 cycles of 10 s rest, 20 s pinching task, and 10 s rest were performed for averaging. Therefore, there is an interval of 20 s between 2 pinching tasks.

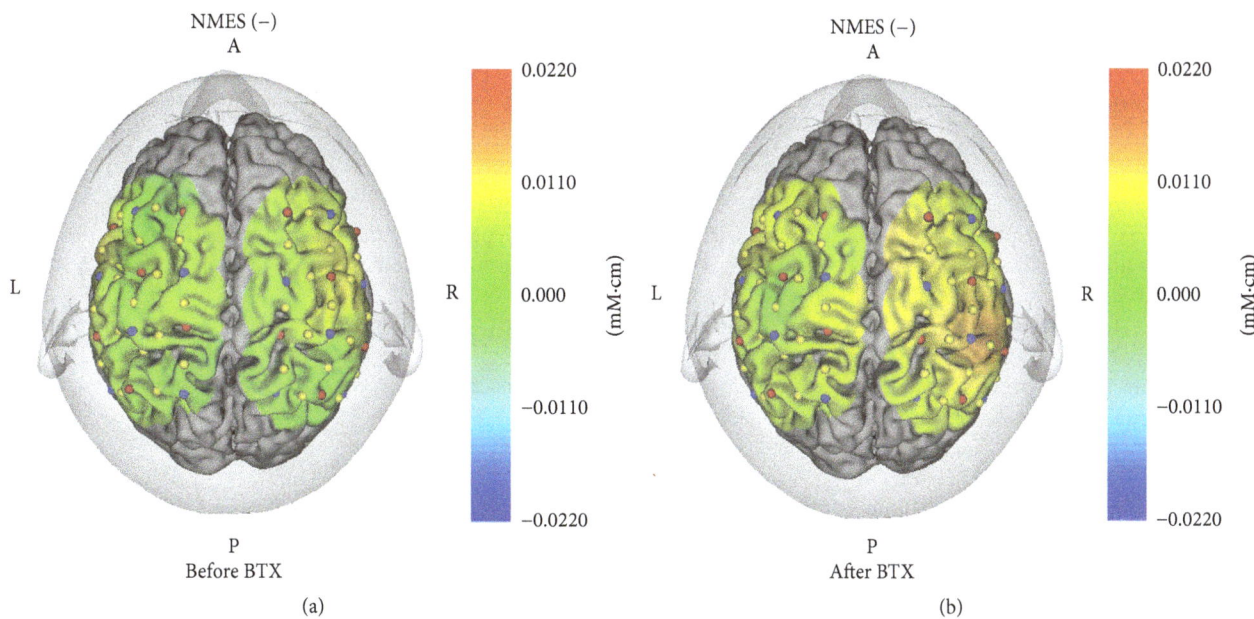

FIGURE 7: Three-dimensional maps of hemodynamic responses (changes in the oxy-Hb concentration) in the brain while the patient performed finger pinching with the left hand before BTX-A treatment (a) and after BTX-A treatment (b). There was an increase in activation in the ipsilesional SMC after BTX-A treatment compared with that before BTX-A treatment.

this sensory gate for motor control is lost in dystonia [17]. In our patient, the putaminal lesion could have altered this delicate balance, leading to distorted afferent cortical information. Before BTX-A treatment, electrical stimulation of the left forearm activated a wide area in both cerebral cortices on NIRS. It is possible that this was due to abnormal sensorimotor integration [18], and the patient performed pinching with great effort.

Intramuscular injection of BTX-A was performed to treat muscle spasticity and dystonia. The therapeutic effects of BTX-A seemed to be due not only to partial denervation of extrafusal muscles but also to fusimotor denervation of

intrafusal fibers that tonically control the sensitivity of spindle sensory afferents [19–21]. Consequently, BTX-A may induce changes in the alpha-gamma linkage of volitional control [22]. In addition, BTX-A applied periphery may directly induce central plasticity in spinal cord via retrograde axonal transport, especially at high doses [21]. It is not yet clear that this direct central effect is induced at therapeutic dose such as in our case report.

Continuous electrical stimulation of the wrist and finger extensor muscles after BTX-A treatment could also inhibit antagonistic muscles such as the flexor muscles of the wrist and finger. Brain activity in the ipsilesional SMC and

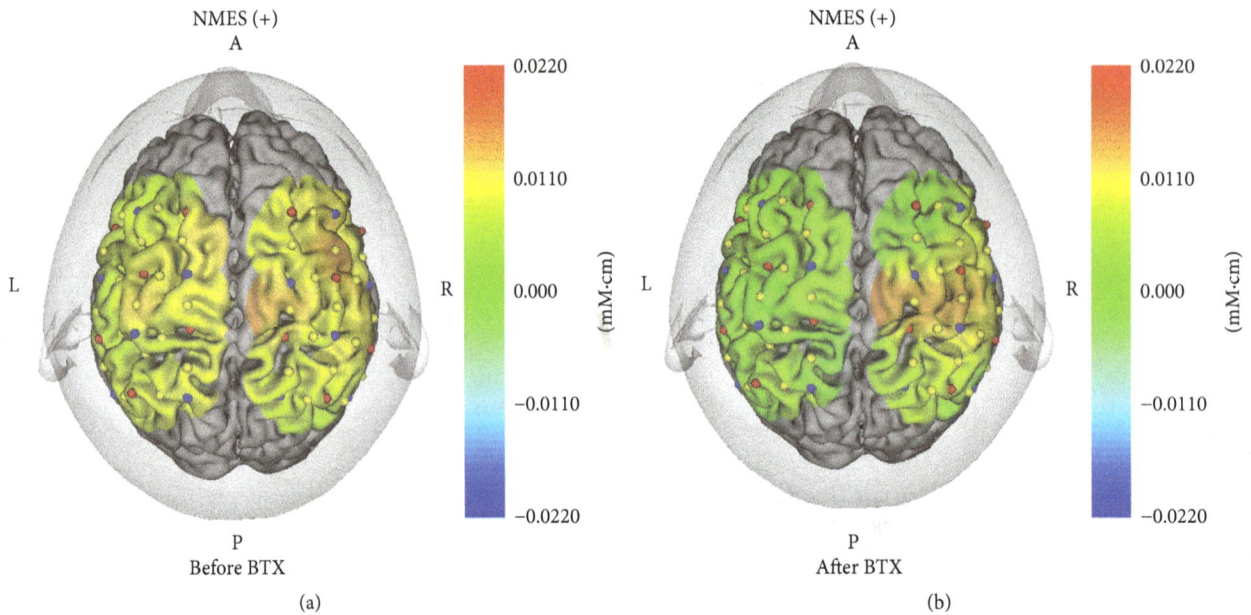

FIGURE 8: Three-dimensional maps of hemodynamic responses (changes in the oxy-Hb concentration) in the brain while the patient performed pinching with the left hand under continuous electrical stimulation of the extensor side of the forearm before BTX-A treatment (a) and after BTX-A treatment (b). There was activation in both SMC and ipsilesional PFC before BTX-A treatment, and the activation area was more localized at the ipsilesional SMC after BTX-A treatment.

MFC areas was more improved with continuous electrical stimulation while pinching, as examined by NIRS. Furthermore, activities in the contralesional hemisphere during continuous electrical stimulation appeared to be suppressed after BTX-A treatment (Figure 8(b)). This suppression might also contribute to the present recovery because activities in contralesional M1 sometimes disturb motor recovery by abnormal interhemispheric interactions during voluntary movement of the paretic hand [23–25].

In our patient, we considered that the frontal lobe did not suppress the grasp reflex or involuntary movement induced by sensory input to the left hand. However, BTX-A treatment combined with NMES improved voluntary movements. This improvement may have been due to not only a decrease in peripheral spasticity, but also a decrease in the excitement from the muscle spindle to the afferent nerve fibers to the spinal cord, and this indirectly influenced the cerebral cortex and improved the cerebral balance to make it easy to perform voluntary movement. Electrically mediated repetitive movement may facilitate the neuroplasticity of motor learning.

5. Conclusions

The grasp reflex of the hemiplegic left upper limb of a patient who suffered infarction of the right putamen and temporal lobe was significantly improved by BTX-A treatment combined with both RFE and object-related training under NMES. This improvement of the grasp reflex by BTX-A consisted of not only the improvement of spasticity but also the improvement of motor control of finger movement. Further research on BTX-A treatment combined with NMES is needed in patients with the grasp reflex that is not improved with ordinary treatment.

Competing Interests

The authors declare no potential conflicts of interests.

References

[1] A. Albanese, M. P. Barnes, K. P. Bhatia et al., "A systematic review on the diagnosis and treatment of primary (idiopathic) dystonia and dystonia plus syndromes: report of an EFNS/MDS-ES task force," *European Journal of Neurology*, vol. 13, no. 5, pp. 433–444, 2006.

[2] P. Greene, H. Shale, and S. Fahn, "Analysis of open-label trials in torsion dystonia using high dosages of anticholinergics and other drugs," *Movement Disorders*, vol. 3, no. 1, pp. 46–60, 1988.

[3] D. M. Simpson, A. Blitzer, A. Brashear, C. Comella, R. Dubinsky, and M. Hallett, "Therapeutics and Technology Assessment Subcommittee of the American Academy of Neurology, Assessment: botulinum neurotoxin for the treatment of movement disorders (an evidence-based review): report of the Therapeutics and Technology Assessment Subcommittee of the American Academy of Neurology," *Neurology*, vol. 13, pp. 1699–1706, 2008.

[4] K. Kawahira, T. Noma, J. Iiyama, S. Etoh, A. Ogata, and M. Shimodozono, "Improvements in limb kinetic apraxia by repetition of a newly designed facilitation exercise in a patient with corticobasal degeneration," *International Journal of Rehabilitation Research*, vol. 32, no. 2, pp. 178–183, 2009.

[5] M. Shimodozono, T. Noma, Y. Nomoto et al., "Benefits of a repetitive facilitative exercise program for the upper paretic

extremity after subacute stroke: a randomized controlled trial," *Neurorehabilitation and Neural Repair*, vol. 27, no. 4, pp. 296–305, 2013.

[6] T. Noma, S. Matsumoto, S. Etoh, M. Shimodozono, and K. kawahira, "Anti-spastic effects of the direct application of vibratory stimuli to the spastic muscles of hemiplegic limbs in post-stroke patients," *Brain Injury*, vol. 23, no. 7-8, pp. 623–631, 2009.

[7] K. Shindo, H. Oba, J. Hara, M. Ito, F. Hotta, and M. Liu, "Psychometric properties of the simple test for evaluating hand function in patients with stroke," *Brain Injury*, vol. 29, no. 6, pp. 772–776, 2015.

[8] R. W. Bohannon and M. B. Smith, "Interrater reliability of a modified Ashworth scale of muscle spasticity," *Physical Therapy*, vol. 67, no. 2, pp. 206–207, 1987.

[9] K. Kawahira, M. Shimodozono, S. Etoh, K. Kamada, T. Noma, and N. Tanaka, "Effects of intensive repetition of a new facilitation technique on motor functional recovery of the hemiplegic upper limb and hand," *Brain Injury*, vol. 24, no. 10, pp. 1202–1213, 2010.

[10] M. Shimodozono, T. Noma, S. Matsumoto, R. Miyata, S. Etoh, and K. Kawahira, "Repetitive facilitative exercise under continuous electrical stimulation for severe arm impairment after subacute stroke: a randomized controlled pilot study," *Brain Injury*, vol. 28, no. 2, pp. 203–210, 2014.

[11] M. L. Schroeter, M. M. Bücheler, K. Müller et al., "Towards a standard analysis for functional near-infrared imaging," *NeuroImage*, vol. 21, no. 1, pp. 283–290, 2004.

[12] J. M. Schott and M. N. Rossor, "The grasp and other primitive reflexes," *Journal of Neurology, Neurosurgery and Psychiatry*, vol. 74, no. 5, pp. 558–560, 2003.

[13] Y. Futagi, Y. Toribe, and Y. Suzuki, "The grasp reflex and moro reflex in infants: hierarchy of primitive reflex responses," *International Journal of Pediatrics*, vol. 2012, Article ID 191562, 10 pages, 2012.

[14] E. De Renzi and C. Barbieri, "The incidence of the grasp reflex following hemispheric lesion and its relation to frontal damage," *Brain*, vol. 115, no. 1, pp. 293–313, 1992.

[15] A. M. Smith, D. Bourbonnais, and G. Blanchette, "Interaction between forced grasping and a learned precision grip after ablation of the supplementary motor area," *Brain Research*, vol. 222, no. 2, pp. 395–400, 1981.

[16] R. Kaji, R. Urushihara, N. Murase, H. Shimazu, and S. Goto, "Abnormal sensory gating in basal ganglia disorders," *Journal of Neurology*, vol. 252, supplement 4, pp. iv13–iv16, 2005.

[17] M. Tinazzi, A. Priori, L. Bertolasi, E. Frasson, F. Mauguière, and A. Fiaschi, "Abnormal central integration of a dual somatosensory input in dystonia. Evidence for sensory overflow," *Brain*, vol. 123, no. 1, pp. 42–50, 2000.

[18] G. Abbruzzese and A. Berardelli, "Sensorimotor integration in movement disorders," *Movement Disorders*, vol. 18, no. 3, pp. 231–240, 2003.

[19] P. P. Urban and R. Rolke, "Effects of botulinum toxin type A on vibration induced facilitation of motor evoked potentials in spasmodic torticollis," *Journal of Neurology, Neurosurgery and Psychiatry*, vol. 75, no. 11, pp. 1541–1546, 2004.

[20] C. Trompetto, M. Bove, L. Avanzino, G. Francavilla, A. Berardelli, and G. Abbruzzese, "Intrafusal effects of botulinum toxin in post-stroke upper limb spasticity," *European Journal of Neurology*, vol. 15, no. 4, pp. 367–370, 2008.

[21] M. Caleo, F. Antonucci, L. Restani, and R. Mazzocchio, "A reappraisal of the central effects of botulinum neurotoxin type A: by what mechanism?" *Journal of Neurochemistry*, vol. 109, no. 1, pp. 15–24, 2009.

[22] R. L. Rosales, K. Arimura, S. Takenaga, and M. Osame, "Extrafusal and intrafusal muscle effects in experimental botulinum toxin-a injection," *Muscle & Nerve*, vol. 19, no. 4, pp. 488–496, 1996.

[23] N. S. Ward and L. G. Cohen, "Mechanisms underlying recovery of motor function after stroke," *Archives of Neurology*, vol. 61, no. 12, pp. 1844–1848, 2004.

[24] N. Murase, J. Duque, R. Mazzocchio, and L. G. Cohen, "Influence of interhemispheric interactions on motor function in chronic stroke," *Annals of Neurology*, vol. 55, no. 3, pp. 400–409, 2004.

[25] M. L. Harris-Love, E. Chan, A. W. Dromerick, and L. G. Cohen, "Neural substrates of motor recovery in severely impaired stroke patients with hand paralysis," *Neurorehabilitation and Neural Repair*, vol. 30, no. 4, pp. 328–338, 2016.

Hypothermia in Multiple Sclerosis: Beyond the Hypothalamus?

Francesco Berti ⓘ,[1] Zeeshan Arif ⓘ,[1] Cris Constantinescu ⓘ,[1,2] and Bruno Gran ⓘ[2]

[1]*Division of Clinical Neuroscience, University of Nottingham School of Medicine, Nottingham, UK*
[2]*Department of Neurology, Nottingham University Hospitals NHS Trust, Nottingham, UK*

Correspondence should be addressed to Bruno Gran; bruno.gran@nuh.nhs.uk

Academic Editor: Isabella Laura Simone

Hypothermia is a rare and poorly understood complication of Multiple Sclerosis (MS). We report on a 66-year-old patient currently with Secondary Progressive MS (SP-MS) who developed unexplained hypothermia associated with multiple hospitalisations and we review the literature on this topic. In our case, magnetic resonance imaging (MRI) of the brain failed to highlight hypothalamic disease, but spinal MRI identified a number of spinal cord lesions. Given the incidence and clinical significance of spinal involvement in MS and the hypothermic disturbances observed in high Spinal Cord Injury (SCI), we hypothesise that upper spinal cord pathology, along with hypothalamic and brainstem dysfunctions, can contribute to hypothermia.

1. Introduction

Multiple Sclerosis (MS) is the most common demyelinating disease and the major cause of neurological disability among young adults, affecting at least 2.5 million persons worldwide [1].

The cause of MS is unknown, but strong evidence suggests it is an autoimmune disorder of the central nervous system (CNS) where a chronic inflammatory response develops against myelin autoantigens leading to demyelination, scarring, and neuronal loss [2]. The multifocal nature of the disease implies that it can occur anywhere within the white and grey matter of the brain and spinal cord; thus its symptomatology can markedly differ based on the localisation of the lesions [1].

Radiological detection of multiple plaques and areas of atrophy is suggestive of MS, but the clinical correlation is often weak, with the absence of such findings failing to explain some dysfunctions [3]. Clinical hypothermia, defined as a core body temperature below 35.0°C [4], is an example of a rare and puzzling manifestation associated with MS. Hypothalamic pathology is considered its main cause but has been radiologically identified in very few of such MS patients.

In this article, we report on an hypothermic MS patient and review the literature on this subject, focusing on exploring whether extrahypothalamic dysfunctions along the thermoregulatory network may contribute to the development of this complication.

2. Case Presentation

A 66-year-old lady with a 21-year history of clinically definite MS, currently in the Secondary Progressive MS (SP-MS) phase, was admitted to hospital 14 times within a two-year period. On 10 occasions this was due to unexplained symptoms such as fatigue, confusion, worsening mobility, and dysarthria associated with hypothermia and suspected urinary tract infections (UTIs) (see Table 1).

Before these admissions, the patient was clinically stable with an Expanded Disability Status Scale (EDSS) score of 6.5 and had been hospitalised only once in the previous eight years, for cellulitis in the legs. At the time, she was suffering from limb weakness (mostly in the legs), spasticity, severe fatigue, reduced hand dexterity, and blepharospasm, but no other comorbidity. She could walk for 20 metres with a supporting frame but was otherwise wheelchair dependent. Since 2005, she had been receiving Botulinum Toxin injections for lower limb spasticity and blepharospasm and was on a trial of low-dose Naltrexone. The patient was also suffering from

TABLE 1: Summary of patient admissions to hospital between March 2013 and March 2015.

Admission date	Main complaint(s)	Temperature at admission (°C)	New finding(s)	Confirmed diagnosis	Treatment(s)	Disease course	Neuroimaging
24 March 2013	Confusion, dysarthria, reduced mobility, and recent falls	34.6	GCS (10/15) Leukopaenia Hyponatraemia (Na+ 131 mmol/l), mildly deranged LFTs Normal LP, CXR, and abdominal USS	No ?SUO ?SIADH	IV antibiotics, naltrexone discontinued because of LFTs	Discharged in 3 weeks (homeothermic) with care package and rehabilitation	Head CT and brain MRI. No acute findings. Bilateral, white-matter changes and generalised atrophy. No hypothalamic involvement
18 July 2013	Urinary incontinence, oedema, and cellulitis	35.8	No	No ?UTI	Antibiotics	Discharged	No
18 October 2013	Confusion lethargy, dysarthria, worsening movements, and decreased taste	33.5	Nystagmus Diplopia Decreased limb power Hyponatraemia (127 mmol/l), normokalaemia (4.4 mmol/l) Hyposmolarity (serum osmolality: 269 mOsm/kg; Urine Osmolality: 368 mOsm/kg)	No ?SIADH	Supportive	Discharged in 5 days while still hypothermic (T: 34.3°C)	No
7 November 2013	Dizziness on standing	33.0	No	No	Supportive	Discharged	No
31 December 2013	Lethargy, unwell, dysarthria, and limb weakness	33.0	Bradycardia, normal liver autoimmune screen, Vitamin D, TFTs, prolactin, PTH, calcium, and random cortisol	No ?UTI	Antibiotics	Discharged in 2 weeks (T: 34.0°C)	Brain MRI: no acute findings. Heavy demyelinating disease burden and a likely incidental small frontal meningioma. No hypothalamic involvement
16 March 2014	Feeling cold, unwell, and dysarthria	32.8	RUQ tenderness Murphy's +ve. Abdominal USS: cholelithiasis and contracted gall bladder	No	Antibiotics then supportive	Discharged in 2 weeks	No
22 May 2014	Weakness	33.1	Positive MSU, CRP 41	UTI	Antibiotics	Discharged the next day	No
27 May 2014	Feeling cold and weakness	33.7	No	No	Supportive	Discharged in 3 days	No
15 September 2014	Right flank pain	32.7	Urinalysis (positive for leukocites and blood +++)	UTI	Antibiotics	Discharged in a week	No

TABLE 1: Continued.

Admission date	Main complaint(s)	Temperature at admission (°C)	New finding(s)	Confirmed diagnosis	Treatment(s)	Disease course	Neuroimaging
2 October 2014	Right flank pain, urinary incontinence, confusion, and persistently low temperatures	34.0	No	AKI and ?UTI	Antibiotics	Discharged in 6 days	No
12 October 2014	Dysarthria, fatigue, confusion, weakness, and decreased power	NK	Hyponatraemia, hyperkalaemia (Na+ 125 mmol/l, K+ 5.8 mmol/l), eGFR 59, urea 8.4 mmol/l MSU (positive for leukocytes) Mixed growth, possible contamination	UTI	Antibiotics 3 days of IV steroids	Discharged in 2 weeks	Brain and spinal MRI Extensive demyelinating lesions with evidence of recent callosal involvement. Spinal imaging revealed diffuse, patchy, T2 hyperintense lesions involving the majority of the cervical cord and T9-10 with associated atrophy
24 October 2014	Neck pain, fatigue, and weakness	37.4	No	No ?UTI	Antibiotics	NK	No
23 March 2015	Lethargy	31.0	No	No? UTI	Supportive	Discharged on same day	No
25 March 2015	Lethargy and high-temperature	37.0	Dysmetric saccades. Cerebellar signs. Worsening power with bilateral upgoing plantar reflexes. Bilateral lower leg oedema.	No	Supportive	Discharged 2 days later	No

Not known (NK); Glasgow Coma Scale (GCS); acute kidney injury (AKI); mid-stream urine (MSU); C-reactive protein (CRP); right upper quadrant (RUQ); sepsis of unknown origin (SUO); liver function tests (LFTs); lumbar puncture (LP); chest X-ray (CXR); ultrasonography (USS); thyroid function tests (TFTs); parathyroid hormone (PTH); estimated glomerular filtration rate (eGFR); Syndrome of Inappropriate Anti-Diuretic Hormone (SIADH).

chronic urinary retention and constipation, for which she was taking an osmotic laxative. She had established normocytic anaemia and mildly elevated liver enzymes.

After repeated admissions with hypothermia, she developed chronically low body temperature (T: 34.0–36.0°C) and by March 2015, she had become bed-bound for most of the day (EDSS = 8.5) and was practising intermittent self-catheterisation.

She was first found hypothermic in March 2013 after an admission for confusion (GCS 10/15), dysarthria, and reduced mobility (see Table 1). The patient had progressively deteriorated in the preceding weeks and had suffered two falls. On admission, her temperature was 34.6°C, but respiratory rate (RR), heart rate (HR), blood pressure (BP), and O_2 saturations were unremarkable. Of note, no shivering or cold sensations were mentioned. Blood tests showed leukopenia, mild hyponatraemia (131 mmol/l) with normal K+ levels (4.6 mmol/l), and acutely elevated Liver Function Tests (LFTs) with particularly high aminotransferases. Clotting tests and spinal fluid analysis (lumbar puncture; LP) results were within normal ranges. Chest X-ray (CXR) and abdominal ultrasonography (USS) were unremarkable. Computerised tomography (CT) scan of the head showed no evidence of acute findings.

Magnetic resonance imaging (MRI) of the brain using a 3 Tesla (T) scanner was performed with and without contrast. No old brain scans were available for comparison; however bilateral, white-matter changes and generalised atrophy consistent with MS were reported. No hypothalamic involvement was detected and spinal MRI was not performed.

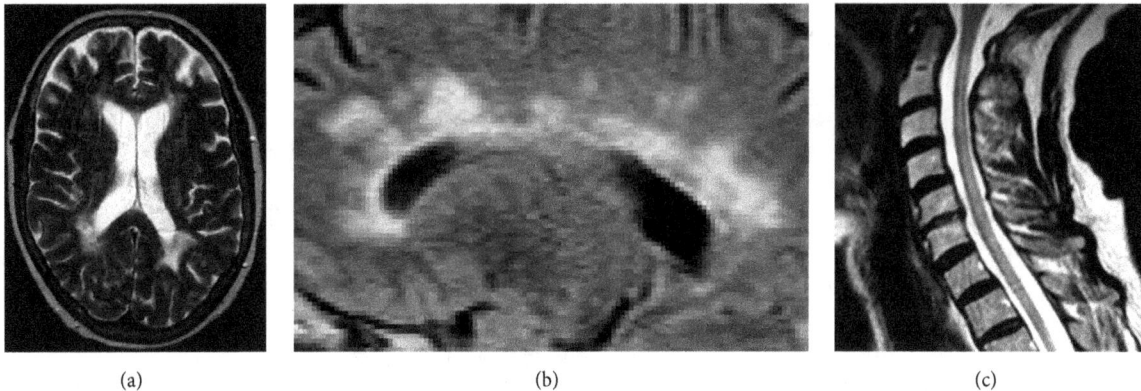

FIGURE 1: Brain and spinal MRI of the patient following admission on 12 October 2014. (a) Brain T2W axial MRI (1.5 T) demonstrating the characteristic periventricular lesions of MS. (b) Magnification of brain FLAIR sagittal MRI showing involvement of the corpus callosum. (c) Sagittal T2W spinal MRI of the cervical cord with diffuse, patchy lesions. T2W: T-2 weighted; FLAIR: Fluid-Attenuated Inversion Recovery; T: Tesla.

The cause of her symptoms was not identified and the patient was treated prophylactically for Sepsis of Unknown Origin (SUO) with IV tazocin for five days. She was reviewed by general medicine and neurology and a diagnosis of Syndrome of Inappropriate Anti-Diuretic Hormone (SIADH) secretion with impaired temperature regulation secondary to MS was considered. Naltrexone was discontinued in consideration of her elevated liver enzymes. The patient gradually improved over the next three weeks and was transferred to rehabilitation services before being discharged in June with a care package.

In July 2013, she was rehospitalised because of symptoms of urinary incontinence, leg oedema, and cellulitis and was treated prophylactically for a Urinary Tract Infection (UTI) (see Table 1).

In October, she presented to the hospital with confusion, lethargy, dysarthria, worsening of movements, and decreased taste in her mouth and was found hypothermic a second time (T: 33.5°C) (see Table 1). Her blood results showed hyponatraemia (127 mmol/l), normokalaemia (4.4 mmol/l), decreased serum osmolality (269 mOsm/kg) with a urine osmolality of 368 mOsm/kg, and no evidence of extracellular space depletion. Her general status gradually improved while still hypothermic (T: 34.3°C) and after five days she was discharged. Regular monitoring of her electrolyte levels was arranged.

After the third hospitalisation with unexplained hypothermia, our patient was readmitted a fourth time in December with lethargy, dysarthria, and limb weakness (see Table 1). Once again she was found hypothermic (T: 33.0°C) and bradycardic. She was treated empirically for urosepsis with IV tazocin, which was then switched to nitrofurantoin as blood tests did not suggest an infectious cause. Thyroid function tests (TFTs), cortisol, Vitamin D, prolactin, parathyroid hormone (PTH), and Ca^{2+} levels were within range and a liver autoimmune screen was negative. A second brain MRI (1.5 T) showed heavy demyelinating disease burden, but no hypothalamic involvement and a likely incidental small frontal meningioma. She was discharged after two weeks, asymptomatic while still hypothermic (T: 34.0°C).

Between March 2014 and March 2015, our patient was hospitalised nine more times (see Table 1). Confusion, lethargy, fatigue, dysarthria, and motor weakness were the most common symptoms and associated hypothermia was registered on at least six admissions. Interestingly, on two occasions, she presented with relatively abnormal high temperatures (T: 37.4°C and T: 37.0°C).

UTI was considered the likely cause of her symptoms in six instances and antibiotics were prescribed. A three-day course of intravenous methylprednisolone was added once, with no apparent benefits and in most cases the patient recovered spontaneously. In the light of only two positive urinary samples, the absence of typical UTI symptoms, and a negative cystoscopy, urology recommended intermittent self-catheterisation due to increased residual urine volume.

Following admission in October 2014, a repeat brain MRI with contrast was performed at 1.5 T that demonstrated recent callosal involvement (see Figure 1). A spinal MRI (1.5 T) was also arranged and revealed diffuse, patchy, T2 hyperintense lesions involving the majority of the cervical cord and T9-10 with associated atrophy (see Figure 1). These findings were discussed at the neuroradiology multidisciplinary team meeting and considered consistent with spinal MS rather than neuromyelitis optica spectrum disorder (NMOSD). This was confirmed by serology tests for anti-aquaporin 4 (AQP4) and anti-myelin oligodendrocyte glycoprotein (MOG) antibodies, which were both negative.

3. Discussion

Our patient developed clinical hypothermia ($T < 35°C$) associated with SP-MS. In the literature, this has been reported for 23 other MS cases (16 females) (see Table 2).

Most patients experienced deteriorations in cognition and consciousness (confusion, lethargy, or even stupor and coma) often accompanied by dysarthria (slurred speech) and worsening motor symptoms associated with hypothermia. On admission, their temperature ranged from 29.0°C to 35.0°C (see Table 2). In over half of these cases hypothermia had occurred after >20 years since diagnosis and was

TABLE 2: Review of the literature: summary of the 1st presentation of patients with hypothermia in Multiple Sclerosis (MS) and the clinical course of the disease.

References	Patient details	Disease duration; MS-type; EDSS	Main complaint(s) before admission	Temperature at admission (°C)	Cognitive symptoms at admission	New neurological signs and symptoms	Dysarthria and/or dysphagia	Haematological abnormalities and onset	Hyponatremia and plasma/urinary osmolalities	Neuroimaging and/or autopsy studies	Suspected diagnosis and disease course	Type of hypothermia and (number of hypothermic episodes)
[7]	61 F	NK; NK; NK	Lethargy, anorexia, poor fluid intake	29.4	NK	NK	NK	Hb 12.9 g/dl; MCV 84 fl Platelets 19×10^9/l Bone marrow aspirate: erythroid hypoplasia	NK	No	Death	Acute (1)
[8]	41 F	7 years; NK; EDSS: 7.0	3 weeks confusion, apathy	32.6	Confusion, Stupor	Marked rigidity in all limbs	No	After 1/52: Anaemia (Hb 7.9 g/dl) Thrombocytopenia (61×10^9/l)	No	Head CT: no abnormality detected	Treated with passive rewarming. Full clinical recovery in 6 days	Chronic: (1)
[8]	52 F	24 years; NK; EDSS: 8.0	3 weeks: confusion, lethargy	31.0	Coma	No	No	Thrombocytopenia (50×10^9/l) at admission, peaking after 5 days (28×10^9/l) and anaemia (Hb 7.4 g/dl)	Yes: (Na+ 107 mmol/l) (?SIADH)	No	Treated with steroids, passive rewarming, hypertonic saline, and furosemide. Full clinical recovery in 5 days	Chronic: (1)

TABLE 2: Continued.

References	Patient details	Disease duration; MS-type; EDSS	Main complaint(s) before admission	Temperature at admission (°C)	Cognitive symptoms at admission	New neurological signs and symptoms	Dysarthria and/or dysphagia	Haematological abnormalities and onset	Hyponatremia and plasma/urinary osmolalities	Neuroimaging and/or autopsy studies	Suspected diagnosis and disease course	Type of hypothermia and (number of hypothermic episodes)
[9]	55 F	24 years; NK; EDSS: 6.0	1 week: confusion, lethargy, visual hallucinations	33.0	Confusion	Generalised myoclonus neck stiffness	No	8 days after: pancytopenia Hb 9.2 g/dl, Platelet 80×10^9/l, Leukocytes 2.9×10^9/l	No	Head CT: no abnormality detected. Brain autopsy: multiple old plaques at various locations (incl. basal ganglia, corpus callosum, occipital white matter, and right upper cerebellar peduncle). No hypothalamic lesions except some recent axon swellings and cell loss	Developed bronchopneumonia. Treated with antibiotics. Full clinical recovery	Acute: (4)
[9]	55 F	22 years; NK; NK	4 weeks: confusion, bradyphrenia, incontinence	NK	NK	Augmented paraparesis	No	No	No	Brain MRI and CT performed after the 2nd admission with hypothermia. Brain MRI and head CT: Important lesions in periventricular and posterior part of corpus callosum No hypothalamic lesions	Developed bronchopneumonia. Treated with antibiotic and passive rewarming. Full clinical recovery.	Acute: (2)
[9]	58 M	16 years; NK; EDSS: 7.0	2 weeks: lethargy, dysarthria, dysphagia	<35	Memory deficit	Tetraparesis, bilateral central nystagmus	Dysarthria, dysphagia	Thrombocytopenia: 100×10^9/l	No	Brain MRI performed after the 4th admission with hypothermia. Brain MRI: several periventricular plaques. No hypothalamic lesions	Developed bronchopneumonia. Treated with antibiotics and passive rewarming recovered in days. Some motor deterioration remained	Acute: (4)

Table 2: Continued.

References	Patient details	Disease duration; MS-type; EDSS	Main complaint(s) before admission	Temperature at admission (°C)	Cognitive symptoms at admission	New neurological signs and symptoms	Dysarthria and/or dysphagia	Haematological abnormalities and onset	Hyponatremia and plasma/urinary osmolalities	Neuroimaging and/or autopsy studies	Suspected diagnosis and disease course	Type of hypothermia and (number of hypothermic episodes)
[10]	52 M	14 years; NK; NK	Augmented motor deficits	32.8	Confusion	Augmented motor paresis	No	No	Yes: (Na+ 114 mEq/l), plasma hyposmolarity (? SIADH)	Brain MRI: No hypothalamic lesions	Treatment with NaCl infusion and fluid restrictions. Hypothermia self-resolved. Clinical full recovery	Acute: (3)
[11]	63 F	25 years; NK; NK	Visual disturbances, depression paranoid, unable to stand up without help	32.4	Confusion	Worsening neurological signs: bilateral Babinski sign, paraparesis, paresthesia, and ataxia in the right arm and mild postural tremor	Dysarthria	Deranged LFTs (ALT and AST mildly raised with hypoalbuminaemia, 31.7 g/l)	No	Brain MRI: diffuse white matter lesions No hypothalamic lesions	Treated with passive rewarming and parenteral thiamine (? Wernicke Encephalopathy) Normothermia in 3 weeks	Acute (1)
[11]	68 F	32 years; NK; NK	3 weeks: gait abnormalities, dysarthria	31.6	Confusion, drowsiness	Severe paraparesis, bilateral Babinski sign, asterixis, partial right lateral rectus palsy, cerebellar signs	Dysarthria	Severe hypoalbuminaemia (18.9 g/l), decreased folic acid	No	Brain MRI: multiple periventricular lesions. No hypothalamic lesions	Treated with parenteral thiamine (? Wernicke Encephalopathy). Full recovery within 1 month	Acute (1)

TABLE 2: Continued.

References	Patient details	Disease duration; MS-type; EDSS	Main complaint(s) before admission	Temperature at admission (°C)	Cognitive symptoms at admission	New neurological signs and symptoms	Dysarthria and/or dysphagia	Haematological abnormalities and onset	Hyponatremia and plasma/urinary osmolalities	Neuroimaging and/or autopsy studies	Suspected diagnosis and disease course	Type of hypothermia and (number of hypothermic episodes)
[12]	53 F	NK; NK; NK	5 days: lethargy, dysphagia, dysarthria	29.0	Confusion	Spastic tetraparesis with bilateral extensor plantar but depressed reflexes	Dysarthria	Thrombocytopenia: platelets 79 × 10⁹/l. Increased APTT ?DIC Raised amylase (321 IU/l)	No.	Brain and spine autopsy: multiple plaques in the brain and spinal cord. A large hypothalamic plaque was found with evidence of current activity and demyelination	Passive rewarming, antibiotics, and atropine. Developed bronchopneumonia, pancreatitis, and died	Acute (1)
[13]	44 F	10 years; PR-MS; NK	Few days: confusion, disorientation, hallucinations	33.3	Confusion	Flaccid paraplegia and cerebellar syndrome (not augmented)	No	No	No	Brain MRI: T2W hyperintensities in the periventricular white matter	Passive rewarming and full clinical recovery within 10 days	NK
[14]	48 M	5 years; NK; EDSS: 6.0	3 weeks: confusion, disorientation, dysarthria deteriorating mobility, drowsiness, cold lower extremities	Initially 36.0 then 31.0	Stupor	Initially flaccid paraparesis and increased tone in the upper limbs. Deterioration over 48 h. He developed repetitive facial twitching, neck stiffness, left lower motor facial weakness, and decerebrate posturing	Dysarthria	Thrombocytopenia: 27 × 10⁹/l. Anaemia: Hb 12.7 g/dl. Increased PT and APTT and low folate	No	CT head: moderate brain atrophy. Previous MRIs had been normal. Brain MRI: after 1st and 2nd admissions with hypothermia: multiple high signals in periventricular white matter. No hypothalamic lesions. Brain autopsy: plaques in periventricular, midbrain, pons, medulla and hypothalamus (incl. posterior hypothalamic nucleus)	Initially treated with IV methylprednisolone for MS relapse, then with antibiotics for ?UTI. Then, passive rewarming. Normothermia after further 48 h. Packed cells, platelets, and plasma proteins transfusion for bleeding. Discharged in 30 days. Residual spastic paraparesis, incoordination, mild upper limb weakness, and sensory deficit after T12	Acute then chronic: (2)

TABLE 2: Continued.

References	Patient details	Disease duration; MS-type; EDSS	Main complaint(s) before admission	Temperature at admission (°C)	Cognitive symptoms at admission	New neurological signs and symptoms	Dysarthria and/or dysphagia	Haematological abnormalities and onset	Hyponatremia and plasma/urinary osmolalities	Neuroimaging and/or autopsy studies	Suspected diagnosis and disease course	Type of hypothermia and (number of hypothermic episodes)
[14]	59 M	30 years; NK; EDSS: 7.0	4 weeks: increasing fatigue, lethargy, confusion, then drowsiness, dysphagia, and dysarthria	33.0	Stupor	NK	Dysphagia, dysarthria	Thrombocytopenia 95×10^9/l	No	NK	Passive rewarming and IV fluids. Normothermia in 36 hours. Paranoid psychosis and confusion, MI and severe LVF. Residual cognitive impairment	Acute (2)
[14]	57 F	20 years; NK; EDSS: 7.0	Decreased mobility, lethargy, dysphagia,	35.0	Oriented (initially)	Bilateral optic atrophy and absent oculocephalic response, neck stiffness, rigidity, spastic tetraparesis	Dysarthria, dysphagia	Thrombocytopenia when normothermic (141) then 99×10^9/l. Raised APTT time. Raised platelets antibodies	Yes: (Na+ 130 mmol/l)	Head CT: bilateral periventricular low density lesions	Rewarming, IV fluids and IV methylpred-nisolone and antibiotics for ?UTI and respiratory infections were given. Normothermia within 24 hours. Full clinical recovery in 4 weeks	Acute: (2)
[14]	64 F	30 years; NK; EDSS: 9.0	Deterioration of motor function, speech disturbance, peripheral oedema, fluctuating consciousness	34.7	Confusion	Periorbital oedema, augmented tetraparesis, impaired palatal movements	Dysarthria	No	Yes: (Na+ 130 mmol/l) corrected with fluid restriction. Normal plasma and urinary osmolalities	NK	Passive rewarming. Normothermia in 24 hours. Full clinical recovery in 7 days	Acute (1)

TABLE 2: Continued.

References	Patient details	Disease duration; MS-type; EDSS	Main complaint(s) before admission	Temperature at admission (°C)	Cognitive symptoms at admission	New neurological signs and symptoms	Dysarthria and/or dysphagia	Haematological abnormalities and onset	Hyponatremia and plasma/urinary osmolalities	Neuroimaging and/or autopsy studies	Suspected diagnosis and disease course	Type of hypothermia and (number of hypothermic episodes)
[14]	47 F	No previous MS (diagnosed in retrospective); EDSS: 3.0	Withdrawal and lethargy	29.0	Coma	Neck stiffness, generalised hypertonia. After 3 days: bilateral extensor plantar responses, mild paraparesis, optic disc pallor	NK	Thrombocytopenia: $33 \times 10^9/l$ Anemia: Hb 10.2	No	Brain MRI: diffuse cortical atrophy, T2W hyperintense periventricular lesions. No hypothalamic lesions	Rewarming. Normothermia in 3 days. Residual physical and cognitive deficits	Acute: (2)
[15]	NK F	NK; NK; NK	Motor and cognitive decline	NK	Drowsiness	Augmented flaccid paresis	Dysarthria	Thrombocytopenia	NK	Head CT and brain MRI: No hypothalamic lesions	NK	Chronic with acute episode: (2)
[15]	NK F	NK; NK; NK	Motor and cognitive decline	NK	Drowsiness	Augmented flaccid paresis	Dysarthria	Thrombocytopenia	NK	Head CT and brain MRI: No hypothalamic lesions.	NK	Chronic with acute episodes (NK)

TABLE 2: Continued.

References	Patient details	Disease duration; MS-type; EDSS	Main complaint(s) before admission	Temperature at admission (°C)	Cognitive symptoms at admission	New neurological signs and symptoms	Dysarthria and/or dysphagia	Haematological abnormalities and onset	Hyponatremia and plasma/urinary osmolalities	Neuroimaging and/or autopsy studies	Suspected diagnosis and disease course	Type of hypothermia and (number of hypothermic episodes)
[16]	45 F	28 years; SP- MS; EDSS: 8.0	4 weeks: hypothermia (32-33°C), stupor, hypotension, hyponatraemia, and hypoglycaemia	33.4	Stupor	No	Dysarthria	Chronic normocytic anaemia. Elevated APTT (61 s). Raised CRP with negative blood cultures. Hypoglycaemia	Yes: (124 mmol/l). ?CSW syndrome	Head CT and brain MRI: known right parietal defect (previous brain abscess), generalised atrophy, periventricular white matter lesions, particularly in the callosum and a hyperintense lesion in the septal region of right thalamus. No hypothalamic lesions	Antibiotics, IV fluids. Initially recovered then further deterioration within a week (33.1°C) stupor and severe hypotension. Within 2 weeks a 3rd episode of hypothermia (31.2°C), bradycardia, and hypotension. She was treated with droxidopa and then discharged once normothermic and stable	Acute: (6)
[4]	61 F	30 years; SP-MS; NK	Confusion, agitation	33.9	Confusion, agitation	No	No	No	No	Brain MRI performed after 3rd hypothermic episode. Periventricular and brain stem plaques were seen with small vessel ischaemia in the ganglionic regions. No hypothalamic involvement	Spontaneous improvement and discharge with a T of 35.2°C	Chronic with acute episodes (6)

TABLE 2: Continued.

References	Patient details	Disease duration; MS-type; EDSS	Main complaint(s) before admission	Temperature at admission (°C)	Cognitive symptoms at admission	New neurological signs and symptoms	Dysarthria and/or dysphagia	Haematological abnormalities and onset	Hyponatremia and plasma/urinary osmolalities	Neuroimaging and/or autopsy studies	Suspected diagnosis and disease course	Type of hypothermia and (number of hypothermic episodes)
[17]	41 M	7 years; NK; NK	3 weeks: slurred speech, hypothermia, dysarthria, paranoid delusions, auditory, visual and tactile hallucinations	30.0	Confusion then coma	Bilateral facial droop, miosis, paraplegia (also present before), and bilateral upper extremities weakness	Dysarthria	Platelets: 113000/mm^3	No	Brain MRI: increased overall lesions and new T2W hypothalamic hyperintensity	Passive rewarming. Then antibiotics and respiratory assistance for ?SUO. Full clinical recovery in 6 weeks. Five monthly IV methylpred-nisolone infusions (1 g/month)	Acute (6)
[18]	39 M	24 years; SP-MS; EDSS: 6.5	Few weeks: augmented spasticity, cognitive decline, confusion	31.0	Stupor	Spastic tetraparesis	Dysarthria, dysphagia	Thrombocytopenia (75 × 10^9/l) Leukopenia (0.7 × 10^9/l) Elevated APTT (37 s) Raised ALT and AST	No	Brain MRI: T2W multiple white matter lesions and atrophy of corpus callosum. Hypothalamic involvement with bilateral nonenhancing preoptic lesions. After 1 year MRI showed no longer signs	Full clinical recovery	NK
[18]	49 M	32 years; PP-MS; EDSS: 7.5	Confusion	32.4	Psychomotor slowing	Augmented tetraparesis, bilateral pyramidal syndrome, right cerebellar syndrome	Dysarthria, dysphagia	Thrombocytopenia (79 × 10^9/l) Raised AST and ALT	No	Brain MRI: T2W white matter lesions. No hypothalamic involvement	Antibiotics for sepsis and 3 steroid injections. Full clinical recovery within days	Acute (1)

Expanded Disability Status Scale (EDSS); Primary Progressive MS (PP-MS); Secondary Progressive MS (SP-MS); not known (NK); aspartate transaminase (AST); alanine transaminase (ALT); disseminated intravascular coagulation (DIC); activated partial thromboplastin time (APTT); Syndrome of Inappropriate Anti-Diuretic Hormone (SIADH); mean corpuscular volume (MCV); T-2 weighted (T2W).

associated with severe disability (see Table 2). At least 12 of these patients suffered from more than one of such episodes (see Table 2).

Our patient developed more numerous episodes of hypothermia, superimposed on a chronic hypothermic state, than patients in previous reports. Chronic hypothermia was defined by the authors of this article as sustained hypothermia, typically lasting months. This had been previously reported in 5 other MS patients (see Table 2). In another case, chronic temperature changes were milder (35.0–36.5°C); hence this did not match the clinical definition of hypothermia [14].

Most MS patients achieved full or partial recovery after the first admission with hypothermia (see Table 2). Two deaths were associated with the initial episode [7, 12] and other two with subsequent ones [15, 17]. Transient haematological abnormalities were recorded in 16 patients during their first episode. Most commonly, these included thrombocytopenia and anaemia (see Table 2). Our anaemic patient, however, did not experience fluctuations of haematological parameters during admissions.

Previous cases of transiently deranged LFTs in hypothermic MS patients have been reported (see Table 2). In our case, mild, chronic LFT abnormalities could have been caused by Naltrexone-induced hepatic damage. Hyponatraemia was also reported in 5 of the previous cases (see Table 2). Cerebral salt wasting syndrome (CSW) and Syndrome of Inappropriate Anti-Diuretic Hormone (SIADH) both present with hyponatraemia and hyposmolality and while SIADH was suspected in this case, it was not formally confirmed. Irrespective of hypothermia, SIADH had been previously reported in MS and associated with the presence of periventricular and/or hypothalamic lesions [19, 20].

More controversial is the pathophysiology of hypothermia in MS, partly because of our limited understanding of thermoregulation. Recently, however, the anatomical basis of the thermoregulatory pathways has been further characterised, mostly in rodents, which share strong similarities on thermal reflexes with humans [5]. An understanding of the current model is helpful to elucidate the importance of different areas in thermoregulation (see Figure 2).

Most of the reports on hypothermic MS patients describe deficits along the thermoregulatory circuit described (see Figure 2). For instance, our patient mentioned to be "feeling cold" only twice and, in the other 23 cases, this symptom is rarely mentioned, suggesting an impairment of the afferent tracts. Similarly, shivering and sympathetic activation (leading to CVC, BAT, and an increase in RR, HR, and BP) are considered physiological responses to mild hypothermia (32–35°C) [4] which were absent in our patient. In one of the early reports, two MS patients suffering from hypothermia were placed in a climatic chamber with a paraplegic pathological control subject [8]. They were exposed, in sequence, to environmental air temperatures of 27.0, 15.0, and 35.0°C for periods of 30–50 minutes [8]. Upon cold exposure, MS patients demonstrated cold awareness but impaired shivering and cutaneous vasoconstriction (CVC) and a small increase in the metabolic rate which resulted in a fall in core body temperature [8]. In the same conditions, the paraplegic

control subject showed marked shivering and peripheral CVC, a more significant metabolic increase, and maintained core body temperature, as would be expected normally [8]. While no formal autonomic tests were arranged in our patient, no significant alterations of respiratory rate or heart rate were detected clinically or recorded in the observation charts.

Given that the hypothalamus is considered a key centre for thermoregulation, the focus of previous reports on hypothermia in MS was often on identifying hypothalamic lesions. In this case, a 3 T MRI and, subsequently, two 1.5 T MRI scans with contrast failed to detect hypothalamic involvement. Brain MRI was recorded in 15 other hypothermic MS patients, but radiological evidence for hypothalamic involvement was poor (n = 2; 13%) and in both cases it involved the preoptic area (POA) [17, 18]. Out of three brains which were examined postmortem, hypothalamic pathology was evident in two [9, 12, 14] (see Table 2). Previous to autopsy, brain MRI had been performed in one of such cases but had failed to detect hypothalamic changes, despite identifying periventricular lesions [14]. Independently, an MRI study on 105 Caucasian patients, with clinically definite MS without hypothermia and typical lesions, revealed a similar (13%) frequency of radiologically-detectable hypothalamic changes, using a 1.5 Tesla MRI scanner, with conventional protocols [21]. Instead, a postmortem study on 17 nonhypothermic MS patients found hypothalamic lesions in 16 brains (97%), 60% of which showed active inflammation [22]. Different factors may explain this disparity in results. Firstly, poor radiological sensitivity, particularly in the earlier reports on hypothermia in MS, may account for the low presence of hypothalamic lesions. Secondly, the patient cohorts of Qiu et al. [21] and Huitinga et al. [22] were different, with the latter having a greater mean age of disease duration which was statistically associated with a greater number of active hypothalamic lesions [22]. Although, using the current MR technology, we are unable to exclude very small hypothalamic lesions, we are mindful that the latter have not been found in other reported cases [14] and by contrast, they can be present in MS patients not affected by hypothermia.

Together with hypothalamic changes, callosal, brainstem, and spinal cord lesions were also detected at autopsy in hypothermic MS patients (see Table 2). All these areas have been previously associated with the development of hypothermic episodes and both the brainstem and the upper spinal cord are known as important thermoregulatory centres [4, 5, 14] (see Figure 2).

Brain callosal involvement, for instance, was detected in our case (see Figure 1) and in other four hypothermic MS patients via MRI or autopsy (see Table 2). In one instance, this was associated with hypothalamic disease [18]. In another report, MRI hyperintensities in the right posterior thalamus were associated with generalised atrophy, displaying clinical similarities to Shapiro's syndrome [16]. This is characterised by the congenital agenesis of the corpus callosum, hyperhidrosis, and recurrent hypothermia [23].

Brainstem lesions were associated with hypothermia in two other MS cases [4, 14]. In addition, a mesodiencephalic haematoma has been reported to be associated with hypothermia in a non-MS patient [24].

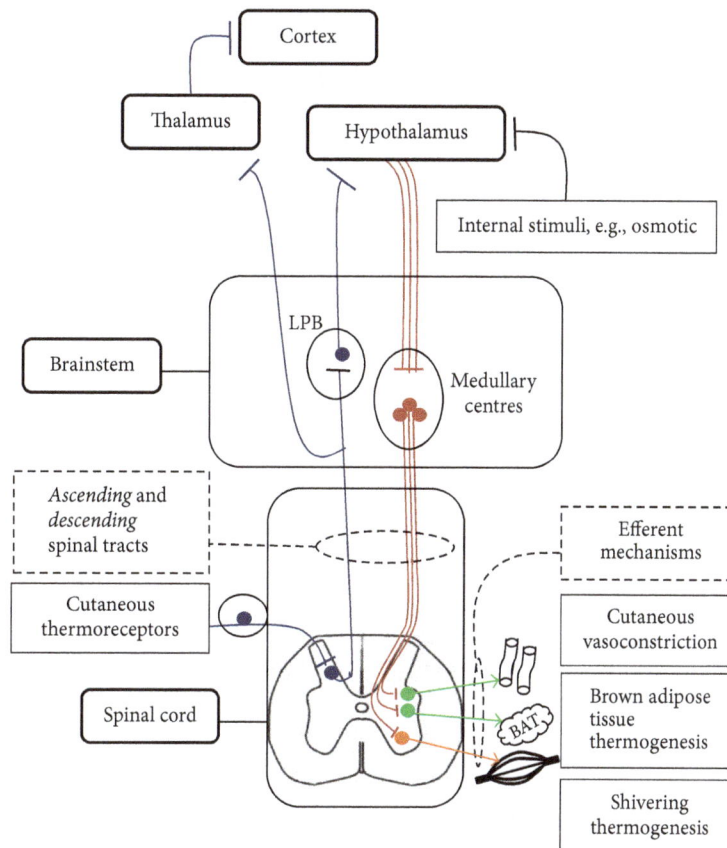

FIGURE 2: A schematic view of the main components of the thermoregulatory pathway according to the current main model [5, 6]. It is thought that cool and warm-sensitive cutaneous thermoreceptors detect changes in skin temperature. These are relayed via parallel *ascending* spinal cords tracts, to the pontine lateral parabrachial nucleus (LPB) [5]. In turn, the LPB transmits these to the anterior hypothalamus [5]. Afferent information is also separately sent to the cortex (thalamocortical tract) [5]. The hypothalamus integrates these signals with sensory information from other areas like visceral thermoreceptors and osmoreceptors to generate an effector response. In physiological conditions, after an increase in cutaneous cool signals is detected by the hypothalamic median preoptic subnucleus (MnPO) of the Preoptic Area (POA), disinhibition of the efferent pathways (in red color) leads to the activation of the three main heat-maintenance/producing mechanisms [5]. The rostral ventromedial medulla, including the rostral raphe pallidus nucleus (rRPa), is considered a key supraspinal area which regulates cutaneous vasoconstriction (CVC) and brown adipose tissue (BAT) thermogenesis (sympathetic (in green color)) and shivering thermogenesis (somatic (in orange color)) [5, 6].

Upper spinal cord pathology in MS could also be associated with hypothermia. Spinal involvement of the cervical region is particularly common in MS and involves both white and grey matter, interneurons and motoneurons [25, 26]. Similarly to brainstem lesions, upper spinal cord changes could impair both ascending and descending tracts of the thermoregulatory circuit (see Figure 2). Extensive spinal cord lesions associated with brain and hypothalamic involvement were found at autopsy in one MS patient [12] and were radiologically detected in ours (see Figure 1). In the previously reported cases, however, spinal MRI was never reported and in ours it was only performed once, after repeated episodes of hypothermia. Hence, our ability to directly estimate the impact of spinal lesions on the development of hypothermia in MS is limited.

Given the prominent spinal involvement, the differential diagnosis of neuromyelitis optica spectrum disorder (NMOSD) was discussed at a neuroradiology meeting but was ruled out on the basis of clinical presentation,

radiological features (multiple, confluent patchy lesions rather than longitudinally extensive lesions), and serology results (anti-AQP4 and anti-MOG antibody negative) [27].

Of note, hypothermia with autonomic impairment is commonly observed after upper Spinal Cord Injury (SCI) [28, 29]. A retrospective study of 50 tetraplegic patients found that subnormal core body temperatures (35.0–36.4°C) were present in all patients and clinical hypothermia was recorded in 15 [30]. Similarities between dysfunctional sympathetic sudomotor skin responses were also identified among patients with transection of the SC at different levels and MS patients [31]. In spite of these resemblances and the frequent involvement of the spinal cord in MS, spinal lesions have not been reported to cause hypothermia in MS. This may be because, similarly to other lesions, a critical impairment of conduction is required before symptoms become manifest and in MS, unlike after SCI, this process is progressive and difficult to monitor.

Interestingly, our patient developed two episodes of abnormally high temperatures (above 36.5°C), associated with admissions (see Table 1). A clinical decay at high temperatures has been previously documented in MS patients ("Uhthoff's phenomenon") but, to our knowledge, was never reported to cause admissions in hypothermic individuals. This effect likely stems from decreased axonal conduction in damaged nerves at higher temperatures [32, 33]. Why this phenomenon occurs at lower temperatures in chronically hypothermic MS patients is controversial. This may indicate a more severe axonal damage or simply the resetting of the body thermostat at a new lower point where these higher temperatures are considered extreme [4, 17].

Regardless of the causative mechanisms, no effective strategies have been devised to treat and prevent the development of hypothermic episodes in MS patients. Antibiotic treatment, in the absence of signs of infection, did not show any objective benefit for our patient and is known to promote antimicrobial resistance. Spontaneous recovery was commonly reported [18]. Treatment with steroids was shown to be potentially beneficial [17] but in our experience did not lead to substantial improvements. Our patient used an electrical blanket to control her body temperature at home, but the usefulness of this measure has not been systematically assessed. However, its use seems logical to prevent hypothermia since the neurological impairments along the thermoregulatory circuit.

4. Conclusion

In summary, hypothermia in MS patients remains a poorly understood phenomenon. The anatomical location of the causative lesions remains controversial and, based on the available evidence [4–6], we hypothesise that upper spinal cord, as well as brain stem lesions, may be involved in its pathogenesis in MS, independently of hypothalamic pathology. Given the disseminated nature of the disease, multiple, anatomically distinguished lesions, as opposed to a large single lesion, may also contribute to the development of this advanced complication by disrupting the thermoregulatory network at different levels [18]. In our opinion, in hypothermic MS patients, spinal MRI should be added to brain MRI to verify the presence of spinal involvement, due to its clinical importance. With the development of more sensitive neuroimaging and follow-up scans, anticipating the clinical course of hypothermia in these patients may be possible. Currently, in fact, the development of chronic hypothermia remains unpredictable.

Conflicts of Interest

The authors declare that there are no conflicts of interest regarding the publication of this article.

Acknowledgments

In loving memory of our patient, who passed away at Nottingham University Hospitals on 15 December 2017, the authors wish to thank her and her family for their support and encouragement.

References

[1] C. A. Dendrou, L. Fugger, and M. A. Friese, "Immunopathology of multiple sclerosis," *Nature Reviews Immunology*, vol. 15, no. 9, pp. 545–558, 2015.

[2] M. M. Goldenberg, "Multiple Sclerosis Review," http://www.pubmedcentral.nih.gov/articlerender.fcgi?artid=3351877&tool=pmcentrez&rendertype=abstract.

[3] M. M. Vellinga, J. J. G. Geurts, E. Rostrup et al., "Clinical correlations of brain lesion distribution in multiple sclerosis," *Journal of Magnetic Resonance Imaging*, vol. 29, no. 4, pp. 768–773, 2009.

[4] J. E. Alty and H. L. Ford, "Multi-system complications of hypothermia: A case of recurrent episodic hypothermia with a review of the pathophysiology of hypothermia," *Postgraduate Medical Journal*, vol. 84, no. 992, pp. 282–286, 2008.

[5] S. F. Morrison, "Central neural control of thermoregulation and brown adipose tissue," *Autonomic Neuroscience: Basic & Clinical*, vol. 196, pp. 14–24, 2016.

[6] K. Nakamura, "Central circuitries for body temperature regulation and fever," *American Journal of Physiology-Regulatory, Integrative and Comparative Physiology*, vol. 301, no. 5, pp. R1207–R1228, 2011.

[7] H. O'Brien, J. A. Amess, and D. L. Mollin, "Recurrent thrombocytopenia, erythroid hypoplasia and sideroblastic anaemia associated with hypothermia," *British Journal of Haematology*, vol. 51, Article ID 7104229, pp. 451–456, 1982, http://www.ncbi.nlm.nih.gov/entrez/query.fcgi?cmd=Retrieve&db=PubMed&dopt=Citation&list_uids=7104229.

[8] F. Sullivan, M. Hutchinson, S. Bahandeka, and R. E. Moore, "Chronic hypothermia in multiple sclerosis," *Journal of Neurology, Neurosurgery & Psychiatry*, vol. 50, no. 6, pp. 813–815, 1987.

[9] M. Lammens, F. Lissoir, and H. Carton, "Hypothermia in three patients with multiple sclerosis," *Clinical Neurology and Neurosurgery*, vol. 91, no. 2, pp. 117–121, 1989.

[10] F. Ghawche and A. Destée, "Hypothermia and multiple sclerosis. A case with 3 episodes of transient hypothermia," in *Nature Reviews Neurology*, vol. 146, pp. 767–769, 1990.

[11] C. Geny, P. F. Pradat, J. Yulis, S. Walter, D. Cesaro, and J. D. Degos, "Hypothermia, Wernicke encephalopathy and multiple sclerosis," *Acta Neurologica Scandinavica*, vol. 86, no. 6, pp. 632–634, 1992.

[12] S. Edwards, G. Lennox, K. Robson, and A. Whiteley, "Hypothermia due to hypothalamic involvement in multiple sclerosis," *Journal of Neurology, Neurosurgery & Psychiatry*, vol. 61, no. 4, pp. 419–420, 1996.

[13] P. Mouton, F. Woimant, and O. Ille, "Hypothermia and the nervous system. Review of the literature apropos of 4 cases," *Annales De Medecine Interne*, vol. 147, pp. 107–114, 1996.

[14] K. D. White, D. J. Scoones, and P. K. Newman, "Hypothermia in multiple sclerosis," *Journal of Neurology, Neurosurgery & Psychiatry*, vol. 61, no. 4, pp. 369–375, 1996.

[15] W. Feneberg and N. H. König, "Two cases of hypothermia in multiple sclerosis," *Journal of Neurology*, vol. 253, no. S1, pp. i37–i37, 2006.

[16] R. A. Linker, A. Mohr, L. Cepek, R. Gold, and H. Prange, "Core hypothermia in multiple sclerosis: Case report with magnetic resonance imaging localization of a thalamic lesion," *Multiple Sclerosis Journal*, vol. 12, no. 1, pp. 112–115, 2006.

[17] N. Weiss, D. Hasboun, S. Demeret et al., "Paroxysmal hypothermia as a clinical feature of multiple sclerosis," *Neurology*, vol. 72, no. 2, pp. 193–195, 2009.

[18] A. Darlix, G. Mathey, and M-L. Monin, "Hypothalamic involvement in multiple sclerosis," *Nature Reviews Neurology*, vol. 168, pp. 434–443, 2012.

[19] E. Ishikawa, S. Ohgo, K. Nakatsuru et al., "Syndrome of Inappropriate Secretion of Antidiuretic Hormone (SIADH) in a Patient with Multiple Sclerosis," *Japanese Journal of Medicine*, vol. 28, no. 1, pp. 75–79, 1989.

[20] G. Liamis and M. Elisaf, "Syndrome of inappropriate antidiuresis associated with multiple sclerosis," *Journal of the Neurological Sciences*, vol. 172, Article ID 0033989706, pp. 38–40, 2000, http://www.scopus.com/inward/record.url?eid=2-s2.0-00339-89706&partnerID=40&md5=5aa44931a75f7f11bbc08886a00d-943c%255Cn.

[21] W. Qiu, S. Raven, J. Wu et al., "Hypothalamic lesions in multiple sclerosis," *Journal of Neurology, Neurosurgery & Psychiatry*, vol. 82, no. 7, pp. 819–822, 2011.

[22] I. Huitinga, C. J. De Groot, P. Van der Valk, W. Kamphorst, F. J. Tilders, and D. F. Swaab, "Hypothalamic lesions in multiple sclerosis," *Journal of Neuropathology & Experimental Neurology*, vol. 60, no. 12, pp. 1208–1218, 2001.

[23] W. R. Shapiro, G. H. Williams, and F. Plum, "Spontaneous recurrent hypothermia accompanying agenesis of the corpus callosum," *Brain*, vol. 92, no. 2, pp. 423–436, 1969.

[24] G. Gaymard, H. Cambon, D. Dormont, A. Richard, and C. Derouesne, "Hypothermia in a mesodiencephalic haematoma," *Journal of Neurology, Neurosurgery & Psychiatry*, vol. 53, no. 11, pp. 1014-1015, 1990.

[25] C. P. Gilmore, J. J. G. Geurts, N. Evangelou et al., "Spinal cord grey matter lesions in multiple sclerosis detected by post-mortem high field MR imaging," *Multiple Sclerosis Journal*, vol. 15, no. 2, pp. 180–188, 2009.

[26] C. Lukas, M. H. Sombekke, B. Bellenberg et al., "Relevance of spinal cord abnormalities to clinical disability in multiple sclerosis: MR imaging findings in a large cohort of patients," *Radiology*, vol. 269, no. 2, pp. 542–552, 2013.

[27] D. M. Wingerchuk, B. Banwell, J. L. Bennett et al., "International consensus diagnostic criteria for neuromyelitis optica spectrum disorders," *Neurology*, vol. 85, no. 2, pp. 177–189, 2015.

[28] M. Menard and G. Hahn, "Acute and chronic hypothermia in a man with spinal cord injury: environmental and pharmacologic causes," *Archives of Physical Medicine and Rehabilitation*, vol. 72, pp. 421–424, 1991.

[29] S. C. Colachis III, "Hypothermia associated with autonomic dysreflexia after traumatic spinal cord injury," *American Journal of Physical Medicine & Rehabilitation*, vol. 81, no. 3, pp. 232–235, 2002.

[30] S. Khan, M. Plummer, A. Martinez-Arizala, and K. Banovac, "Hypothermia in patients with chronic spinal cord injury," *The Journal of Spinal Cord Medicine*, vol. 30, no. 1, pp. 27–30, 2007.

[31] T. Yokota, T. Matsunaga, R. Okiyama et al., "Sympathetic skin response in patients with multiple sclerosis compared with patients with spinal cord transection and normal controls," *Brain*, vol. 114, no. 3, pp. 1381–1394, 1991.

[32] W. Uhthoff, "Untersuchungen über die bei der multiplen Herd-sklerose vorkonimenden Augenstörungen," *Archiv für Psychiatrie und Nervenkrankheiten*, vol. 21, no. 2, pp. 305–410, 1890.

[33] S. L. Davis, T. C. Frohman, C. G. Crandall et al., "Modeling Uhthoff's phenomenon in MS patients with internuclear ophthalmoparesis," *Neurology*, vol. 70, no. 13, pp. 1098–1106, 2008.

3

A Pediatric Tumor Found Frequently in the Adult Population: A Case of Anaplastic Astroblastoma in an Elderly Patient

Christopher Payne,[1] **Ali Batouli,**[2] **Kristen Stabingas,**[1]
Dunbar Alcindor,[1] **Khaled Abdel Aziz,**[1] **Cunfeng Pu,**[3] **Elizabeth Tyler-Kabara,**[4]
Robert Williams,[2] **and Alexander Yu**[1]

[1]*Department of Neurosurgery, Allegheny General Hospital, Pittsburgh, PA, USA*
[2]*Department of Radiology, Allegheny General Hospital, Pittsburgh, PA, USA*
[3]*Department of Pathology, Allegheny General Hospital, Pittsburgh, PA, USA*
[4]*Department of Neurological Surgery, Children's Hospital of Pittsburgh, University of Pittsburgh, Pittsburgh, PA, USA*

Correspondence should be addressed to Christopher Payne; paynech@tcd.ie

Academic Editor: Norman S. Litofsky

Astroblastomas are rare, potentially curable primary brain tumors which can be difficult to diagnose. We present the case of astroblastoma in a 73-year-old male, an atypical age for this tumor, more classically found in pediatric and young adult populations. Through our case and review of the literature, we note that this tumor is frequently reported in adult populations and the presentation of this tumor in the elderly is well described. This tumor is an important consideration in the differential diagnosis when managing both pediatric and adult patients of any age who present with the imaging findings characteristic of this rare tumor.

1. Introduction

Astroblastomas are uncommon tumors of neuroepithelial origin first described by Bailey and Cushing in 1926 [1]. These tumors are found in the cerebral hemispheres, most commonly seen in children and young adults, with a reported incidence of 0.45–2.8% [2]. A bimodal distribution of cases has been reported with peak prevalence between 5 and 10 years of age and 21 and 30 years [3]. Astroblastomas present with signs of increased intracranial pressure and currently do not have unified diagnostic criteria [4, 5]. Furthermore, they have similar radiologic and histopathologic features as other glial tumors and because of this may be easily misdiagnosed [6–8].

The rarity of this tumor and, as a result, the limited knowledge surrounding the unique histological and radiological characteristics which differentiate this tumor type complicate our ability to obtain a prompt and accurate diagnosis. Such difficulty is furthermore complicated when a rare tumor presents outside the expected patient demographic. This was the case in the patient we present, an unusual case of a 73-year-old male with an anaplastic astroblastoma.

2. Case Report

2.1. History. A 73-year-old male presented after a fall with complaints of headaches and memory loss over the past year. The patient had a history of hypertension, hypothyroidism, and prostate cancer treated 22 years priorly. On presentation the patient was mildly confused but otherwise had no focal neurologic signs or symptoms.

2.2. Imaging. Computed tomography (CT) of the head demonstrated a well-circumscribed partially hemorrhagic mass in the left temporal-occipital region. The mass caused effacement of the occipital horn and atrium of the left lateral ventricle as well as trapping of the temporal horn (Figure 1).

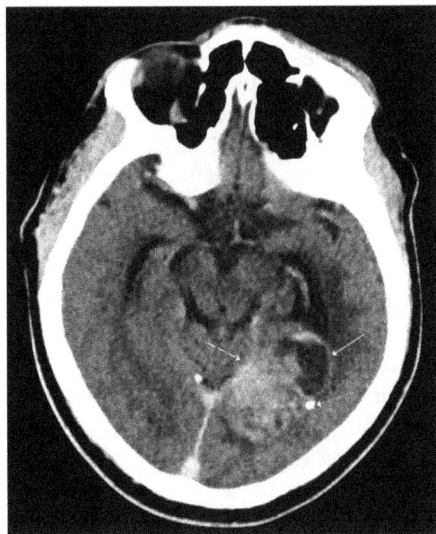

FIGURE 1: Noncontrast axial computed tomography image shows a mixed solid (dashed white arrow) and cystic (solid white arrow) temporooccipital mass with a hyperattenuating solid component and a punctate calcification peripherally (dotted white arrow).

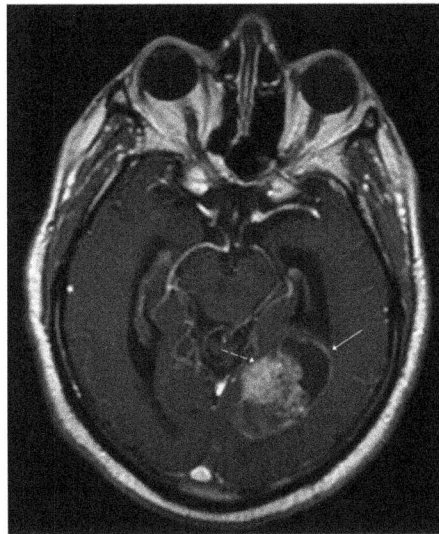

FIGURE 3: Postcontrast axial T1 weighted MR image demonstrates avid heterogeneous enhancement in the solid component (dashed white arrow) with rim enhancement of the cystic component.

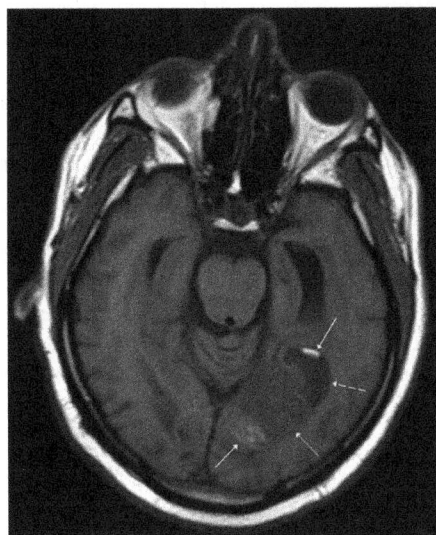

FIGURE 2: Precontrast axial T1 weighted image shows the solid component (dotted white arrows) to be hypointense to grey matter with small areas of T1 hyperintensity (solid white arrows) seen peripherally within the cystic (dashed white arrow) and solid components, likely representing areas of focal hemorrhage.

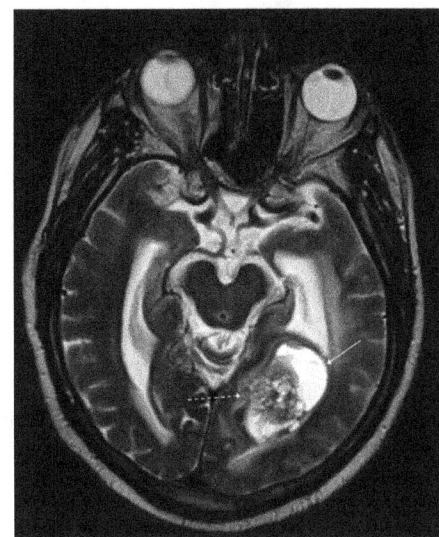

FIGURE 4: T2 weighted axial image shows a mixed solid (dashed white arrow) and cystic (solid white arrow) temporooccipital mass with a heterogeneous, bubbly appearance of the solid component.

MRI of the brain revealed a heterogeneously enhancing, mixed cystic and solid mass (Figures 2, 3, and 4). At this time, a differential diagnosis of glioblastoma multiforme or metastasis was proposed. A metastatic workup with CT of the chest, abdomen, and pelvis however was unremarkable. The patient and his family wanted a biopsy performed first for tissue diagnosis before they would decide on proceeding with a gross resection. A stereotactic biopsy was subsequently performed.

2.3. Histology. Sections of the tumor showed a solid tumor comprised of epitheliod cuboidal-to-columnar cells with abundant eosinophilic cytoplasm and large nuclei with moderate to marked atypia. These cells demonstrated perivascular distribution in a pseudorosette pattern with broad cytoplasmic processes radiating toward the centrally placed blood vessels (Figure 5). The tumor however was nearly completely devoid of any fibrillarity. A papillary appearance was noted in multiple foci. Areas of geographic necrosis and high mitotic index of up to 11 mitotic figures per high power field were noted.

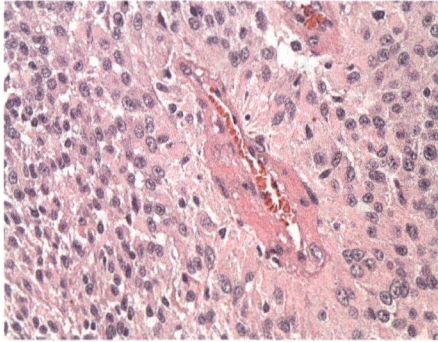

FIGURE 5: H&E stain demonstrating a perivascular pseudorosette with blunted end foot plates of the tumor cells directed toward a central blood vessel (40x).

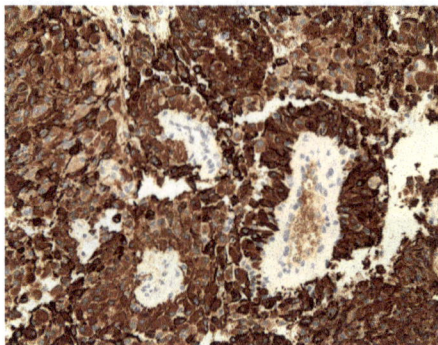

FIGURE 6: Glial fibrillary acidic protein (GFAP) stain shows positive staining demonstrating the glial origin of tumor cells (20x). Again, we can appreciate the tumor cells arranged in a perivascular pseudorosette with tumor cells directed toward the central blood vessel and the lack of fibrillarity.

Immunohistochemical stains performed showed neurofilament protein and NeuN stains to be negative within the tumor, consistent with a solid pattern of growth. The glial fibrillary acidic protein (GFAP) stain showed extensive cytoplasmic positivity (Figure 6). The CAM 5.2 immunostain was negative and epithelial membrane antigen (EMA) was expressed in a membrane and focally dot-like pattern in a subset of tumor cells. The tumor was negative for IDH (R132H) mutant protein expression. A Ki67 immunohistochemical stain showed a labeling index of 9.8%. A D2-40 immunostain showed strong cytoplasmic positivity and CD99 was extensively expressed in a membranous pattern. Patchy OLIG2 staining was also noted. These histologic and immunohistochemical findings were consistent with a diagnosis of anaplastic astroblastoma.

2.4. Postoperative Course. Three weeks after the initial biopsy, a left occipital craniotomy for gross total resection was performed. The tumor was cystic, rubbery, and tan-yellow in appearance and demonstrated extension into the lateral ventricle. Histological analysis again demonstrated a solid tumor comprised of epitheliod cells with abundant eosinophilic cytoplasm, large nuclei, and a lack of fibrillarity.

Numerous examples of tumor cells arranged in perivascular pseudorosettes were again noted. The immunohistochemical staining pattern was consistent with that observed from the tissue obtained during the stereotactic biopsy, confirming the diagnosis of anaplastic astroblastoma. Adjuvant radiotherapy of 60 gray in 30 fractions was administered to the patient. Clinically, the patient improved, demonstrating mild confusion with an otherwise nonfocal neurological exam. Two years after the initial resection however, the patient presented with worsening mental status and was found to have recurrence of this tumor. Repeat resection was performed which again demonstrated tissue consistent with anaplastic astroblastoma. During his postoperative course his mental status continued to remain poor. He was discharged to hospice care and later expired.

3. Discussion

Astroblastomas are almost exclusively supratentorial; they frequently show calcification and are peripherally located. They have both solid and a multicystic component giving the distinctive bubbly appearance, characteristic of this tumor [4, 7, 9–11]. On MRI, they have relatively little peritumoral T2 hyperintensity despite their large size, suggesting a lack of tumor infiltration into local tissue [7]. Due to the relative difficulty in differentiating between astroblastomas and ependymomas on histology, it is recommended that radiologic findings demonstrating a suspicion for astroblastoma be communicated to the pathologist [12, 13]. In comparison to astroblastomas, ependymomas are frequently observed in the posterior fossa and do not commonly show the bubbly appearance characteristic of astroblastomas [11]. Radiologic imaging in the case we present was consistent with many of the features described above, such as the supratentorial location of these tumors and the characteristic solid and cystic, bubbly appearance with little surrounding T2 hyperintensity (Figure 4).

The histogenesis of anaplastic astroblastoma is controversial; however tanycytes, glial precursor cells, have been suggested as a potential tissue of origin [14–16]. The diagnosis requires a well-defined margin with the presence of perivascular pseudorosettes with thick and short, blunted tumor cells which do not taper as they project toward the central blood vessel [7, 9, 10, 17, 18]. The perivascular structures can be uniform or loosely scattered structures with round to oval nuclei and may exhibit chromatin aggregation [12]. Hyalinization and fibrotic vessel walls can be visible with occasional areas of infarcted brain tissue [10, 19]. In comparison to astroblastomas, ependymomas show some subtle but very important histological differences. The pseudorosettes of ependymomas have cell processes which taper toward the central blood vessel compared with the cell processes of astroblastomas which do not taper in this manner. True rosettes and areas of fibrillarity may be observed in ependymomas while astroblastomas are characteristically devoid of fibrillarity and do not have true rosettes [11, 13, 17]. Astroblastomas show reactivity to S-100, GFAP, and their cell membranes may be EMA reactive [2, 6, 10, 18, 20].

The Ki-67 proliferation indices range from 1% to 18%; however this does not correlate with outcome [10, 21]. A number of chromosomal aberrations have been described in small series and include gains of chromosomes 19 and 20q [10, 17, 22, 23]. There are two variants, anaplastic or high-grade astroblastoma and well differentiated or low-grade astroblastoma. The anaplastic variant displays atypical cells, more obvious mitotic activity, necrosis, and disorganized cell architecture [6, 19]. Pathological assessment of our specimen demonstrated the anaplastic variant.

Astroblastomas show a slight female predominance and are often noted in the literature to be a pediatric tumor [4, 5, 7, 24–26] with congenital lesions also reported [17, 18, 27–29]. In our review however we note many reports of this tumor presenting in adult patients and the incidence of this is well described [3–5, 7, 9, 16, 17, 24, 30–32]. Ahmed et al., for example, carried out the largest retrospective analysis that we identified in the literature and out of 239 cases, 168 were above 21 years of age. With this shift in thinking, the tumor may be considered more frequently in the differential diagnosis of adults of all ages presenting with primary brain tumors who have imaging studies characteristic for this type of tumor. Our case of an astroblastoma in a 73-year-old was uncharacteristic of this tumor type but these tumors by no means appear to be limited to a pediatric and young adult population.

The treatment of astroblastoma is not well-established owing to its rarity but surgery continues to play a vital role in the management of this condition. Complete resection is curative in low-grade cases [30, 31, 33]. In contrast to this, high-grade astroblastomas have a worse prognosis due to higher recurrence rates and more rapid progression and invasion of local brain regions [16, 19]. More aggressive treatment and close follow-up are warranted in these cases [8, 22, 30, 33, 34]. It is also suggested that the extent of peritumoral edema or peritumoral T2 hyperintensity associated with an astroblastoma on MRI may also be a feature predictive of recurrence, independent of the grade of tumor [35]. Radiotherapy has been recognized as an important adjuvant therapy in a number of high-grade astroblastoma cases [19, 29, 32], as well as following the recurrence of a low-grade lesion [30]. This differs from the treatment of ependymoma where the current standard of treatment utilizes radiotherapy in all cases, not just high-grade or recurrent cases, further highlighting the importance of accurately differentiating these two tumor types [13].

Ahmed et al. performed a retrospective analysis involving two hundred and thirty-nine patients with astroblastoma and noted a median overall survival of 55 months in patients receiving treatment. They also noted a decreased survival associated with increasing age at presentation. Though not yet proven, it is suggested that this may be associated with genetic differences in these tumors akin to the differences observed between glioblastoma cases seen in pediatric versus adult populations [5]. Though the majority of astroblastomas present in a supratentorial location, infratentorial tumors were shown to have a better prognosis [5].

4. Conclusion

Astroblastomas are rare, potentially curable primary brain tumors which can be difficult to diagnose. The literature often refers to this as a tumor frequently found in pediatric and young adult populations; however our patient presented with this tumor at 73 years of age. In our review we note many cases of astroblastoma reported which present in adults with some series showing a higher incidence in the adult population. The occurrence of this tumor in the elderly is also well described. We propose that this tumor is better referred to as a primary brain tumor presenting frequently in both pediatric and adult populations. This change in thinking will favor considering astroblastoma in the differential diagnosis when assessing adult patients who present with imaging findings characteristic of this rare tumor. In doing so, we may avoid any possible delays in diagnosis or misdiagnosis that might occur when overlooking this tumor as a potential primary brain neoplasm affecting adults.

Competing Interests

All authors certify that they have no affiliations with or involvement in any organization or entity with any financial interest (such as honoraria; educational grants; participation in speakers' bureaus; membership, employment, consultancies, stock ownership, or other equity interest; and expert testimony or patent-licensing arrangements) or nonfinancial interest (such as personal or professional relationships, affiliations, knowledge, or beliefs) in the subject matter or materials discussed in this manuscript.

Acknowledgments

The authors would like to thank Dr. Arie Perry from the Department of Pathology, University of California, San Francisco, for his assistance in histological examination and diagnosis in this case.

References

[1] P. Bailey and H. Cushing, *A Classification of the Tumors of the Glioma Group on a Histogenetic Basis with a Correlated Study of Prognosis*, Lippincott, Philadelphia, Pa, USA, 1926.

[2] B. L. Pizer, T. Moss, A. Oakhill, D. Webb, and H. B. Coakham, "Congenital astroblastoma: an immunohistochemical study. Case report," *Journal of Neurosurgery*, vol. 83, no. 3, pp. 550–555, 1995.

[3] G. Bahadur and P. Hindmarsh, "Age definitions, childhood and adolescent cancers in relation to reproductive issues," *Human Reproduction*, vol. 15, no. 1, pp. 227–230, 2000.

[4] M. E. Sughrue, J. Choi, M. J. Rutkowski et al., "Clinical features and post-surgical outcome of patients with astroblastoma," *Journal of Clinical Neuroscience*, vol. 18, no. 6, pp. 750–754, 2011.

[5] K. A. Ahmed, P. K. Allen, A. Mahajan, P. D. Brown, and A. J. Ghia, "Astroblastomas: a surveillance, epidemiology, and end results (SEER)-based patterns of care analysis," *World Neurosurgery*, vol. 82, no. 1-2, pp. e291–e297, 2014.

[6] V. Agarwal, R. Mally, D. Palande, and V. Velho, "Cerebral astroblastoma: a case report and review of literature," *Asian Journal of Neurosurgery*, vol. 7, no. 2, pp. 98–100, 2012.

[7] J. W. Bell, A. G. Osborn, K. L. Salzman, S. I. Blaser, B. V. Jones, and S. S. Chin, "Neuroradiologic characteristics of astroblastoma," *Neuroradiology*, vol. 49, no. 3, pp. 203–209, 2007.

[8] R. Kemerdere, R. Dashti, M. O. Ulu et al., "Supratentorial high grade astroblastoma: report of two cases and review of the literature," *Turkish Neurosurgery*, vol. 19, no. 2, pp. 149–152, 2009.

[9] A. Alaraj, M. Chan, S. Oh, E. Michals, T. Valyi-Nagy, and T. Hersonsky, "Astroblastoma presenting with intracerebral hemorrhage misdiagnosed as dural arteriovenous fistula: review of a rare entity," *Surgical Neurology*, vol. 67, no. 3, pp. 308–313, 2007.

[10] D. J. Brat, Y. Hirose, K. J. Cohen, B. G. Feuerstein, and P. C. Burger, "Astroblastoma: clinicopathologic features and chromosomal abnormalities defined by comparative genomic hybridization," *Brain Pathology*, vol. 10, no. 3, pp. 342–352, 2000.

[11] J. D. Port, D. J. Brat, P. C. Burger, and M. G. Pomper, "Astroblastoma: radiologic-pathologic correlation and distinction from ependymoma," *American Journal of Neuroradiology*, vol. 23, no. 2, pp. 243–247, 2002.

[12] N. Kurwale, D. Agrawal, and B. Sharma, "Astroblastoma: a radio-histological diagnosis," *Journal of Pediatric Neurosciences*, vol. 3, no. 2, pp. 160–162, 2008.

[13] D. J. Duff and D. C. Miller, "Ependymomas," *Pathology Case Reviews*, vol. 18, no. 5, pp. 221–230, 2013.

[14] L. J. Rubinstein and M. M. Herman, "The astroblastoma and its possible cytogenic relationship to the tanycyte—an electron microscopic, immunohistochemical, tissue-and organ-culture study," *Acta Neuropathologica*, vol. 78, no. 5, pp. 472–483, 1989.

[15] T. Kubota, K. Sato, H. Arishima, H. Takeuchi, R. Kitai, and T. Nakagawa, "Astroblastoma: immunohistochemical and ultrastructural study of distinctive epithelial and probable tanycytic differentiation," *Neuropathology*, vol. 26, no. 1, pp. 72–81, 2006.

[16] M. Kujas, T. Faillot, Lalam, B. Roncier, M. Catala, and J. Poirier, "Astroblastomas revisited. Report of two cases with immunocytochemical and electron microscopic study. Histogenetic considerations," *Neuropathology and Applied Neurobiology*, vol. 26, no. 3, pp. 295–298, 2000.

[17] K.-S. Eom, J.-M. Kim, and T.-Y. Kim, "A cerebral astroblastoma mimicking an extra-axial neoplasm," *Journal of Korean Neurosurgical Society*, vol. 43, no. 4, pp. 205–208, 2008.

[18] D. S. Kim, S. Y. Park, and S. P. Lee, "Astroblastoma: a case report," *Journal of Korean Medical Science*, vol. 19, no. 5, pp. 772–776, 2004.

[19] J. M. Bonnin and L. J. Rubinstein, "Astroblastomas: a pathological study of 23 tumors, with a postoperative follow-up in 13 patients," *Neurosurgery*, vol. 25, no. 1, pp. 6–13, 1989.

[20] A. Cabello, S. Madero, A. Castresana, and R. Diaz-Lobato, "Astroblastoma: electron microscopy and immunohistochemical findings: case report," *Surgical Neurology*, vol. 35, no. 2, pp. 116–121, 1991.

[21] M. Kaji, H. Takeshima, Y. Nakazato, and J.-I. Kuratsu, "Low-grade astroblastoma recurring with extensive invasion: case report," *Neurologia Medico-Chirurgica*, vol. 46, no. 9, pp. 450–454, 2006.

[22] I. Chopra, F. Roncaroli, V. Apostolopoulos, J. Moss, D. Peston, and K. O'Neill, "October 2006: a 37-year old male with headache," *Brain Pathology*, vol. 17, no. 2, pp. 251–252, 2007.

[23] H. Hirano, S. Yunoue, M. Kaji, M. Tsuchiya, and K. Arita, "Consecutive histological changes in an astroblastoma that disseminated to the spinal cord after repeated intracranial recurrences: a case report," *Brain Tumor Pathology*, vol. 25, no. 1, pp. 25–31, 2008.

[24] L. Denaro, M. Gardiman, M. Calderone et al., "Intraventricular astroblastoma: case report," *Journal of Neurosurgery: Pediatrics*, vol. 1, no. 2, pp. 152–155, 2008.

[25] M. I. A. El Hag, A. Hdeib, P. D. S. C. Ciarlini, and M. L. Cohen, "Astroblastoma and other predominantly pediatric supratentorial papillary/epithelioid gliomas," *Pathology Case Reviews*, vol. 18, no. 6, pp. 244–252, 2013.

[26] L. M. Tumialán, D. J. Brat, A. J. Fountain, and D. L. Barrow, "An astroblastoma mimicking a cavernous malformation: case report," *Neurosurgery*, vol. 60, no. 3, pp. E569–E570, 2007.

[27] A. M. Stark, S. Modlich, A. Claviez, A. van Baalen, H.-H. Hugo, and H. M. Mehdorn, "Congenital diffuse anaplastic astrocytoma with ependymal and leptomeningeal spread: case report," *Journal of Neuro-Oncology*, vol. 84, no. 3, pp. 325–328, 2007.

[28] K. Uchida, M. Mukai, H. Okano, and T. Kawase, "Possible oncogenicity of subventricular zone neural stem cells: case report," *Neurosurgery*, vol. 55, no. 4, pp. 977–978, 2004.

[29] E. Unal, Y. Koksal, I. Vajtai, H. Toy, Y. Kocaogullar, and Y. Paksoy, "Astroblastoma in a child," *Child's Nervous System*, vol. 24, no. 2, pp. 165–168, 2008.

[30] P. P. L. Lau, T. M. M. Thomas, P. C. W. Lui, and A. T. Khin, "'Low-grade' astroblastoma with rapid recurrence: a case report," *Pathology*, vol. 38, no. 1, pp. 78–80, 2006.

[31] C. Notarianni, M. Akin, M. Fowler, and A. Nanda, "Brainstem astroblastoma: a case report and review of the literature," *Surgical Neurology*, vol. 69, no. 2, pp. 201–205, 2008.

[32] M. Salvati, A. D'Elia, C. Brogna et al., "Cerebral astroblastoma: analysis of six cases and critical review of treatment options," *Journal of Neuro-Oncology*, vol. 93, no. 3, pp. 369–378, 2009.

[33] E. Caroli, M. Salvati, V. Esposito, E. R. Orlando, and F. Giangaspero, "Cerebral astroblastoma," *Acta Neurochirurgica*, vol. 146, no. 6, pp. 629–633, 2004.

[34] M. Kantar, Y. Ertan, T. Turhan et al., "Anaplastic astroblastoma of childhood: aggressive behavior," *Child's Nervous System*, vol. 25, no. 9, pp. 1125–1129, 2009.

[35] C. Janz and R. Buhl, "Astroblastoma: report of two cases with unexpected clinical behavior and review of the literature," *Clinical Neurology and Neurosurgery*, vol. 125, pp. 114–124, 2014.

4

Neuroendoscopic Removal of Acute Subdural Hematoma with Contusion: Advantages for Elderly Patients

Ryota Tamura, Yoshiaki Kuroshima, and Yoshiki Nakamura

Department of Neurosurgery, Tokyo Medical Center, 2-5-1 Higashigaoka, Meguro-ku, Tokyo 152-8902, Japan

Correspondence should be addressed to Ryota Tamura; moltobello-r-610@hotmail.co.jp

Academic Editor: Dominic B. Fee

Background. Large craniotomy for acute subdural hematoma is sometimes too invasive. We report good outcomes for two cases of neuroendoscopic evacuation of hematoma and contusion by 1 burr hole surgery. *Case Presentation.* Both patients arrived by ambulance at our hospital with disturbed consciousness after falling. Case 1 was an 81-year-old man who took antiplatelet drugs for brain infarction. Case 2 was a 73-year-old alcoholic woman. CT scanning showed acute subdural hematoma and frontal contusion in both cases. In the acute stage, glycerol was administered to reduce edema; CTs after 48 and 72 hours showed an increase of subdural hematoma and massive contusion of the frontal lobe. Disturbed consciousness steadily deteriorated. The subdural hematoma and contusion were removed as soon as possible by neuroendoscopy under local anesthesia, because neither patient was a good candidate for large craniotomy considering age and past history. 40%~70% of the hematoma was removed, and the consciousness level improved. *Conclusion.* Neuroendoscopic removal of acute subdural hematoma and contusion has advantages and disadvantages. For patients with underlying medical issues or other risk factors, it is likely to be effective.

1. Introduction

Hematoma evacuation by large craniotomy is the standard treatment for acute subdural hematoma (ASDH) with brainstem compression. Craniotomy in general is known to impose a significant burden on patients due to the large amount of bleeding, large skin incision, and long operation time. It also requires general anesthesia, which adds to the burden. Therefore, there are many patients who are considered unsuitable for large craniotomy, because of antiplatelet or anticoagulation drugs, hepatic cirrhosis, or older age. In contrast, neuroendoscopy hematoma evacuation is a minimally invasive procedure, requiring only a 4 cm skin incision and 1 burr hole. It can be performed under local anesthesia and mild sedation. Here we report good outcomes for two patients who underwent neuroendoscopic procedure for hematoma and contusion evacuation.

To our knowledge, there are no previous reports of this procedure performed for ASDH with concomitant contusion.

2. Case Presentations

2.1. Case 1. An 81-year-old man presented to our hospital by ambulance with disturbed consciousness after falling. He was taking the antiplatelet drug cilostazol for brain infarction. The admission Glasgow Coma Scale (GCS) score was 13 (E4V4M5). Computed tomography (CT) scanning revealed left ASDH and bilateral frontal contusion with a thickness of 14 mm and a midline shift (MLS) of 8 mm (Figure 1(a)). Our initial plan was to give conservative treatment. In the acute stage, tranexamic acid (2000 mg) was administered to staunch the bleeding. But CT 24 hours later revealed worsening (thickness 16 mm, MLS 8 mm). Contusion in the left frontal lobe became especially apparent. Glycerol (1600 mL/day) was administered to reduce edema, but the 72-hour CT showed massive contusion of the left frontal lobe and the MLS had increased to 9 mm (Figure 1(b)). The GCS score deteriorated steadily to E2V2M4. At this point, decision to perform surgery was made. As for the method of surgery, neuroendoscopy under local anesthesia and mild sedation

(a)

(b)

(c)

(d)

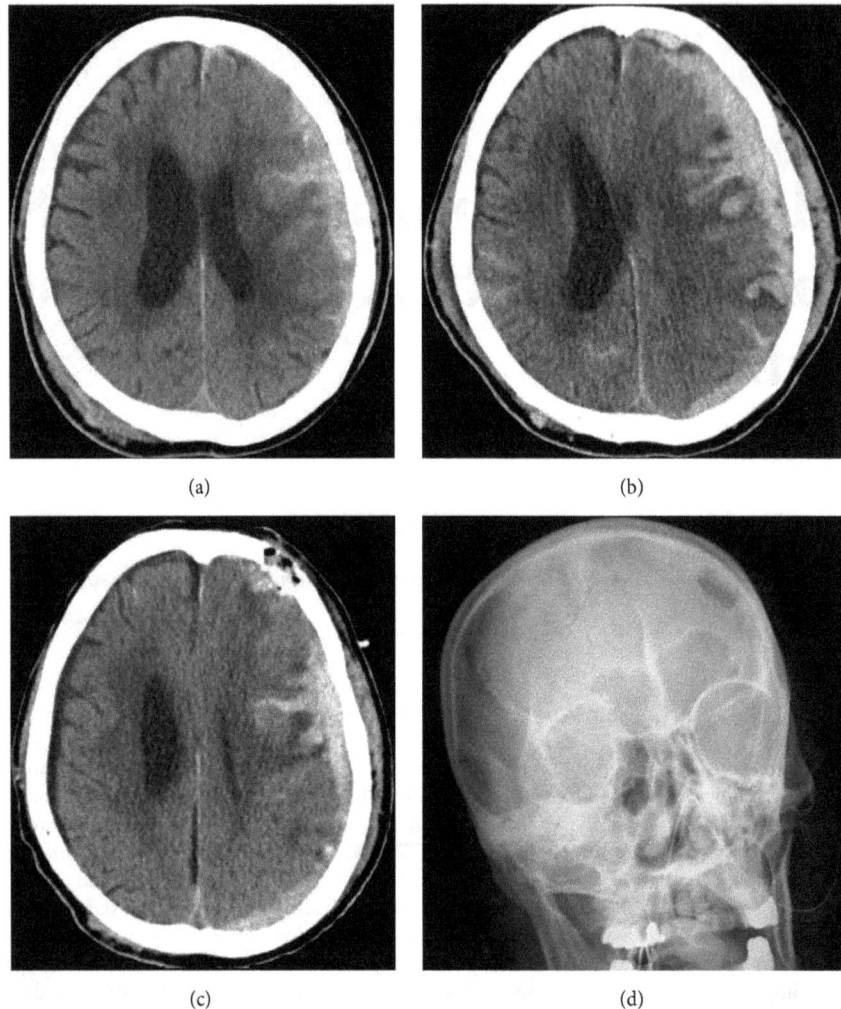

FIGURE 1: (a) Axial plain CT scan at the time of admission shows left acute subdural hematoma and bilateral frontal contusion with thickness of 14 mm and midline shift of 8 mm. There is a bruised area in the right parietal region without bone fracture. (b) Axial plain CT scan 72 hours after admission shows worsened acute subdural hematoma with thickness of 16 mm and midline shift of 9 mm. Massive contusion of the left frontal lobe has occurred. (c) Radiographic frontal view shows the location of the burr hole 4 cm above the left eyebrow. (d) Axial plain CT scan after surgery shows reduced hematoma. Midline shift had improved to 4 mm. There is a small amount of air in the subdural space. Burr hole is covered by bone powders.

was chosen, since the patient was not a good candidate for large craniotomy considering his age and the use of antiplatelet drug. A 4 cm skin incision was made along the shriveled skin of the left forehead 4 cm above the eyebrow in the hairline, and 1 burr hole was made using a hand drill. We then formed the hole into an earthenware mortar shape and made a cross-dural incision to expose the brain surface. A 10 mm diameter sheath (Neuroport, Olympus Corp.) was inserted into the brain and the contusion was removed first using a rigid scope (0°, 2.7 mm). We then guided the Neuroport to the subdural space and removed the subdural hematoma as completely as possible.

In total, 40% of the hematoma was removed, and the MLS was improved to 4 mm after the procedure (Figures 1(c) and 1(d)). Tranexamic acid (250 mg) was administered to prevent postoperative oozing.

The consciousness level started to improve right after the operation and eventually improved to E4V3M5 20 days after operation. The patient could eat without assistance by this time. Kampo (goreisan) was prescribed to prevent chronic subdural hematoma.

2.2. Case 2. A 73-year-old woman presented to our hospital by ambulance with disturbed consciousness after drinking alcohol and falling. Her past medical history was diabetes and alcohol abuse. Her admission GCS score was 14 (E4V4M6). CT scanning showed right ASDH and right frontal and temporal contusion with a thickness of 10 mm and an MLS of 6 mm (Figure 2(a)). Our initial plan was to give conservative treatment. In the acute stage, tranexamic acid (2000 mg) and glycerol were administered, as with Case 1. But the CT after 48 hours showed edema around the contusion and uncal

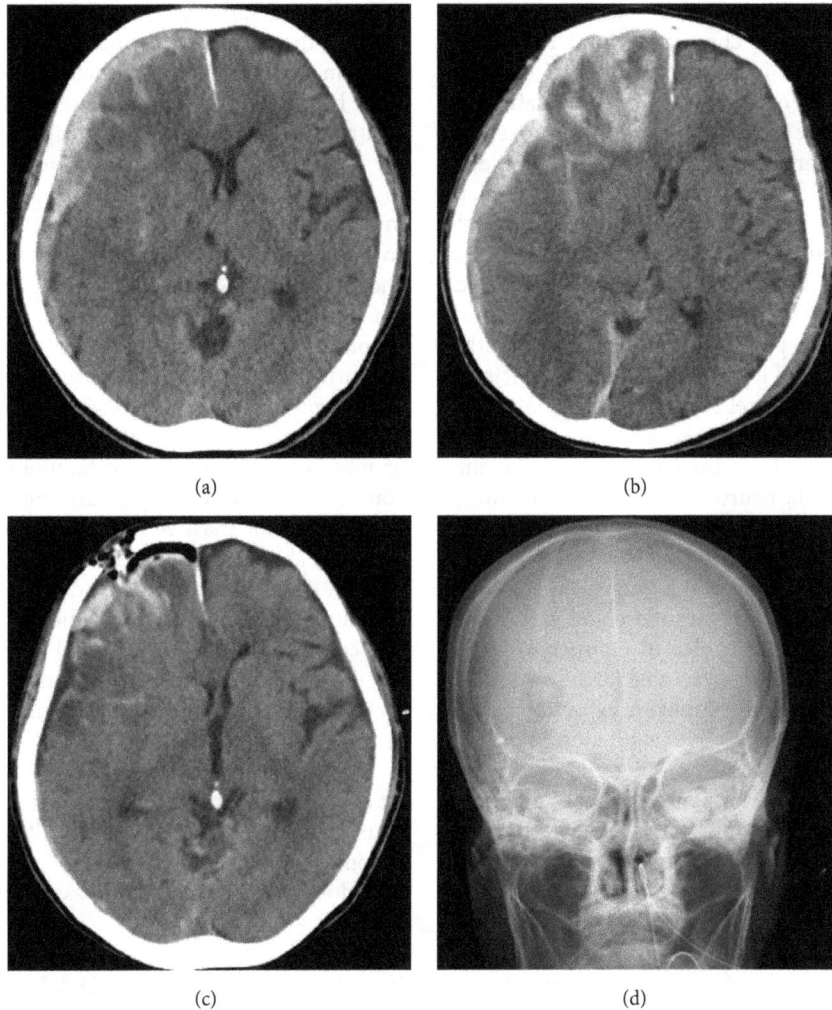

FIGURE 2: (a) Axial plain CT scan at the time of admission shows right acute subdural hematoma and right frontal and temporal contusion with thickness of 10 mm and midline shift of 6 mm. There is a bruised area in the left temporal region without bone fracture. (b) Axial plain CT scan 48 hours after admission showed massive contusion and uncal herniation. The midline shift has worsened to 9 mm. (c) Most hematoma was removed and midline shift was completely resolved. The massive contusion in the right frontal lobe was reduced. The information drain was inserted into the subdural space. (d) Radiographic frontal view shows location of the burr hole 3 cm above the right eyebrow.

herniation with anisocoria (Figure 2(b)). Since the massive contusion in the frontal lobe exerted a mass effect, removal of contusion was considered.

We removed the subdural hematoma and contusion to the furthest extent possible by neuroendoscopy under local anesthesia and mild sedation, as with Case 1. We placed a 4 cm incision on the forehead outside of the hairline in order to remove the massive contusion together with the subdural hematoma. Considering cosmetic outcomes, incision was made parallel to the wrinkle lines and 5-0 nylon suture was used for skin closure. In total, 70% of the hematoma was removed, and the MLS improved completely (Figures 2(c) and 2(d)). Tranexamic acid (250 mg) was administered to prevent postoperative oozing.

The consciousness level started to improve right after the operation and eventually improved to E4V4M6 27 days after the operation. The skin incision was hardly noticeable after suture removal.

3. Discussion

3.1. Indications. Surgical treatment often considered for ASDH is large craniotomy hematoma evacuation. However, craniotomy in general imposes a significant burden on patients due to the large amount of bleeding, large question mark skin incision, and long operation time under general anesthesia. Therefore, the procedure may be inadvisable for patients with medical conditions such as liver cirrhosis, older age, and the use of antiplatelet/anticoagulation drugs.

In contrast, neuroendoscopic surgery is a minimally invasive technique that can be performed under local anesthesia and therefore can be applied to patients who may not endure craniotomy. For example, it is considered suitable for elderly patients with complications such as heart failure. In such cases, reduction of antiedema drugs will become possible after the surgery, thus preventing the exacerbation of heart failure. However, there are few reports of neuroendoscopic surgery on ASDH. Although there are increasing reports on neuroendoscopic removal of chronic subdural hematoma (CSDH), removal of ASDH is considered difficult because of its gelatinous nature as opposed to the serous nature of CSDH [1–3]. Our literature research revealed only one report of neuroendoscopic surgery for pure ASDH. It was a case of ASDH (width 15 mm, MLS 14 mm) of an 84-year-old woman with GCS of E1VTM6 who fell a week before the surgery. Hematoma was removed through 2 perforating burr holes at the front and back of the convexity, using a 0-degree and a 30-degree rigid scope. The operation took 2 hours, and blood loss was 150 mL. The patient was discharged 2 months later without any sequelae [4, 5]. We found no reports of neuroendoscopy performed to relieve ASDH with contusion. The probable reason for this is that there are some difficulties with stopping the bleeding from the contusion and oozing from the brain surface via neuroendoscopy. Due to these hemostatic problems, large craniotomy, which allows better hemostatic control, is usually selected for cases that need decompression from the moment of injury.

From our experience of two cases presented earlier, we would like to recommend the choice of neuroendoscopic surgery on cases of ASDH that are able to be observed clinically without immediate surgery but are expected to gain better outcomes (e.g., efficiency of rehabilitation) through surgical intracranial pressure reduction. For such cases, we also recommend the wait time, if possible, of about 48 hours before surgery for better hemostatic control.

In our cases, it was not our original intent to wait for 48 hours after the traumatic accident. Our initial plan was to give conservative treatment, but since the patients' consciousness level gradually deteriorated, we decided to switch to surgical treatment. As for the method of surgery, neuroendoscopy was chosen because the patients were elderly with multiple complications. During the surgery, we did not experience any difficulty in hemostasis; this is why we considered that 48 hours of wait time may have brought a natural hemostasis and thus resulted in a safer endoscopic surgery. However, it goes without saying that continuous assessment of consciousness and frequent follow-up CT examinations are required during the wait time. Surgical treatment should immediately be applied to patients when deterioration of consciousness is observed. For our cases, we also did a careful checkup of coagulation factors during the wait time because the use of tranexamic acid may slightly increase the risk of thromboembolic events.

Endoscopic surgery performed under local anesthesia is much less invasive compared to the traditional surgery, resulting in a faster postoperative recovery. As for our two patients, their conditions improved soon after the operation and both followed a good postoperative course. Thus, we consider that the 48–72 hours of wait time did not affect their clinical outcome. The reason for the increased hospital stay in our cases was that the patients lived alone with no family and therefore took longer time to be transferred to a rehabilitation hospital. Although the hematoma removal was incomplete for both cases, we consider that this was not related to the increased hospital stay. Total removal of hematoma is considered unnecessary if partial removal of hematoma is sufficient enough to alleviate the mass effect because the remaining hematoma gets absorbed naturally. Even in large craniotomy, there are cases when we leave some hematomas untouched, especially ones that are located around the skull base and the bridging vein.

There may be some concerns over the removal of contusion, since the contusion is normally reserved in order to improve functional outcomes. However, when a contusion is so massive that it forms an intracerebral hematoma over 30 cc and exerts a mass effect, removal of contusion (=intracerebral hematoma) needs to be considered. For such cases, a simple decompressive surgery may not be sufficient to decrease the intracranial pressure, and thus removal of intracerebral hematoma may be required. As for the method of surgery, we often have no choice but to perform craniotomy for cases of massive contusion in the temporal lobe, because those contusions produce early brainstem compression. On the other hand, for massive contusions in the frontal lobe, we are often able to take a wait-and-see approach, so these are possible candidates for neuroendoscopic surgery. In our case, the patient had an intracerebral hematoma caused by a massive contusion in the right frontal lobe. We planned to control the intracranial pressure by removing the massive intracerebral hematoma together with the subdural hematoma under endoscopic surgery.

Last but not least, we would like to point out that although we are currently unable to perform neuroendoscopic surgery at an acute stage due to the difficulty of hemostasis, it may become possible in the future in response to the development of endoscopic hemostatic devices.

3.2. Technical Methodology. We make 1 burr hole in the direction of the long axis of the ASDH. We do not make it on the convexity, because that location imposes a limitation for neuroendoscopy. We locate the burr hole in front of the contusion if the patient has massive contusion with ASDH. We can remove both ASDH and the contusion by doing it this way.

When we remove the hematoma by neuroendoscopy through the forehead, it is easy to remove the contusion, but it is important to guide the Neuroport to the subdural space in a skillful manner. Firstly, we guide the Neuroport into the subdural space after removing the contusion omnidirectionally. Then, we move the Neuroport to the outside and continuously feed it into the subdural space beyond the contusion. After that, we can advance the Neuroport for about 6 cm. Gradually, we manage to recognize the Sylvian vein. Further aspiration would lead to bleeding, so we suggest not advancing further after recognition of the Sylvian vein.

This is technical advice, but deep lying hematoma in the brain can easily be suctioned, since there are very few vessels in the deep matter. However, vessels are rich in the subpial space, and frequent electrocoagulation using suction coagulation device is necessary. In addition, we do not recommend the use of a flexible scope, because its suction effect is somewhat lacking. We recommend using a suction instrument to reduce the hematoma through a rigid scope. A flexible scope can cause impairment of the brain directly. In contrast, we can use the Neuroport attached to the rigid scope as the brain retractor.

For safety, we recommend the placement of an information drain into the subdural space in order to check the postoperative bleeding, because we cannot stop bleeding completely insomuch as does a large craniotomy.

In terms of cosmesis of Case 2, it would have been better for the incision to be placed in the hairline like Case 1. However, Case 2 was an exceptional case in which a massive intracerebral hematoma on the right frontal lobe exerted a mass effect on the brain. There was a necessity to make the skin incision on the middle of the forehead in order to remove the intracerebral hematoma together with the subdural hematoma. We placed a 4 cm incision parallel to the wrinkle line and used 5-0 nylon suture for skin closure. In this way, we managed to make the scar hardly noticeable after suture removal. In case of a complication, additional scar would have been required in order to perform craniotomy in Case 2, but it should be noted that this was an exceptional case due to the location of hematoma. If the incision can be placed on the hairline as in Case 1, it is possible to connect the incision with a regular craniotomy incision.

4. Conclusion

For patients with underlying medical issues or other risk factors, craniotomy could be unbearably invasive. For those patients, after hemostasis is complete, neuroendoscopic removal of the hematoma and brain contusion is likely to be an effective emergency procedure.

Conflict of Interests

The authors declare that there is no conflict of interests regarding the publication of this paper.

References

[1] D. Hellwig, T. J. Kuhn, B. L. Bauer, and E. List-Hellwig, "Endoscopic treatment of septated chronic subdural hematoma," *Surgical Neurology*, vol. 45, no. 3, pp. 272–277, 1996.

[2] R. Mobbs and P. Khong, "Endoscopic-assisted evacuation of subdural collections," *Journal of Clinical Neuroscience*, vol. 16, no. 5, pp. 701–704, 2009.

[3] G. S. Rodziewicz and W. C. Chuang, "Endoscopic removal of organized chronic subdural hematoma," *Surgical Neurology*, vol. 43, no. 6, pp. 569–573, 1995.

[4] P. J. Codd, A. S. Venteicher, P. K. Agarwalla, K. T. Kahle, and D. H. Jho, "Endoscopic burr hole evacuation of an acute subdural hematoma," *Journal of Clinical Neuroscience*, vol. 20, no. 12, pp. 1751–1753, 2013.

[5] S. Son, C. J. Yoo, S. G. Lee, E. Y. Kim, C. W. Park, and W. K. Kim, "Natural course of initially non-operated cases of acute subdural hematoma: the risk factors of hematoma progression," *Journal of Korean Neurosurgical Society*, vol. 54, no. 3, pp. 211–219, 2013.

5

Nivolumab-Induced Autoimmune Encephalitis in Two Patients with Lung Adenocarcinoma

Suma Shah ⓘ,[1] Anastasie Dunn-Pirio,[1] Matthew Luedke,[1] Joel Morgenlander,[2] Mark Skeen,[1] and Christopher Eckstein ⓘ[1]

[1]*Duke University Department of Neurology, USA*
[2]*Duke University Departments of Neurology and Orthopedic Surgery, USA*

Correspondence should be addressed to Suma Shah; suma.shah@duke.edu

Academic Editor: Dominic B. Fee

Immune checkpoint inhibitors have improved patient survival outcomes in a variety of advanced malignancies. However, they can cause a number of immune-related adverse effects (irAEs) through lymphocyte dysregulation. Central nervous system (CNS) irAEs are rare, but as the number of indications for checkpoint inhibitors increases, there has been emergence of CNS immune-mediated disease among cancer patients. Given the relatively recent recognition of checkpoint inhibitor CNS irAEs, there is no standard treatment, and prognosis is variable. Therefore, there is a great need for further study of checkpoint inhibitor-induced CNS irAEs. Here, we present two unique cases of nivolumab-induced autoimmune encephalitis in patients with non-small cell lung cancer and review the available literature.

1. Introduction

Immune checkpoints are built-in regulatory mechanisms of the adaptive immune system that function to maintain self-tolerance and attenuate physiologic immune responses [1]. Tumors can evade immune surveillance by manipulating immune checkpoints to establish more favorable environments for their growth [2]. Landmark clinical trials of immune checkpoint inhibitors targeting cytotoxic T-lymphocyte associated protein 4 (CTLA4) and the programmed cell death protein 1 (PD-1)/programmed death-ligand 1 (PD-L1) pathway have demonstrated improved survival rates in a variety of advanced malignancies [3].

Although checkpoint inhibitors have proven efficacy and are welcomed alternatives to traditional cytotoxic chemotherapy, they can cause immune-related adverse events (irAEs) due to their interference with lymphocyte regulation. Commonly described irAEs include rash, pruritus, colitis, hepatitis, and various endocrinopathies, such as thyroiditis and hypophysitis [4]. Neurologic irAEs are far less frequent and most often involve the peripheral nervous system [5, 6]. Here, we present two unique cases of central nervous system (CNS) irAEs following treatment with PD-1 inhibitor, nivolumab.

2. Case 1

A 66-year-old Caucasian woman with stage IIIb lung adenocarcinoma developed right hemiballismus and dysarthria following four months of nivolumab administration. The hemiballismus then evolved to bilateral ballismus in all extremities over a two-week period. Neurologic examination revealed hypophonic and dysarthric speech, orobuccolingual dyskinesias, and severe bilateral arm and leg ballismus.

Initial brain magnetic resonance imaging (MRI) with and without gadolinium showed symmetric T2 hyperintense and T1 hypointense basal ganglia abnormalities [Figures 1(a) and 1(b)]. Cerebrospinal fluid (CSF) analysis demonstrated a normal cell count and glucose level, a mildly elevated protein concentration of 56mg/dL (15-50mg/dL), and negative cytology. There were 16 oligoclonal bands present in the CSF compared to 2 in the serum. A CSF paraneoplastic antibody assay revealed a novel, unclassified antibody. A repeat brain MRI three weeks later redemonstrated symmetric T2 hyperintense basal ganglia but with a transition to T1 hyperintensities in the same location [Figures 1(c) and 1(d)].

Despite the consensus of an immune-mediated etiology, the patient was refractory to 5 days of intravenous (IV)

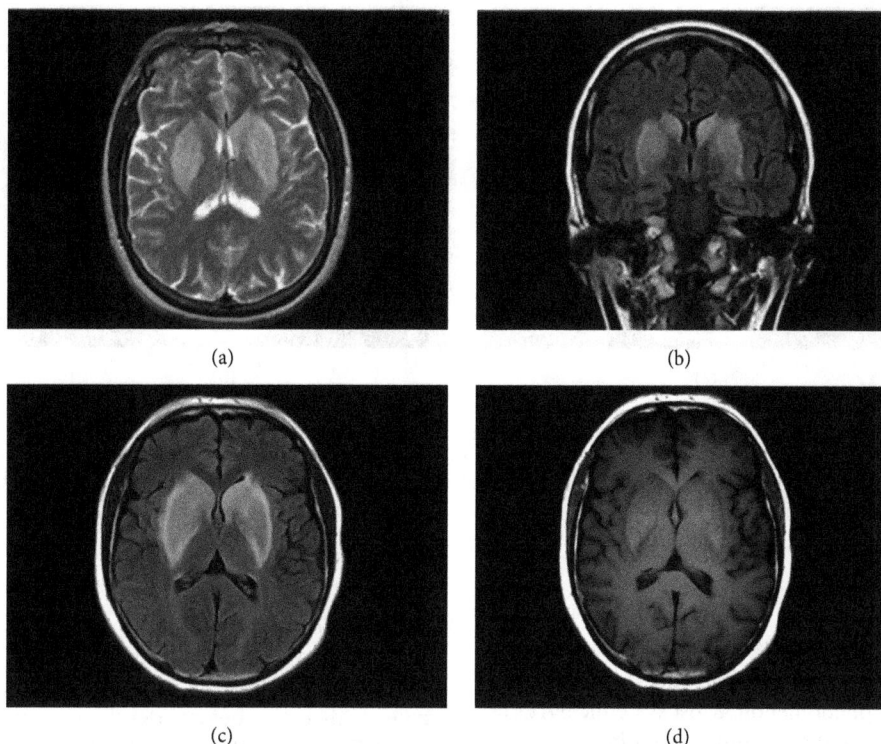

FIGURE 1: Initial and follow-up MRI brain for Case 1. (a) Initial MRI: axial T2-weighted image with hyperintensities in the bilateral basal ganglia. (b) Initial MRI: coronal FLAIR-weighted image with hyperintensities in the bilateral basal ganglia. (c) Follow-up MRI: axial FLAIR-weighted image with hyperintensities in the bilateral basal ganglia. (d) Follow-up MRI: axial T1-weighted image with hyperintensities in the bilateral basal ganglia.

methylprednisolone (1000mg/day) and 5 plasma exchanges. Haloperidol and olanzapine also did not offer symptomatic relief. She continued to decline despite subsequent trials of IV immunoglobulin (IVIg) (total dose of 2.5g/kg), prednisone, rituximab (1000mg once), and tetrabenazine (20mg, 3x/day). Due to continued clinical decline, she was eventually transitioned to comfort-only care and inpatient hospice.

3. Case 2

A 44-year-old Caucasian woman with type 1 diabetes mellitus (DM1) diagnosed at age 30 and stage IV lung adenocarcinoma treated with 5 cycles of nivolumab (3 mg/kg, every 2 weeks) developed several days of progressive altered mental status, nausea, and vomiting. She then presented to the emergency department following a first time seizure. Upon initial evaluation, she exhibited abnormal tongue movements, inappropriate laughter, and rhythmic movements of her right arm that improved with lorazepam.

An electroencephalogram revealed left temporal slowing and frequent interictal discharges. Brain MRI with and without gadolinium demonstrated T2 signal hyperintensities of the bilateral mesial temporal lobes compatible with limbic encephalitis. Additionally, there were 2 enhancing foci within the left occipital and right temporal lobes, concerning for metastatic disease [Figure 2]. CSF analysis detected 19 nucleated cells (97% lymphocytes) and normal protein and glucose

levels. There were 7 oligoclonal bands in the CSF and 3 in the serum. CSF cytology was negative. A CSF autoimmune encephalitis panel (Mayo Medical Laboratories) demonstrated the presence of glutamic acid decarboxylase 65-isoform (GAD65) antibodies: 2.70nmol/L (<= 0.02nmol/L). Serum GAD65 antibodies were also detected: 275nmol/L (<= 0.02nmol/L).

The patient was diagnosed with GAD65 antibody positive autoimmune encephalitis. She received IV methylprednisolone (1000mg/day) for 5 days followed by 5 plasma exchanges. However, she continued to experience refractory seizures despite treatment with multiple antiepileptic drugs and developed worsening ataxia, vertigo, and gait impairment. Therefore, she was given IV rituximab (1000mg) during the hospitalization. Upon discharge, seizures were under control and mental status improved. The patient currently receives maintenance rituximab (1000mg) every 6 months and remains seizure-free but with severe residual vertigo and moderate gait ataxia. Her most recent brain MRI demonstrated interval resolution of enhancing foci and abnormal T2 signal in the temporal lobes [Figure 2]. Following discontinuation of nivolumab, she was transitioned to brigatinib (a multikinase inhibitor with activity against anaplastic lymphoma kinase (ALK) as well as EGFR deletions and point mutations) for lung cancer treatment and remains oncologically stable.

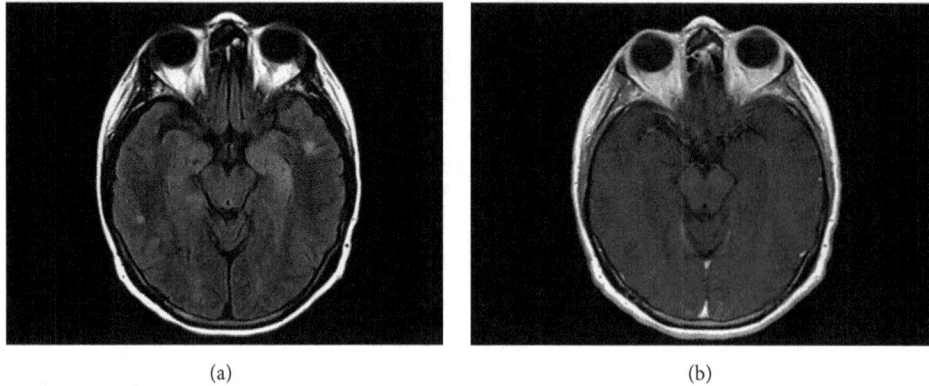

(a)   (b)

FIGURE 2: MRI brain imaging for Case 2. (a) MRI brain FLAIR imaging. This image demonstrates mildly expansile T2 signal hyperintensity of the left greater than right mesial temporal lobes. Additional small regions of cortical and subcortical T2 signal hyperintensity are noted in the temporal lobes of both hemispheres. (b) MRI brain, T1 sequence with contrast. There is no enhancement noted in the affected areas after administration of gadolinium contrast.

4. Discussion

Systemic irAEs secondary to immune checkpoint blockade are a well-recognized phenomenon. Most systemic irAEs are successfully managed by discontinuing the offending agent alone or in combination with temporary immunosuppressive therapy such as corticosteroids and/or tumor necrosis factor-alpha (TNF-α) inhibitors [4]. In contrast, neurological irAEs occur less frequently, estimated in < 1% of individuals receiving immune checkpoint inhibitors. They can have more aggressive clinical courses and often involve the peripheral nervous system, especially the neuromuscular junction [6, 7]. In fact, clinical trial data indicate that autoimmune encephalitis occurs in as few as 0.1 to <1% of patients receiving checkpoint inhibition [8].

To the best of our knowledge, our cases represent the first descriptions of nivolumab-induced autoimmune encephalitis manifesting as choreiform movements as well as a GAD65 antibody positive autoimmune encephalitis. Each case entailed an aggressive neurological disease course, with the patient in the former case ultimately succumbing to the irAE. This is particularly troubling because development of nivolumab-induced irAEs in patients with non-small cell lung cancer (NSCLC) may predict a favorable oncologic treatment response [9].

It is to be determined whether these cases represent checkpoint inhibitor-induced de novo autoimmunity or the unmasking of a preexisting subclinical disorder. In oncology, the study of PD-1/PD-L1 signaling has largely focused on PD-L1 expression within the tumor microenvironment resulting in PD-1+T-lymphocyte inhibition and subsequent tumor escape. However, the role of PD-1/PD-L1 interactions extends beyond cell-mediated immunity and into humoral immunity. Specifically, PD-1+ follicular helper T cells (T_{FH} cells) are critical for germinal center function and antibody production. It was recently demonstrated that PD-L1+ regulatory B cells negatively regulate T_{FH} cells and thus attenuate humoral responses [10]. Therefore, it is possible that disruption of the PD-1/PD-L1 interaction at the level of the germinal center

may have led to the de novo formation of aberrantly directed antibodies to self-antigens found in the CNS.

We suspect that the patient in Case 2, who was a known type 1 diabetic before developing nivolumab-associated GAD65 autoimmune encephalitis, was already at risk for developing CNS autoimmunity. As GAD65 is located on both pancreatic islet cells and CNS gamma-amino-butyric acid (GABA-ergic) neurons, there is an association between GAD65 antibody positive CNS autoimmune disease and DM1. Antibodies against GAD65 are detectable in roughly 70-80% of individuals with DM1 but typically at lower titers than in individuals who have coexisting neurologic autoimmunity [11, 12]. If the patient had preexisting GAD65 antibodies, it is plausible that nivolumab exposure simply exacerbated her condition. If more GAD65 antibody positive CNS autoimmunity are reported in patients with type 1 diabetes following immune checkpoint blockade, then screening for preexisting GAD65 antibodies prior to cancer immunotherapy may be clinically useful.

As the development of irAEs from nivolumab in patients with NSCLC has been correlated with improved cancer-related outcomes it is crucial to aggressively manage irAEs as well as supporting patients through the acute immune-mediated illness so they can continue with appropriate cancer treatment. Unlike the more common systemic irAEs, CNS irAEs are rare, and, therefore, optimal treatment is not as well established. In addition to establishing more efficacious treatments for CNS irAEs, developing biomarkers to predict risk of developing CNS irAEs is also warranted.

Conflicts of Interest

The authors declare that they have no conflicts of interest.

Authors' Contributions

Dr. Shah and Dr. Dunn-Pirio were responsible for acquisition of data, analysis and interpretation, and drafting the manuscript for intellectual content. Dr. Luedke was responsible for analysis and interpretation. Dr. Morgenlander was responsible for study concept and design. Dr. Skeen was responsible for study concept and design and study supervision. Dr. Eckstein was responsible for critical revisions of the manuscript for important intellectual content and study supervision. Drs. Shah and Dunn-Pirio contributed equally to the manuscript.

Acknowledgments

Dr. Skeen has received honoraria from Biogen, Novartis, Celgene, and Mallinckrodt.

References

[1] D. M. Pardoll, "The blockade of immune checkpoints in cancer immunotherapy," *Nature Reviews Cancer*, vol. 12, no. 4, pp. 252–264, 2012.

[2] Y. Diesendruck and I. Benhar, "Novel immune check point inhibiting antibodies in cancer therapy—Opportunities and challenges," *Drug Resistance Updates*, vol. 30, pp. 39–47, 2017.

[3] R. A. M. Wilson, T. R. J. Evans, A. R. Fraser, and R. J. B. Nibbs, "Immune checkpoint inhibitors: New strategies to checkmate cancer," *Clinical & Experimental Immunology*, vol. 191, pp. 133–148, 2018.

[4] M. A. Postow, R. Sidlow, and M. D. Hellmann, "Immune-related adverse events associated with immune checkpoint blockade," *The New England Journal of Medicine*, vol. 378, no. 2, pp. 158–168, 2018.

[5] J. Naidoo, D. B. Page, B. T. Li et al., "Toxicities of the anti-PD-1 and anti-PD-L1 immune checkpoint antibodies," *Annals of Oncology*, vol. 26, no. 12, pp. 2375–2391, 2015.

[6] D. Makarious, K. Horwood, and J. I. G. Coward, "Myasthenia gravis: An emerging toxicity of immune checkpoint inhibitors," *European Journal of Cancer*, vol. 82, pp. 128–136, 2017.

[7] J. Larkin, B. Chmielowski, C. D. Lao et al., "Neurologic serious adverse events associated with nivolumab plus ipilimumab or nivolumab alone in advanced melanoma, including a case series of encephalitis," *The Oncologist*, vol. 22, no. 6, pp. 709–718, 2017.

[8] S. Schneider, S. Potthast, P. Komminoth, G. Schwegler, and S. Böhm, "PD-1 checkpoint inhibitor associated autoimmune encephalitis," *Case Reports in Oncology*, vol. 10, no. 2, pp. 473–478, 2017.

[9] K. Sato, H. Akamatsu, E. Murakami et al., "Correlation between immune-related adverse events and efficacy in non-small cell lung cancer treated with nivolumab," *Lung Cancer*, vol. 115, pp. 71–74, 2018.

[10] A. R. Khan, E. Hams, A. Floudas, T. Sparwasser, C. T. Weaver, and P. G. Fallon, "PD-L1hi B cells are critical regulators of humoral immunity," *Nature Communications*, vol. 6, article no. 5997, 2015.

[11] A. McKeon and J. A. Tracy, "GAD65 neurological autoimmunity," *Muscle & Nerve*, vol. 56, no. 1, pp. 15–27, 2017.

[12] A. L. Notkins and Å. Lernmark, "Autoimmune type 1 diabetes: Resolved and unresolved issues," *The Journal of Clinical Investigation*, vol. 108, no. 9, pp. 1247–1252, 2001.

6

Auditory Hallucinations as a Rare Presentation of Occipital Infarcts

Firas Ido ⓘ**, Reina Badran, Brandon Dmytruk, and Zain Kulairi** ⓘ

Wayne State University School of Medicine, 1101 W. University Drive, 2 South, Rochester, MI 48307, USA

Correspondence should be addressed to Firas Ido; firasido85@gmail.com

Academic Editor: Jacqueline A. Pettersen

A stroke is a clinical syndrome characterized by a focal neurologic deficit that can be attributed to a vascular territory within the brain. The presenting features of an acute stroke depends on the area of the brain affected. Although unusual, the presenting feature may include psychosis with auditory and/or visual hallucinations. A 56-year-old female was admitted to the psychiatric unit after threatening her husband with a knife. She reported experiencing altered sensorium for one week with suicidal and homicidal command hallucinations. Given the acute onset, brain images were obtained to rule out an organic etiology. A brain MRI revealed an acute right occipital lobe infarct with hemorrhagic transformation. The patient's symptoms were self-limited, resolving without antipsychotic medications. Psychosis with auditory hallucinations is not commonly reported following stroke. Since histologic and functional alterations in the occipital lobe appear to play a significant role in psychosis of schizophrenics, it is likely that ischemia in the same area may cause similar changes. Familiarity with this rare presentation is important, as it prevents a delay in diagnosis, which may negatively impact the outcome.

1. Background

Stroke is the fourth leading cause of mortality in the US affecting both men and women [1]. It is a clinical syndrome characterized by a focal neurologic deficit that can be attributed to a vascular territory within the brain. Stroke is organized primarily as ischemic or hemorrhagic, occurring in 85% and 15% of all cases, respectively, which can be distinguished with brain imaging [2]. The pathophysiology of ischemic stroke may involve a cardioembolic phenomenon, large artery emboli, large/small artery atherosclerosis with thrombus formation, and small artery arteriosclerosis in the setting of hypertension leading to lacunar infarcts. In contrast, hemorrhagic infarcts occur more commonly in the setting of a ruptured intracerebral aneurysm or trauma [3].

The presenting features of an acute stroke depend on the area of the brain affected by the vascular insult. Based on arterial anatomy, anterior and middle cerebral involvement commonly present with hemiparesis, hemiplegia, facial droop, dysarthria, aphasia, and gaze preference. Posterior circulatory infarcts affect the cerebellum and occipital lobe which can manifest as vertigo, ataxia, and visual disturbances [3].

Although poststroke mood and emotional disturbances such as depression, anxiety, and anger are common, psychiatric manifestations as a presenting feature of stroke are rare and limited in number of reported cases [4]. When present, psychiatric symptoms may differ depending on the area of the brain involved. Symptoms of hallucinations and delusions are uncommon but have been reported in strokes involving the caudate and thalamus [5]. Even more discrete changes in behavior from baseline such as increased sleep and not attending work were documented in a basal ganglia stroke [6]. The frontal lobe, being the primary focus for executive function, has been linked to personality changes such as emotional instability, impulsivity, and apathy [7]. In addition, the presence of visual and auditory hallucinations were noted to be a presenting feature of a right frontal stroke [8]. In a retrospective analysis, 7% of patients that presented with altered mental status were found to have an acute stroke

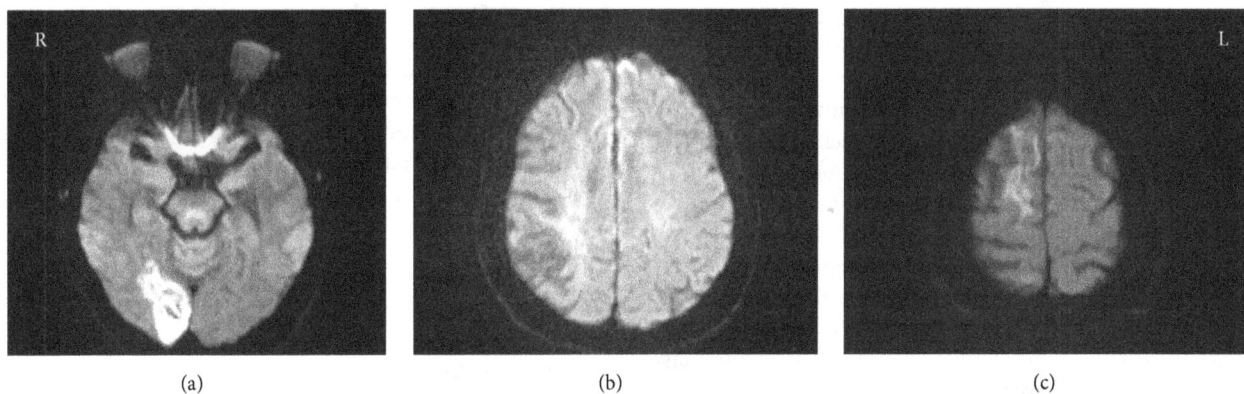

FIGURE 1: (a) Diffuse weighted/TRACE-acute right occipital infarct with hemorrhagic transformation. (b) Diffuse weighted/TRACE-encephalomalacia of the right posterior parietal lobe. (c) Diffuse weighted/TRACE-encephalomalacia of the superior frontal lobe.

in the frontoparietal, occipital, frontal, and right pontine areas of the brain [9]. Right temporal lobe strokes have been associated with the 5 behavioral phenomena (hypergraphia, atypical sexuality, intensified mental life, circumstantiality, and hyperreligiosity) which are the components of Geschwind syndrome [10]. Finally, strokes involving the temporooccipital regions have been documented to present with excessive talkativeness and repetitiveness, termed logorrhea [11].

Although unusual, the presenting feature of a stroke may rarely include psychosis with auditory and/or visual hallucinations in the absence of somatic alterations [12]. In the rare circumstance that the stroke does present with psychosis as the predominating symptom, this may result in a delay in diagnosis. Given the time sensitivity of imaging and early medical therapy in stroke, this delay in diagnosis may negatively impact the outcome.

2. Case Report

A 56 year-old female was transported to the emergency department by EMS after physically threatening her husband with a knife. According to the patient, she experienced altered sensorium for one week prior to presentation, primarily resulting in suicidal and homicidal command hallucinations instructing her to overdose on NSAIDs and kill her husband. She denied any headaches, vertigo, fevers, head trauma, urinary symptoms, or use of illicit substances. There was no history of psychosis, schizophrenia, mania, or depression and a review of her medication list for any potential hallucinogenic agents did not indicate a pharmacologic etiology. Her past medical history was comprised of two prior strokes, the most recent being two years ago that involved the right frontal lobe. MRI of the brain at the time also showed evidence of an old right parietal lobe infarct. An echocardiogram during that hospitalization revealed a severely decreased left ventricular function and the patient was initiated on warfarin for anticoagulation. Since the two prior cerebral infarcts, the patient and her husband denied noting any behavioral changes, cognitive impairment, or any focal neurologic deficits. On presentation, she appeared

disheveled and exhibited a flat affect with minimal verbalization. Physical examination revealed only a left hemianopia without hemiplegia. All cranial nerves were evaluated as well as gait, cerebellar function, and proprioception, which were all found to be normal. The patient was alert and oriented with intact mentation.

She was initially admitted to the psychiatric unit for further evaluation where the patient participated in daily activities and reported no symptoms. Given the acute onset of her symptoms, laboratory studies and brain images were obtained in order to rule out an organic etiology. A complete blood count was normal and a basic metabolic panel revealed normal electrolytes and renal function. Additional labs included liver function tests, lipid panel, cardiolipin antibody, and TSH, which were all normal and RPR was nonreactive. A urine sample was negative for urinary tract infection and 8-panel urine drug screen was negative. An MRI of the brain was obtained, which revealed old ischemic infarcts within the right parietal and frontal lobes along with a new acute right occipital lobe infarct with hemorrhagic transformation (Figure 1). The patient was subsequently transferred to the medical unit for further workup and management.

The patient was placed on telemetry, which showed normal sinus rhythm. Given the involvement of multiple brain territories and circulations, a cardioembolic source of stroke was highly suspected. A cardiologist evaluated the patient and performed a transesophageal echocardiogram that revealed a low ejection fraction of less than 20%. In addition, a bubble study was performed that was positive for a patent foramen ovale. Given her significantly low ejection fraction, the patient underwent placement of an automated implantable cardioverter-defibrillator. The patient's presenting symptom of psychosis, primarily in the form of auditory hallucinations, was self-limited and resolved on day two of hospitalization without requiring the use of antipsychotic medications.

3. Discussion

Psychosis with auditory hallucinations is not a commonly reported behavioral alteration following stroke [13]. These symptoms are more typical features of drug intoxication and psychiatric illnesses including brief psychotic episode, schizophreniform, and schizophrenia. Symptoms of psychosis can be categorized into positive symptoms (hallucinations, delusions, and disorganized speech) and negative symptoms (flat affect and avolition) [14]. Auditory hallucinations, the presence of auditory sensation in the absence of external stimuli, have been described in less than 1% of patients found to have subcortical, brainstem, and temporal infarcts [15]. These hallucinations are described as a dissociative phenomenon of perceiving peers/relatives conversing or hearing one's own voice [16]. Command hallucinations following a stroke are atypical and therefore may be misdiagnosed as a primary psychiatric disorder.

The auditory center, which is primarily located in the temporal lobes, has been linked to psychosis in schizophrenia [17]. Auditory hallucinations in cerebrovascular disease have been observed with infarction involving the bitemporal cerebral cortex [18]. They have also been described in strokes involving the anterior/inferior cerebellar arteries and posterior circulation [18]. Therefore, it is plausible that ischemia to neurons involved in excitatory/inhibitory function may alter the sensorium leading to abnormal behaviors. The areas of the brain most commonly associated with schizophrenia include the frontal lobes, temporal lobes, limbic system, and brain stem. The occipital lobe, which is the primary visual cortex, has not been traditionally associated with auditory function. However, recent evidence regarding the role of the occipital brain in schizophrenia has showed altered volume and histologic changes including changes in density involving gray and white matter within the occipital lobes [19]. Since histologic and functional alterations in the occipital lobe appear to play a significant role in psychosis of schizophrenics, then it is likely that the ischemia that occurs following a cerebral infarct in the same area may cause similar changes.

Our patient did have a history of multiple ischemic infarcts, but did not exhibit any prior behavioral changes. Following her new occipital stroke, her only presenting feature was auditory command hallucinations. These hallucinations were self-limited and resolved the following day without any intervention. In summary, cerebral infarcts presenting with hallucinations along with other symptoms of psychosis are rare and can therefore lead to a delay in diagnosis that can have catastrophic outcomes. Familiarity with behavioral changes as a presenting sign of stroke is very important, as it allows for prompt diagnosis and early treatment. The additional signs of stroke that clinicians should be familiar with include auditory and visual hallucinations. Not only does this allow for time sensitive management to occur, but it also avoids unnecessary psychiatric treatment.

Conflicts of Interest

The authors declare that there are no conflicts of interest regarding the publication of this article.

Authors' Contributions

Firas Ido completed the literature review and drafted and edited the initial manuscript. Reina Badran edited the manuscript and drafted the abstract. Brandon Dmytruk obtained the MRI images and drafted the descriptions. Zain Kulairi was the senior editor and mentor to the case.

References

[1] B. Ovbiagele and M. N. Nguyen-Huynh, "Stroke epidemiology: advancing our understanding of disease mechanism and therapy," *Neurotherapeutics*, vol. 8, no. 3, pp. 319–329, 2011.

[2] P. M. W. Bath and K. R. Lees, "Acute stroke," *Western Journal of Medicine*, vol. 173, no. 3, pp. 209–212, 2000.

[3] T. D. Musuka, S. B. Wilton, M. Traboulsi, and M. D. Hill, "Diagnosis and management of acute ischemic stroke: speed is critical," *Canadian Medical Association Journal*, vol. 187, no. 12, pp. 887–893, 2015.

[4] J. S. Kim, "Post-stroke mood and emotional disturbances:pharmacological therapy based on mechanisms," *Journal of Stroke*, vol. 18, no. 3, pp. 244–255, 2016.

[5] S. Santos, O. Alberti, T. Corbalan, and M. T. Cortina, "Stroke-psychosis: description of two cases," *Actas Españolas de Psiquiatría*, vol. 37, pp. 240–242, 2009.

[6] S. J. Wagner and T. Begaz, "Basal ganglion stroke presenting as subtle behavioural change," *BMJ Case Reports*, 2009.

[7] T. W. Chow, "Personality in frontal lobe disorders.," *Current Psychiatry Reports*, vol. 2, no. 5, pp. 446–451, 2000.

[8] S. Badrin, N. Mohamad, N. A. Yunus, and M. M. Zulkifli, "A brief Psychotic Episode with depressive symptoms in silent right frontal lobe infarct," *Korean Journal of Family Medicine*, vol. 38, no. 6, pp. 380–382, 2017.

[9] S. R. Benbadis, C. A. Sila, and R. L. Cristea, "Mental status changes and stroke," *Journal of General Internal Medicine*, vol. 9, no. 9, pp. 485–487, 1994.

[10] M. Hoffmann, "Isolated right temporal lobe stroke patients present with geschwind gastaut syndrome, frontal network syndrome and delusional misidentification syndromes," *Behavioural Neurology*, vol. 20, no. 3-4, pp. 83–89, 2008.

[11] S. Khanra, N. Paul, and S. Mukherjee, "Early marked behavioral symptoms in bilateral posterior cerebral artery stroke: a disguised presentation," *Journal of Psychological Medicine*, vol. 40, no. 1, pp. 96–98, 2018.

[12] S. Srivastava, M. P. Agarwal, and A. Gautam, "Post stroke psychosis following lesions in basal ganglion," *Journal of Clinical and Diagnostic Research*, vol. 11, no. 5, pp. VD01–VD02, 2017.

[13] R. Kaur, "Post stroke psychosis," *Delhi Psychiatric Journal*, vol. 15, no. 1, pp. 221–222, 2012.

[14] M. K. Larson, E. F. Walker, and M. T. Compton, "Early signs, diagnosis and therapeutics of the prodromal phase of schizophrenia and related psychotic disorders," *Expert Review of Neurotherapeutics*, vol. 10, no. 8, pp. 1347–1359, 2010.

[15] B. Piechowski-Jozwiak and J. Bogusslavsky, *Manifestatios of Stroke*, Karger, Germany, 2012.

[16] Y. Lampl, M. Lorberboym, R. Gilad, M. Boaz, and M. Sadeh, "Auditory hallucinations in acute stroke," *Behavioural Neurology*, vol. 16, no. 4, pp. 211–216, 2005.

[17] D. C. Javitt and R. A. Sweet, "Auditory dysfunction in schizophrenia: integrating clinical and basic features," *Nature Reviews Neuroscience*, vol. 16, no. 9, pp. 535–550, 2015.

7

Open-Label Fosmetpantotenate, a Phosphopantothenate Replacement Therapy in a Single Patient with Atypical PKAN

Yiolanda-Panayiota Christou,[1] George A. Tanteles,[2] Elena Kkolou,[1] Annita Ormiston,[1] Kostas Konstantopoulos,[3] Maria Beconi,[4] Randall D. Marshall,[4] Horacio Plotkin,[4] and Kleopas A. Kleopa[1]

[1]Neurology Clinics, The Cyprus Institute of Neurology and Genetics, Nicosia, Cyprus
[2]Clinical Genetics Clinic, The Cyprus Institute of Neurology and Genetics, Nicosia, Cyprus
[3]European University Cyprus, Nicosia, Cyprus
[4]Retrophin Inc., New York, NY, USA

Correspondence should be addressed to Kleopas A. Kleopa; kleopa@cing.ac.cy

Academic Editor: Isabella Laura Simone

Objective. Pantothenate kinase-associated neurodegeneration (PKAN) is an autosomal recessive disorder with variable onset, rate of progression, and phenotypic expression. Later-onset, more slowly progressive PKAN often presents with neuropsychiatric as well as motor manifestations that include speech difficulties, progressive dystonia, rigidity, and parkinsonism. PKAN is caused by biallelic *PANK2* mutations, a gene that encodes pantothenate kinase 2, a regulatory enzyme in coenzyme A biosynthesis. Current therapeutic strategies rely on symptomatic relief. We describe the treatment of the first, later-onset PKAN patient with oral fosmetpantotenate (previously known as RE-024), a novel replacement therapy developed to bypass the enzymatic defect. *Methods.* This was an open-label, uncontrolled, 12-month treatment with fosmetpantotenate of a single patient with a later-onset, moderately severe, and slowly progressive form of PKAN. *Results.* The patient showed improvement in all clinical parameters including the Unified Parkinson's Disease Rating Scale (UPDRS), Barry-Albright Dystonia Scale, the EuroQol five-dimensional three-level (EQ-5D-3L) scale, timed 25-foot walk test, and electroglottographic speech analysis. Fosmetpantotenate was well-tolerated with only transient liver enzyme elevation which normalized after dose reduction and did not recur after subsequent dose increases. *Conclusions.* Fosmetpantotenate showed promising results in a single PKAN patient and should be further studied in controlled trials.

1. Introduction

Pantothenate kinase-associated neurodegeneration (PKAN) is the most common form of neurodegeneration with brain iron accumulation (NBIA). It is an autosomal recessive disorder resulting from biallelic mutations in the *PANK2* gene on chromosome 20p13 [1, 2] for which there is only symptomatic treatment. PKAN has traditionally been divided into a classic, earlier-onset form and an atypical, later-onset form which typically shows slower progression [2]. The presence however of patients with overlapping features between the two forms is increasingly becoming evident. The majority of PKAN patients are diagnosed in the first 10 years of life with affected children usually losing the ability to walk within 10 to 15

years after disease onset [3]. Clinical manifestations of PKAN have highly variable age of onset and rate of progression and include developmental delay, dystonia sometimes causing intractable pain, choreoathetosis, dysarthria, spasticity, rigidity, parkinsonism with gait freezing and bradykinesia, retinal degeneration, and dysphagia [3, 4]. Age of onset and rate of progression are variable, with some patients progressing rapidly to death within a few years, whereas others may live into later adulthood with more slowly progressive symptoms [3–6]. In most patients, brain MRI reveals the typical "eye-of-the-tiger" sign, resulting from excessive brain iron deposition in the basal ganglia. MRI changes may precede clinical manifestations [2, 3].

The normal product of *PANK2* is a pantothenate kinase which is essential in coenzyme A (CoA) biosynthesis and catalyzes the phosphorylation of pantothenate (vitamin B5) to phosphopantothenic acid (PPA). *PANK2* mutations can generally be divided into null or missense and only a few are recurring. Missense mutations (majority of identified variants) can lead to either early or late onset PKAN forms. Generally, no clear genotype-phenotype correlation has been observed except in the case of homozygous individuals for null alleles who usually present with classic disease [7].

PANK2 mutations are thought to result in deficiency (complete or partial) of pantothenate kinase 2 and accumulation of cysteine-containing cytotoxic substrates [9]. Pantothenate kinase 2 deficiency is also predicted to deplete CoA leading to multiple downstream consequences including defective membrane biosynthesis depending on specific tissue demand [10]. It has been postulated that, in PKAN patients, PPA deficiency leads to decreased CoA levels [5]. A phosphopantothenate replacement therapy to bypass the genetic deficiency in the Pank1−/− mouse model recently showed that administration of selected candidate compounds corrected their deficiency in hepatic CoA [11]. The results provided strong support for PanK as a master regulator of intracellular CoA and illustrated the feasibility of employing PanK bypass therapy to restore CoA levels in genetically deficient mice.

Fosmetpantotenate (previously known as RE-024) was developed by Retrophin, Inc. to bypass this biochemical defect for the treatment of PKAN. It is a novel small molecule precursor of PPA designed to release PPA intracellularly, leading to restoration of CoA levels (Figure 1(a) and Supplementary Figure 1, in Supplementary Material available online at https://doi.org/10.1155/2017/3247034). It has been reported that 4′-phosphopantothenic acid is not permeable to cell membranes, and thus systemic administration of PPA, the enzymatic product of PanK2, to PKAN patients will not be effective. In contrast, fosmetpantotenate has been shown to significantly increase intracellular CoA levels and increase tubulin acetylation in vitro in neuroblastoma cells that have been silenced for PanK2 expression [12, 13], presumably via access to mitochondrial PanK2. When dosed orally in nonhuman primates, microdialysis sampling detected fosmetpantotenate in the brain at levels consistent with meaningful conversion to PPA [13], suggesting similar BBB in humans.

We have in the past reported on a PKAN family in which a novel biallelic missense variant in exon 2 of the *PANK2* gene [c.695A>G(p.Asp232Gly)] was identified [14]. Here, we present the results of the first oral replacement therapy with fosmetpantotenate in a single patient from this family with onset of PKAN symptoms in his early 20s.

2. Case Description and Evaluation Methods

The oral replacement therapy results presented here involve a Cypriot patient affected with later-onset PKAN who was homozygous for the novel c.695A>G (p.Asp232Gly) missense mutation in exon 2 of the *PANK2* gene [14]. He initially presented with gait instability at the age of 22 years and subsequently developed progressive trunk and limb rigidity, more prominent on the right lower limb, impairing his ability to walk unaided, with frequent falls (Supplementary Video). By the age of 27 he presented to a neurology clinic with dysarthria, poor concentration (mild bradyphrenia), palilalia, bradykinesia in both hands, and marked axial rigidity. His gait was characterized by leg spasticity, toe walking, and moderate instability. MRI revealed the "eye-of-the-tiger" sign. He was unable to walk without support having a tendency to fall backwards. He showed a continuous progression and became wheelchair bound for most of the time by the age of 34. There was also worsening of dysarthria, dysphonia with palilalia, and dysphagia along with mild concentration difficulties and obsessive-compulsive behavior. Treatment with fosmetpantotenate was initiated at the age of 35.

After receiving a Named Patient approval for fosmetpantotenate administration from Government Authorities according to national law (Ph.S.5.21.2.1.6), informed consent was obtained, and fosmetpantotenate treatment was initiated with a starting dose of 0.1 mg/kg twice daily orally and it gradually increased over one week to 240 mg (3 mg/kg/day), divided equally as three times daily.

A baseline evaluation was performed with weekly follow-up visits for the first two months and every month thereafter. Clinical evaluation included the Unified Parkinson's Disease Rating Scale (UPDRS/I,II,III) [15], the Barry-Albright Dystonia (BAD) Scale, the EuroQol five-dimensional three-level (EQ-,5D-3L) scale, and the timed 25-foot walk test.

Electroglottographic analysis was performed noninvasively [8] before and two weeks after starting treatment. Variables used for voice analysis included average fundamental frequency and jitter as well as the average time in milliseconds for the production of speech diadochokinesis. The patient was asked to perform a rapid repetition of consonant-vowel pairs sequences on a single breath such as /pʌ/, /tʌ/, and /kʌ/ defined as Alternating Motion Rates (AMRs) and the average time in milliseconds for the production of consonants /p, t, k/ was registered.

Whole blood samples were collected for pharmacokinetic analysis on treatment Day 7 before dose and at 0.0833, 0.25, 0.5, 1, 2, 4, and 8 hours after dose. Samples were acidified immediately upon collection, treated with an enzyme inhibitor, and stored frozen until analysis. Fosmetpantotenate and metabolites were quantified under GLP conditions, by liquid chromatography tandem mass spectrometry (LC-MS/MS), using methods developed and GLP-validated by Nextcea (Worcester, MA) (Figure 1(b)). Metabolites quantified included fosmetpantotenate derivatives containing the intact PPA moiety, PA, and PPA.

3. Results

3.1. Dosing, Tolerance, and Safety. Fosmetpantotenate was well-tolerated with only mild nausea after taking the medication the first 2 days, which resolved without treatment or dose adjustment. At the end of week 2, transaminase increases were noted (2-3-fold) and treatment was stopped on Day 14. Transaminases rapidly decreased, and treatment was restarted on Day 22 at 120 mg daily (1.5 mg/Kg/day;

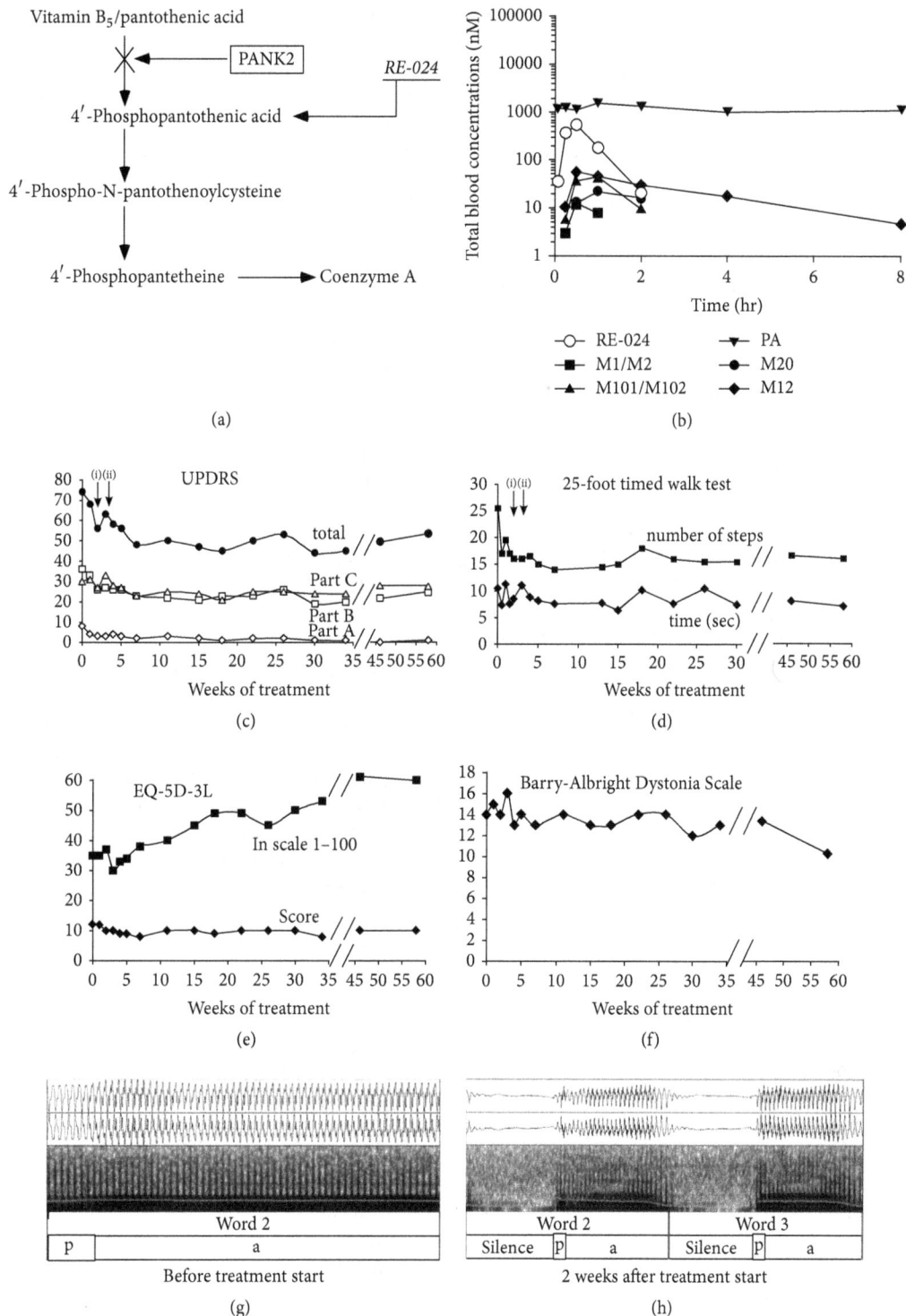

(a)

(b)

(c)

(d)

(e)

(f)

(g)

(h)

FIGURE 1: *Mode of Action, Pharmacokinetics, and Clinical Effects of Fosmetpantotenate.* (a) Diagram showing the metabolic pathway from pantothenic acid to coenzyme A with the pantothenate kinase defect found in PKAN patients and the bypassing effect of fosmetpantotenate. (b) Whole blood concentrations of fosmetpantotenate and metabolites over time following a 1 mg/kg oral dose on Day 7 of treatment. (c–f) Clinical evaluations before and after 58 weeks of treatment with fosmetpantotenate. (c) Unified Parkinson's Disease Rating Scale (UPDRS) including parts C and D and total score. (d) Timed 25-foot gait test including number of steps and time to complete (arrows in diagrams (c) and (d) indicate (i) interruption of treatment; (ii) restarting treatment at half dose). (e) Quality of life scale (EQ-5D-3L). (f) Barry-Albright Dystonia Scale. (g-h) Representative illustrations of electroglottographic analysis [8] before (g) and two weeks after (h) starting treatment showing individual /pa/ segmentation. Before treatment there is an apparent trend to prolong the vowel while after medication there is a significant improvement in the production of /pa/.

half dose). Dosing was gradually increased to 150 mg daily (1.9 mg/kg/day) on Week 15 and gradually to 210 mg daily (2.64 mg/kg/day, divided tid) by Week 40 without any further adverse effects or clinically significant laboratory or electro-cardiogram abnormalities through 12 months of treatment.

3.2. Pharmacokinetic Studies. Following the 1 mg/kg dose, fosmetpantotenate showed a short half-life ($t_{1/2}$ = 0.3 h) and was detectable for 2 hours. Fosmetpantotenate metabolite concentrations were at least 10 times lower than those of fosmetpantotenate but detectable for a longer period of time. The M12 metabolite had the highest C_{max} and was detectable in circulation through 8 hours after dose, with a $T_{1/2}$ of 2.1 hours (Figure 1(b)).

3.3. Clinical Evaluation. Clinical benefit from fosmetpantotenate was observed based on multiple outcome measures, addressing the multiple manifestations of the disease, including continuous improvement of the patient's ability to walk in the first two months of treatment and stabilization thereafter during one year of follow-up. At baseline, the patient required another person's assistance when walking. After treatment, on the timed 25-foot walk test he was able to walk faster with longer steps and for a few meters without assistance (Figure 1(d) and Supplementary Video). Dystonia, parkinsonism, rigidity, and bradykinesia together with overall quality of life (QoL) improved as noted on the UPDRS, BAD, and EQ-5D-3L scales (Figures 1(c)–1(f)). During the one week of dose interruption due to elevated transaminases all clinical scales deteriorated but improved again upon restarting treatment.

3.4. Electroglottographic Analysis. In sustained phonation of the /a/ sound, the average fundamental frequencies of voice and the jitter (cycle-to-cycle variation in fundamental frequency) were lowered after medication (123.77 Hz; jitter 0.50%) as compared to previously (139.97 Hz; jitter 0.64%) (normal for males: around 125 Hz; jitter < 1) [8]. Acoustic analysis of the AMRs showed similar trends in the mean production of the sounds /p, t, k/ (/p/: 0.05 msec before and 0.01 msec after treatment; /t/: 0.02 msec before and 0.01 msec after; /k/: 0.07 msec before and 0.01 msec after treatment) (Figures 1(g) and 1(h)).

3.5. Brain MRI. The baseline brain MRI scan was characterized by bilateral peripheral hypointensity in the globi pallidi with a central focus of gliosis, the typical "eye-of-the-tiger" sign [14]. Follow-up MRI performed after eight months of treatment showed no significant change.

4. Discussion

Despite rapid developments in understanding the genetics, pathophysiology, and clinical presentation of PKAN in the last decade, only symptomatic relief therapies are available [4, 16]. Bilateral deep brain stimulation of the globus pallidus was shown to partially improve dystonia severity in a multicenter retrospective study of 23 PKAN patients [17] and in a cohort of 7 children [18]. Repetitive transcranial magnetic stimulation 1-Hz of premotor cortex was experimentally used in a single patient and resulted in mild transient improvement [19]. A phase II pilot open trial of the iron-chelator deferiprone in 10 PKAN patients for a period of six months showed reduction in pallidal iron content but with no significant clinical improvement [20], whereas a more recent four-year study of six patients with NBIA, including five with PKAN, resulted in clinical stabilization correlating with radiological improvement [21].

In our patient, oral treatment with fosmetpantotenate proved to be safe and well-tolerated with only transient nausea and mild transaminase elevation, which resolved after dosage adjustment and has not recurred with gradually increasing doses. However, safety and tolerability of this treatment remain to be confirmed in larger numbers of patients.

In 2015, Tomić et al. [22] evaluated the clinical features and disease course of nine molecularly confirmed patients with atypical PKAN. The majority of patients reached seven significant clinical milestones in the first 4.6 years during the course of the disease. A long-lasting, relatively stable period of slower progression followed. This period was mostly complicated by skeletal deformities (developing after 7.0 ± 2.8 years) [22]. The study did not show any periods of clear clinical improvement being part of the natural course of the disease.

In our patient clinical benefit from fosmetpantotenate was observed based on multiple outcome measures, addressing the multiple manifestations of this disease, including dystonia, parkinsonism, and speech dysfunction [5]. Our study showed that, following a single oral administration, fosmetpantotenate enters the blood stream. Metabolites of fosmetpantotenate were detectable, but with no change in levels of pantothenic acid (PA), suggesting that PA from fosmetpantotenate is diluted by endogenous pantothenic acid pools to undetectable levels. Its half-life suggests that more than one daily dose may be needed for adequate coverage. In this patient, fosmetpantotenate was administered three times daily. Although it seems unlikely that the drug will reverse neurodegeneration, it may improve function of surviving cells, thereby preventing disease progression. This also underscores the importance of early treatment in future studies.

Since this is a single case we cannot exclude the possibility of a placebo effect or the effect of study participation, especially on the QoL scores. Furthermore, disease progression in this patient, though relentless, was at the slower end of the spectrum, and longer observation periods of over a year may be needed to confirm a lasting effect. Controlled studies will be required to demonstrate a real benefit from this treatment.

In conclusion, this open-label, uncontrolled, 12-month treatment of a single atypical PKAN patient with fosmetpantotenate was associated with transient nausea and mild liver enzyme elevations which resolved with treatment cessation and did not recur upon rechallenge. Most importantly, the treatment was associated with stabilization and persistent improvement of the patient's symptoms. Although symptom stabilization has clearly been reported in the literature, the improvement of symptoms observed in our patient is clinically meaningful and represents something not reported to be part of the natural course of the disease. Controlled studies should evaluate the therapeutic potential of fosmetpantotenate in patients with PKAN.

Conflicts of Interest

The Cyprus Institute of Neurology and Genetics is the recipient of an unrestricted grant from Retrophin, Inc., to support ongoing research on PKAN.

Acknowledgments

The authors would like to thank the family for their support and participation in this study.

References

[1] B. Zhou, S. K. Westaway, B. Levinson, M. A. Johnson, J. Gitschier, and S. J. Hayflick, "A novel pantothenate kinase gene (PANK2) is defective in Hallervorden-Spatz syndrome," *Nature Genetics*, vol. 28, no. 4, pp. 345–349, 2001.

[2] S. J. Hayflick, S. K. Westaway, B. Levinson et al., "Genetic, clinical, and radiographic delineation of Hallervorden-Spatz syndrome," *The New England Journal of Medicine*, vol. 348, no. 1, pp. 33–40, 2003.

[3] A. Gregory, B. J. Polster, and S. J. Hayflick, "Clinical and genetic delineation of neurodegeneration with brain iron accumulation," *Journal of Medical Genetics*, vol. 46, no. 2, pp. 73–80, 2009.

[4] S. A. Schneider, P. Dusek, J. Hardy, A. Westenberger, J. Jankovic, and K. P. Bhatia, "Genetics and pathophysiology of neurodegeneration with brain iron accumulation (NBIA)," *Current Neuropharmacology*, vol. 11, no. 1, pp. 59–79, 2013.

[5] M. Kruer, "Pantothenate-kinase associated neurodegeneration," in *Molecular and Genetic Basis of Neurological and Psychiatric Disease*, R. Rosenberg and J. Pascual, Eds., pp. 473–481, Academic Press, 2014.

[6] T. Klopstock, M. Elstner, C. B. Lücking et al., "Mutations in the pantothenate kinase gene PANK2 are not associated with Parkinson disease," *Neuroscience Letters*, vol. 379, no. 3, pp. 195–198, 2005.

[7] S. Williams, A. Gregory, P. Hogarth, S. J. Hayflick, and M. B. Gillingham, "Metabolism and energy requirements in pantothenate kinase-associated neurodegeneration," *Molecular Genetics and Metabolism*, vol. 110, no. 3, pp. 336–341, 2013.

[8] K. Konstantopoulos, M. Vikelis, J. A. Seikel, and D.-D. Mitsikostas, "The existence of phonatory instability in multiple sclerosis: an acoustic and electroglottographic study," *Neurological Sciences*, vol. 31, no. 3, pp. 259–268, 2010.

[9] E. Y. Yang, A. Campbell, and S. C. Bondy, "Configuration of thiols dictates their ability to promote iron-induced reactive oxygen species generation," *Redox Report*, vol. 5, no. 6, pp. 371–375, 2000.

[10] A. Gregory and S. Hayflick, "Pantothenate kinase-associated neurodegeneration," in *GeneReviews®*, R. Pagon, M. Adam, H. Ardinger et al., Eds., University of Washington, Seattle, Wash, USA, 1993–2016.

[11] S. P. Zano, C. Pate, M. Frank, C. O. Rock, and S. Jackowski, "Correction of a genetic deficiency in pantothenate kinase 1 using phosphopantothenate replacement therapy," *Molecular Genetics and Metabolism*, vol. 116, no. 4, pp. 281–288, 2015.

[12] A. Di Marco, G. Auciello, M. Quinton, A. Vecchi, E. Monteagudo, and M. G. Beconi, "Development of a human neuroblastoma model of pantothenate kinase-associated neurodegeneration," in *Proceedings of the ACMG Annual Clinical Genetics Meeting*, Tampa, Fla, USA, March 2016, http://epostersonline .com/acmg2016/node/2740.

[13] M. G. Beconi, A. Di Marco, E. Monteagudo et al., "RE-024, a phosphopantothenate replacement therapy for PKAN: mechanism of action and efficacy in nonclinical models," in *Proceedings of the ACMG Annual Clinical Genetics Meeting*, Tampa, Fla, USA, March 2016, http://epostersonline.com/acmg2016/ node/2749.

[14] G. A. Tanteles, E. Spanou-Aristidou, C. Antoniou, V. Christophidou-Anastasiadou, and K. A. Kleopa, "Novel homozygous PANK2 mutation causing atypical pantothenate kinase-associated neurodegeneration (PKAN) in a Cypriot family," *Journal of the Neurological Sciences*, vol. 340, no. 1-2, pp. 233–236, 2014.

[15] Movement Disorder Society Task Force on Rating Scales for Parkinson's Disease, "The Unified Parkinson's Disease Rating Scale (UPDRS): status and recommendations," *Movement Disorders*, vol. 18, pp. 738–750, 2003.

[16] S. A. Schneider, J. Hardy, and K. P. Bhatia, "Syndromes of neurodegeneration with brain iron accumulation (NBIA): an update on clinical presentations, histological and genetic underpinnings, and treatment considerations," *Movement Disorders*, vol. 27, no. 1, pp. 42–53, 2012.

[17] L. Timmermann, K. A. M. Pauls, K. Wieland et al., "Dystonia in neurodegeneration with brain iron accumulation: outcome of bilateral pallidal stimulation," *Brain*, vol. 133, no. 3, pp. 701–712, 2010.

[18] R. Mahoney, R. Selway, and J.-P. Lin, "Cognitive functioning in children with pantothenate-kinase-associated neurodegeneration undergoing deep brain stimulation," *Developmental Medicine and Child Neurology*, vol. 53, no. 3, pp. 275–279, 2011.

[19] V. Mylius, A. Gerstner, M. Peters et al., "Low-frequency rTMS of the premotor cortex reduces complex movement patterns in a patient with pantothenate kinase-associated neurodegenerative disease (PKAN)," *Neurophysiologie Clinique*, vol. 39, no. 1, pp. 27–30, 2009.

[20] V. Leoni, L. Strittmatter, G. Zorzi et al., "Metabolic consequences of mitochondrial coenzyme A deficiency in patients with PANK2 mutations," *Molecular Genetics and Metabolism*, vol. 105, no. 3, pp. 463–471, 2012.

[21] G. Cossu, G. Abbruzzese, G. Matta et al., "Efficacy and safety of deferiprone for the treatment of pantothenate kinase-associated neurodegeneration (PKAN) and neurodegeneration with brain iron accumulation (NBIA): results from a four years follow-up," *Parkinsonism and Related Disorders*, vol. 20, no. 6, pp. 651–654, 2014.

[22] A. Tomić, I. Petrović, M. Svetel, V. Dobričić, N. D. Mišković, and V. S. Kostić, "Pattern of disease progression in atypical form of pantothenate-kinase-associated neurodegeneration (PKAN)—prospective study," *Parkinsonism and Related Disorders*, vol. 21, no. 5, pp. 521–524, 2015.

8

Globus Pallidus Internus Deep Brain Stimulation for Disabling Diabetic Hemiballism/Hemichorea

Byung-chul Son,[1,2] **Jin-gyu Choi,**[1] **and Hak-cheol Ko**[1]

[1]*Department of Neurosurgery, Seoul St. Mary's Hospital, College of Medicine, The Catholic University of Korea, Seoul, Republic of Korea*
[2]*Catholic Neuroscience Institute, College of Medicine, The Catholic University of Korea, Seoul, Republic of Korea*

Correspondence should be addressed to Byung-chul Son; sbc@catholic.ac.kr

Academic Editor: Mathias Toft

Unilateral hemichorea/hemiballism (HH) associated with contralateral neuroimaging abnormalities of the basal ganglia, which is characterized by T1 hyperintensity on magnetic resonance imaging (MRI) and is secondary to diabetic nonketotic hyperglycemia, is a rare and unique complication of poorly controlled diabetes mellitus (DM). Although almost all prior reports have documented rapid resolution of HH within days after normalization of blood glucose levels, medically refractory persistent HH has been noted. The experience of surgical intervention for persistent HH is limited. A 46-year-old, right-handed female patient with type 2 DM presented with refractory diabetic HH on the left side of 6 months' duration despite DM control and neuroleptic medication usage. Image-guided deep brain stimulation (DBS) on the right globus pallidus internus (GPi) was performed. A mechanical micropallidotomy effect was observed and chronic stimulation of GPi was quite effective in symptomatic control of diabetic HH until a 16-month follow-up visit. DBS of the GPi can be an effective treatment for medically refractory diabetic HH.

1. Introduction

Hemichorea/hemiballism (HH) is a hyperkinetic movement disorder characterized by acute or subacute onset of high-amplitude, involuntary movements affecting one side of the body [1, 2]. Ischemic/hemorrhagic stroke within the contralateral subthalamic nucleus (STN) and basal ganglia and nonketotic hyperglycemia are the most common causes of HH. Diabetic HH is a unique syndrome characterized by HH, hyperglycemia, and striatal hyperintensity on T1-weighted magnetic resonance image (MRI) [3].

The clinical course of diabetic HH is favorable and the symptoms tend to resolve rapidly with normalization of hyperglycemia in patients who develop diabetic HH secondary to nonketotic hyperglycemia [2, 4]. However, there are rare patients who continue to have persistent HH years after the inciting hyperglycemic crisis [5]. In rare, medically refractory diabetic HH, stereotactic lesioning of the ventrolateral (VL) thalamus [6] and GPi [7] and DBS of the thalamic ventralis oralis (VO) nucleus [8] have been reported to show significant benefit in case reports. Although

GPi DBS was reported to be effective in a patient with HH secondary to vascular insult to the STN and substantia nigra [9], its effectiveness in diabetic HH has not yet been reported. We report the effectiveness of chronic GPi stimulation in a patient suffering refractory diabetic HH and summarized the utility of stereotactic surgery in this rare hyperkinetic movement disorder of metabolic cause.

2. Case Presentation

A 46-year-old, right-handed female patient with an 11-year history of type 2 diabetes mellitus (DM) presented with a continuous, violent choreic/ballistic movement of the left arm, leg, and trunk of 6 months' duration. At the beginning, she experienced vague discomfort in her left arm after a brief episode of heavy lifting. An involuntary choreic movement gradually developed in her arm within several hours. Owing to cramping pain associated with a flinging movement in her left arm and hand, she was initially treated with nonsteroidal anti-inflammatory drugs and physical therapy. However, the choreic movement progressively worsened over the following

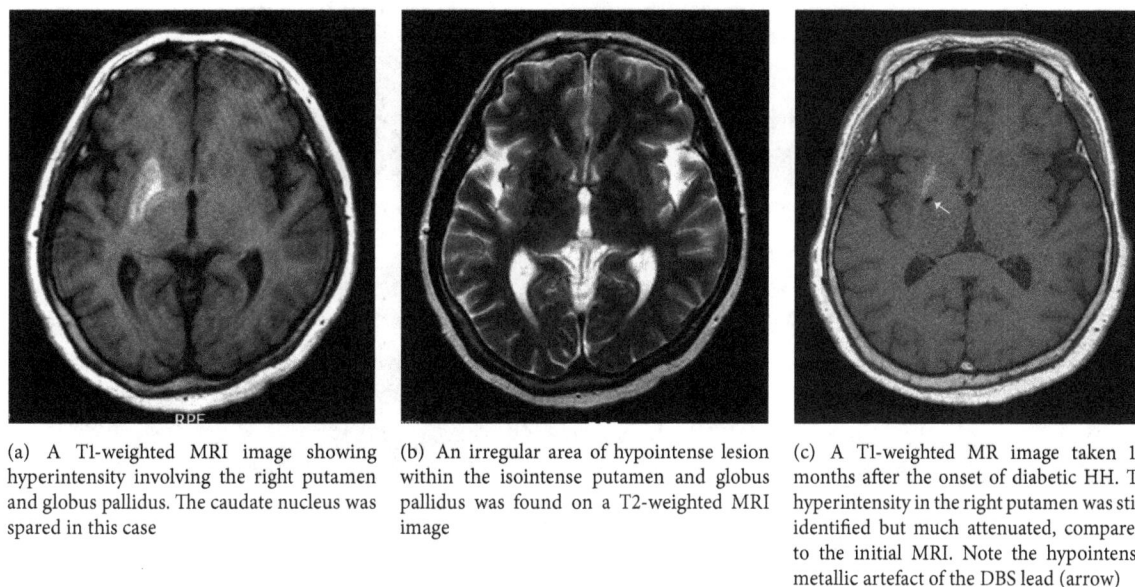

(a) A T1-weighted MRI image showing hyperintensity involving the right putamen and globus pallidus. The caudate nucleus was spared in this case

(b) An irregular area of hypointense lesion within the isointense putamen and globus pallidus was found on a T2-weighted MRI image

(c) A T1-weighted MR image taken 16 months after the onset of diabetic HH. T1 hyperintensity in the right putamen was still identified but much attenuated, compared to the initial MRI. Note the hypointense metallic artefact of the DBS lead (arrow)

FIGURE 1: Magnetic resonance imaging (MRI) findings of diabetic hemichorea/hemiballism.

2 weeks and eventually became ballistic and involved her left arm and leg and had a high amplitude. She was admitted to another hospital via the emergency department for evaluation. Neurologic examination showed facial dyskinesis (grimacing) and a ballistic movement in her left trunk, arm, and legs. The movements could not be suppressed voluntarily but ceased during sleep. Muscle tone and strength in the upper and lower extremities were normal bilaterally. There was no sensory impairment and her cranial nerves were normal. Laboratory studies revealed a fasting blood glucose level of 536 mg/dl, a serum osmolarity of 335 mOsm/kg, and an HbA1c count of 15.7%. Urinalysis was negative for ketones. There was no history of dopamine agonist or estrogen medication use or rheumatic fever/Sydenham's chorea.

A T1-weighted MRI image revealed a region of increased signal intensity restricted to the right putamen and globus pallidus, which was isointense on T2-weighted images (Figure 1). No abnormal enhancement with gadolinium was found. Under a diagnosis of nonketotic hyperglycemic hyperosmolar syndrome, the patient's blood glucose level was controlled with subcutaneous injection of insulin. The severe ballistic movement progressively improved with titration of haloperidol (up to 10 mg/day), clonazepam (6 mg/day), amantadine (300 mg/day), and tiapride (200 mg/day) for HH. Clinical manifestations progressively improved over the course of 3 months of DM control with neuroleptics but did not disappear. She suffered continuous HH, which was most severe in the left leg and foot and involved a severe gait impairment. Finally the patient was referred to our clinic for surgical treatment for chronic, disabling HH at 6 months after the onset of diabetic HH. Considering the chronicity and medical intractability of the situation, GPi DBS was decided upon.

The patient underwent a stereotactic MRI scan (1.5 tesla Archieva®, Philips, Best, The Netherlands), and volumetric T1-weighted three-dimensional images, T2-weighted images,

and proton density images were obtained. The images were transferred to a Framelink® planning station (version 4.1, Medtronic, Minneapolis, MN, USA) so that we could determine the coordinates of the image-guided GPi target and were reformatted for extraventricular trajectory planning (Figure 2(a)) [10, 11]. Implantation of the electrode (model 6149, St. Jude Medical, Plano, Texas, USA) was performed under C-arm fluoroscopy guidance under the general anesthesia. After implantation of the lead, "O-arm" intraoperative CT scan (Medtronic, Minneapolis, MN, USA) was performed and the images were again transferred to the Framelink® planning station and merged with the preoperative volumetric T1-weighted MR images to verify the location of the electrodes (Figure 2(b)). After verification of electrode location, the distal end of the electrode was tunneled subcutaneously for external stimulation. After the patient recovered from anesthesia, an immediate postoperative computed tomography (CT, 1 mm thick axial slices) scan was taken again for verification of the location of the lead with the preoperative T1 MR images and intraoperative O-arm images (Figure 2(c)).

A prominent mechanical effect with significant reduction (50% reduction in intensity) of the choreic and proximal ballistic movements was observed. Bipolar electrical stimulation (100–130 Hz, 1–3 mA, 130 usec, up to 3.5 mA) further suppressed HH, and the hyperkinetic movements became grossly undetectable after 7 days of external stimulation. No stimulation-related side effects such as dysarthria, dysphasia, or motor contraction were observed. A pulse generator (Libra®, St. Jude Medical, Plano, TX, USA) was implanted via a transaxillary subpectoral route after 7 days of external stimulation [12]. The patient returned to her usual activities and became reemployed in her previous job on diabetic medication control and clonazepam (1.5 mg/day). However, she felt continuous cramping pain and an internal sensation of muscular contraction in her lower leg and foot without any grossly visible choreic movements when walking.

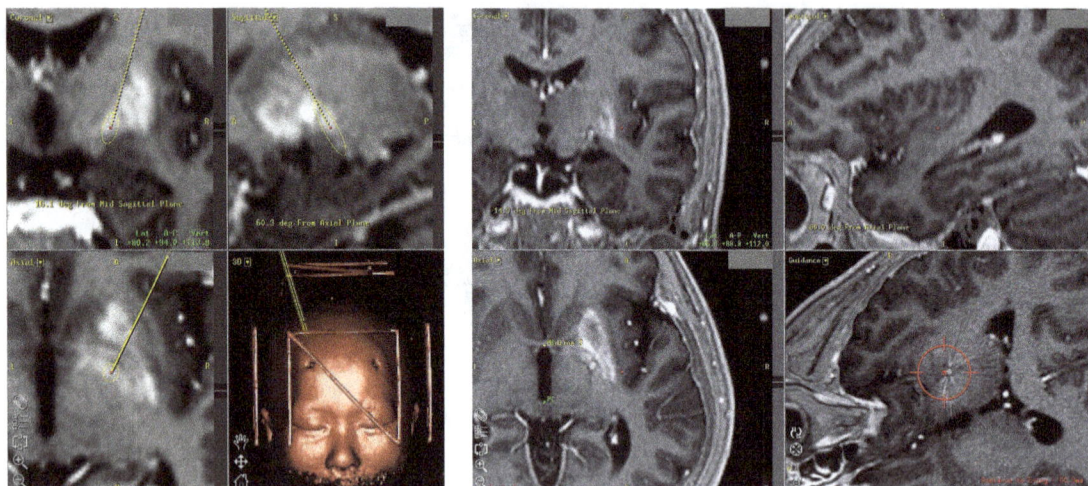

(a) An image in the planning software showing target localization and trajectory planning for right GPi DBS. The target was directed to the posterolateral portion of the GPi which was easily identified owing to hyperintensity in the volumetric T1-weighted MRI images

(b) An image captured from the planning software after fusion of an intraoperative O-arm CT scan with preoperative volumetric T1 images to verify the location of the implanted lead, which was taken with the patient under general anesthesia. Although the electrode was found to be about 1 mm posterior and medial to the initial target point, it was accepted

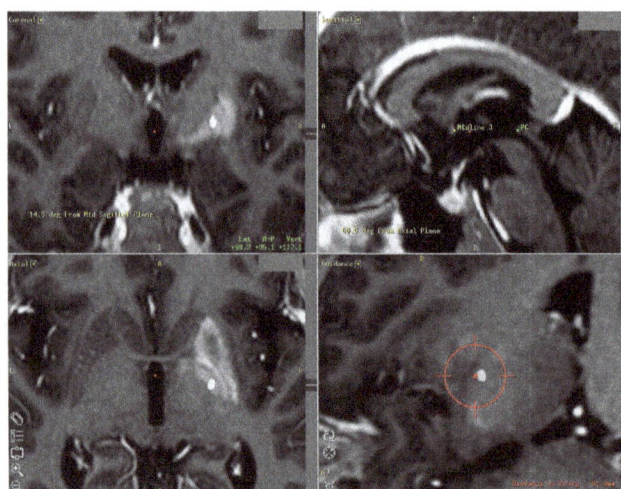

(c) An image captured from the planning software after fusion of the postoperative CT scan with preoperative volumetric T1 images. This image corresponds to the center of the 2nd contact (number 2), which was used as an anode for chronic stimulation

FIGURE 2: Image-guided deep brain stimulation (DBS) of the globus pallidus internus (GPi) for refractory diabetic HH.

Chronic GPi stimulation was performed with regular adjustment of the stimulation parameters (2.6–3.0 mA, 110–130 Hz, 110–120 usec, 1 (−), 2 (+)) every 3 months. At a 16-month postoperative follow-up, the patient was grossly free of HH. However, minimal chorea in the left calf and foot was noted. She was readmitted for an on and off stimulation study and a follow-up MRI examination. After 30-minute off stimulation, the ballistic movements of the left thigh, distal leg, and shoulder returned and gait difficulty was noticed along with chorea in the left foot. After 10 minutes of on stimulation, the HH in her left leg and foot disappeared almost completely. Her fasting blood glucose, serum osmolarity, and HbA1c level were 109 mg/dl, 291 mOsm/kg, and 7.9%, respectively. T1-weighted MRI images again revealed a high signal intensity confined to the right putamen, which was greatly attenuated compared with that seen on the initial preoperative MRI scan (Figures 1(a) and 1(c)).

3. Discussion

3.1. Diabetic HH. Transient chorea/ballism provoked by an episode of nonketotic hyperglycemia has repeatedly been reported over the past couple of decades and is the second most common cause of hemiballism [12]. The blood glucose level in patients with the condition ranges from 500 to 1000 mg/dL during the hyperglycemic precipitating crisis. HH is commonly associated with type 2 DM and is rarely associated with type 1 DM. Although diabetic HH mostly

TABLE 1: Summary of stereotactic surgery for diabetic hemichorea/hemiballism.

Study/year	Number of patients	Age/sex	Timing of surgery	Surgery (lesion/DBS)	Results	follow-up period	Remarks
Takamatsu et al. [6], 1995	1	57/f	1.5 mo.	VL lesion	Excellent	4 years	
Nakano et al. [8], 2005	1	65/m	5 mo.	VO (Voa, Vop) DBS	Effective	9 mo.	Persistent HH in off stimulation
Goto et al. [7], 2010	1	78/f	N/A	GPi lesion	Excellent	12 mo.	HH immediately disappeared
Current case, 2017	1	46/f	6 mo.	GPi DBS	Effective	16 mo.	Persistent HH in off stimulation

GPi: globus pallidus internus; HH: hemichorea/hemiballism; mo: months; VL: ventral lateral nucleus; VO: ventralis oralis; Voa: ventralis oralis anterior; Vop: ventralis oralis posterior.

occurs when patients are in a state of nonketotic hyperglycemia, some patients also have ketotic hyperglycemia [13]. The movements are typically unilateral but can be generalized in rare cases [5]. Description of the movements ranges from mild chorea to severe ballism. According to a review of 53 cases of diabetic HH [4], the average age of onset is 71, and there is a female predominance of 1.8 : 1. Genetic factors may play a role, with an Asian predominance in reported cases [4].

High intensity in the basal ganglia on T1-weighted MRI is a characteristic finding in diabetic HH [2–6, 14, 15]. T1 striatal hyperintensity involves the putamen in all cases, the head of the caudate nucleus in most cases, and the globus pallidus in a minority of cases [14, 15]. In contrast to typical T1 hyperintensity, the findings on T2-weighted images are variable and range from hyper- and iso- to hypointensity. Gradient-echo and gadolinium-enhanced T1-weighted images are reported to be normal. Several mechanisms have been proposed to explain T1 striatal hyperintensity, including acute ischemia, petechial microhemorrhage, injury secondary to hyperviscosity, and vasogenic edema [14]. Currently, hyperviscosity is suggested to be the most plausible mechanism because of the following findings [14]: elevated serum osmolarity at the time of HH, variable T2-weighted MR signal changes that reflect the difference in patterns and severity of hyperviscosity, and elevated myoinositol and choline levels seen on MR spectroscopy that are in line with a finding of abundant gemistocytes with increased protein content [14–17].

The putamen has been suggested to play a central role in diabetic HH [14]. The putamen has abundant medium-sized spiny neurons which store and release gamma amino butyric acid (GABA) [18], and there is universal involvement of the putamen in diabetic HH [14, 15]. Therefore, dysfunction of GABAergic neurons in the putamen may result in a disturbance of output nuclei of the basal ganglia, such as the substantia nigra and GPi [14]; resultant disinhibition of the motor thalamus ensues, leading to hyperkinetic movement disorder.

3.2. Treatment of Diabetic HH. Diabetic HH generally resolves over time, and often no treatment is necessary. Determining the etiology of the condition is a matter of paramount importance and correcting nonketotic hyperglycemia along with long-term diabetic control is the mainstay of treatment [2, 4, 12]. In cases of prolonged diabetic HH, dopamine receptor blocking agents (chlorpromazine or haloperidol),

neuroleptics (olanzapine, clozapine), and dopamine depleting agents (tetrabenazine) have been reported to be beneficial [2]. However, there are some rare patients who continue to have persistent HH years after the inciting hyperglycemic crisis [5]. The exact incidence of medically refractory diabetic HH is unclear. In rare, medically refractory diabetic HH, stereotactic surgery has sporadically been reported in single case reports and we summarized them in Table 1.

Owing to the limited reports on surgical intervention against diabetic HH, the timing and type of surgery, lesioning, or DBS are difficult to determine. However, despite the limited evidence, both lesioning and stimulation in the VL or VO thalamus and GPi showed good results [6–8]. Because diabetic HH is especially prevalent in Asians, all 3 cases regarding surgical treatment came from Japan [6–8]. We chose the GPi as a target of surgical intervention because previous reports regarding GPi lesioning produced uniformly positive results against diabetic HH [7] as well as HH secondary to vascular insults involving the STN and the brain stem [9, 19–21]. In addition, determination of the target within the GPi and trajectory planning was easily done with stereotactic MR images owing to prominent T1 hyperintensity in the GP (Figure 2(a)). A case of DBS of the VO thalamic nucleus was reported to be effective in diabetic HH [8], and we also achieved significant long-term effectiveness with GPi stimulation. Owing to the rarity of diabetic HH, the present case is the first report of GPi DBS for refractory diabetic HH. The present case showed persistent choreiform dyskinesia during off GPi stimulation even after 16 months following the onset of diabetic HH despite long-term continuous diabetic control and medical treatment with much attenuation of T1 hyperintensity in the follow-up MRI. Therefore, timely surgical intervention would be of help in alleviation of disabling motor symptoms in rare patient with persistent diabetic HH.

4. Conclusion

We report the long-term effectiveness of GPi DBS in the treatment of chronic, disabling diabetic HH.

Conflicts of Interest

The authors declare that they have no conflicts of interest regarding this manuscript.

References

[1] J. Jankovic and S. Fahn, "Chorea, ballism, athetosis," in *Principles and Practice of Movement Disorders*, J. Jankovic and S. Fahn, Eds., pp. 401–403, Churchill Livingston Elsevier, Philadelphia, Pa, USA, 1st edition, 2007.

[2] J. S. Hawley and W. J. Weiner, "Hemiballismus: current concepts and review," *Parkinsonism & Related Disorders*, vol. 18, no. 2, pp. 125–129, 2012.

[3] T. Hashimoto, N. Hanyu, H. Yahikozawa, and N. Yanagisawa, "Persistent hemiballism with striatal hyperintensity on T1-weighted MRI in a diabetic patient: A 6-year follow-up study," *Journal of the Neurological Sciences*, vol. 165, no. 2, pp. 178–181, 1999.

[4] S.-H. Oh, K.-Y. Lee, J.-H. Im, and M.-S. Lee, "Chorea associated with non-ketotic hyperglycemia and hyperintensity basal ganglia lesion on T1-weighted brain MRI studya meta-analysis of 53 cases including four present cases," *Journal of the Neurological Sciences*, vol. 200, no. 1-2, pp. 57–62, 2002.

[5] E. J. Ahlskog, H. Nishino, V. G. H. Evidente et al., "Persistent chorea triggered by hyperglycemic crisis in diabetics," *Movement Disorders*, vol. 16, no. 5, pp. 890–898, 2001.

[6] K. Takamatsu, T. Ohta, S. Sato et al., "Two diabetics with hemichorea hemiballism and striatal lesions," *No To Shinkei*, vol. 47, no. 2, pp. 167–172, 1995.

[7] T. Goto, T. Hashimoto, S. Hirayama, and K. Kitazawa, "Pallidal neuronal activity in diabetic hemichorea-hemiballism," *Movement Disorders*, vol. 25, no. 9, pp. 1295–1297, 2010.

[8] N. Nakano, T. Uchiyama, T. Okuda, M. Kitano, and M. Taneda, "Successful long-term deep brain stimulation for hemichorea-hemiballism in a patient with diabetes," *Journal of Neurosurgery*, vol. 102, no. 6, pp. 1137–1141, 2005.

[9] H. Hasegawa, M. Samuel, J. Jarosz, and K. Ashkan, "The treatment of persistent vascular hemidystonia-hemiballismus with unilateral GPi deep brain stimulation," *Movement Disorders*, vol. 24, no. 11, pp. 1967-1968, 2009.

[10] B. C. Son, Y. M. Shon, J. G. Choi et al., "Clinical outcome of patients with deep brain stimulation of the centromedian thalamic nucleus for refractory epilepsy and location of the active contacts," *Stereotactic and Functional Neurosurgery*, vol. 94, no. 3, pp. 187–197, 2016.

[11] B. C. Son, S. H. Han, Y. S. Choi et al., "Transaxillary subpectoral implantation of implantable pulse generator for deep brain stimulation," *Neuromodulation: Technology at the Neural Interface*, vol. 15, no. 3, pp. 260–266, 2012.

[12] R. B. Postuma and A. E. Lang, "Hemiballism: revisiting a classic disorder," *The Lancet Neurology*, vol. 2, no. 11, pp. 661–668, 2003.

[13] Y. Abe, T. Yamamoto, T. Soeda et al., "Diabetic striatal disease: Clinical presentation, neuroimaging, and pathology," *Internal Medicine*, vol. 48, no. 13, pp. 1135–1141, 2009.

[14] N. Kandiah, K. Tan, C. C. T. Lim, and N. Venketasubramanian, "Hyperglycemic choreoathetosis: Role of the putamen in pathogenesis," *Movement Disorders*, vol. 24, no. 6, pp. 915–919, 2009.

[15] C. Battisti, F. Forte, E. Rubenni et al., "Two cases of hemichorea-hemiballism with nonketotic hyperglycemia: A new point of view," *Neurological Sciences*, vol. 30, no. 3, pp. 179–183, 2009.

[16] K. Chu, D. W. Kang, D. E. Kim, S. H. Park, and J. K. Roh, "Diffusion-weighted and gradient echo magnetic resonance findings of hemichorea-hemiballismus associated diabetic hyperglycemia: a hyperviscosity syndrome?" *Archives of Neurology*, vol. 59, no. 3, pp. 448–452, 2003.

[17] D. E. Shan, D. M. Ho, C. Chang, H. C. Pan, and M. M. Teng, "Hemichorea-hemiballismus: an explanation for MR signal changes," *American Journal of Neuroradiology*, vol. 19, pp. 863–870, 1998.

[18] A. M. Graybiel, "Neurotransmitters and neuromodulators in the basal ganglia," *Trends in Neurosciences*, vol. 13, no. 7, pp. 244–254, 1990.

[19] J. I. Suarez, L. Verhagen Merman, S. G. Reich, P. M. Dougherty, M. Hallett, and F. A. Lenz, "Pallidotomy for hemiballismus: Efficacy and characteristics of neuronal activity," *Annals of Neurology*, vol. 42, no. 5, pp. 807–811, 1997.

[20] J. L. Vitek, V. Chockkan, J.-Y. Zhang et al., "Neuronal activity in the basal ganglia in patients with generalized dystonia and hemiballismus," *Annals of Neurology*, vol. 46, no. 1, pp. 22–35, 1999.

[21] K. Yamada, M. Harada, and S. Goto, "Response of postapoplectic hemichorea/ballism to GPi pallidotomy: Progressive improvement resulting in complete relief," *Movement Disorders*, vol. 19, no. 9, pp. 1111–1114, 2004.

9

Neurological Complications of Middle East Respiratory Syndrome Coronavirus

Hussein Algahtani,[1] **Ahmad Subahi,**[2] **and Bader Shirah**[3]

[1]*King Abdulaziz Medical City/King Saud bin Abdulaziz University for Health Sciences, P.O. Box 12723, Jeddah 21483, Saudi Arabia*
[2]*King Saud bin Abdulaziz University for Health Sciences, P.O. Box 12723, Jeddah 21483, Saudi Arabia*
[3]*King Abdullah International Medical Research Center/King Saud bin Abdulaziz University for Health Sciences, P.O. Box 12723, Jeddah 21483, Saudi Arabia*

Correspondence should be addressed to Hussein Algahtani; halgahtani@hotmail.com

Academic Editor: Isabella Laura Simone

Middle East Respiratory Syndrome Coronavirus (MERS-CoV) was first discovered in September 2012 in Saudi Arabia. Since then, it caused more than 1600 laboratory-confirmed cases and more than 580 deaths among them. The clinical course of the disease ranges from asymptomatic infection to severe lower respiratory tract illness with multiorgan involvement and death. The disease can cause pulmonary, renal, hematological, and gastrointestinal complications. In this paper, we report neurological complications of MERS-CoV in two adult patients, and we hypothesize the pathophysiology. The first patient had an intracerebral hemorrhage as a result of thrombocytopenia, disseminated intravascular coagulation, and platelet dysfunction. The second case was a case of critical illness polyneuropathy complicating a long ICU stay. In these cases, the neurological complications were secondary to systemic complications and long ICU stay. Autopsy studies are needed to further understand the pathological mechanism.

1. Introduction

Middle East Respiratory Syndrome Coronavirus (MERS-CoV) was first identified and isolated in Jeddah, Saudi Arabia, in a 60-year-old male who presented with acute pneumonia complicated by renal failure and death [1]. Since that report, more than 1600 laboratory-confirmed cases of infection with MERS-CoV have been documented in 26 countries until the end of 2015. Among them, more than 580 died comprising about 35% of the total number of cases [2]. The syndrome generally presents as lower respiratory tract disease that includes fever, cough, and shortness of breath that may progress to acute respiratory distress syndrome (ARDS), multiorgan failure, and death [3]. Neurological complications of MERS-CoV have been reported only once in the literature in three cases from Riyadh, Saudi Arabia

[4]. Another article from Saudi Arabia reported confusion at presentation among the symptoms of 18 (25.7%) out of 70 confirmed MERS-CoV cases [5]. In this paper, we report two cases of neurological complications of MERS-CoV that affected both the central and peripheral nervous system and we hypothesize the pathophysiology.

2. Method

We retrospectively reviewed all MERS-CoV cases admitted at King Abdulaziz Medical City, Jeddah, since the onset of the epidemic in 2012. We identified a total of 120 confirmed cases of MERS-CoV infection. Two patients with neurological complications of MERS-CoV were the subjects of our study. They were admitted to different wards and were managed by different medical teams prior to admission to the intensive care unit (ICU). The clinical, laboratory, and radiological findings of these cases were reviewed. Testing for MERS-CoV was performed using real-time reverse transcription polymerase chain reaction (RT-PCR). This study was approved by the institutional review board (IRB) of King Abdullah International Medical Research Center (KAIMRC), and since this is an observational study, the consent was waived as per the institutional policy.

3. Patient 1

A thirty-four-year-old female, who was newly diagnosed with diabetes mellitus, presented to the emergency room with a history of high-grade fever of one-day duration. Fever was documented at home and relieved by oral paracetamol. She denied any history of cough or shortness of breath but complained of generalized bone pain and fatigue. Systemic examination showed a febrile ill-looking lady with no lymph node enlargement or skin rash. Chest examination showed decreased air entry bilaterally with crepitation. Neurological examination was normal including higher mental functions, cranial nerves, and motor system, sensory system, and coordination. Laboratory investigations on admission revealed white blood cells of 4.7 with lymphopenia, hemoglobin of 11.3, platelets 203, ESR 47, and CRP 56.5. Chest imaging showed right lung homogenous opacity and the patient was started on intravenous hydration, tazocin, and azithromycin. RT-PCR came back positive for MERS-CoV from sputum. She started to improve, and her condition was stabilized. Unfortunately, two weeks following admission, the patient developed a severe headache, nausea, and vomiting. Few hours later, her consciousness level deteriorated and GCS dropped to 3/15. Urgent CT showed right frontal lobe intracerebral hemorrhage with massive brain edema and midline shift (Figure 1). She was intubated and mechanically ventilated, and she received intravenous mannitol and dexamethasone. Laboratory investigations revealed pictures of disseminated intravascular coagulation including thrombocytopenia and prolonged coagulation profile. Unfortunately, she started to develop multiorgan failure and signs of irreversible brain stem dysfunction and she died two months later.

4. Patient 2

A twenty-eight-year-old male, an orthopedic resident, presented to the emergency room with four-day history of fever, generalized myalgia, dizziness, and productive cough. He gave history of contact with a confirmed case of MERS-CoV. He was admitted to an isolated room as a case of acute viral illness with bronchitis and was started on supportive and symptomatic treatment, azithromycin and oseltamivir. He was fully investigated and on day 13 after admission, RT-PCR for MERS-CoV was positive from respiratory secretions. Since admission, his fever never remitted and respiratory functions were progressively deteriorating with desaturation and requirement of high oxygen supplement. On the 4th day after admission, he was intubated and mechanically ventilated and transferred to the ICU. The patient had a

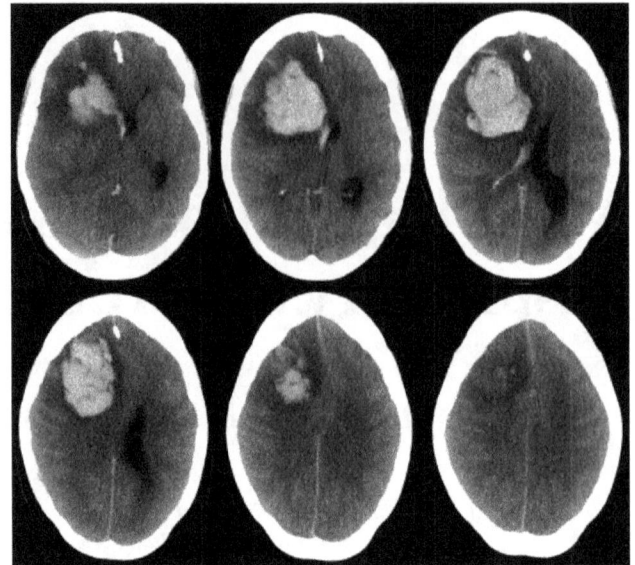

FIGURE 1: CT of the brain showing right frontal lobe intracerebral hemorrhage with massive brain edema, midline shift, and intraventricular extension.

stormy course in the ICU, with secondary bacterial pneumonia for which antibiotics were given in full courses. He eventually improved, extubated, and transferred to the floor. In the floor, neurology consultation was requested because of weakness in both legs and inability to walk with numbness and tingling in stocking distribution. He was investigated throughout including neuroimaging, CSF analysis, nerve conduction velocity (NCV) studies, and EMG. MRI of the whole spine and CSF analysis were normal. NCV studies showed low amplitude with normal latency and conduction velocity especially in the lower extremity, which indicated length dependent axonal polyneuropathy. The final diagnosis was critical illness polyneuropathy complicating a long ICU stay. He received intravenous immunoglobulins 400 mg/kg daily for five days and had his respiratory functions closely monitored. He also received extensive daily physiotherapy and was sent home 40 days after admission. He was seen six months later in the clinic, and he was slowly improving.

5. Discussion

Coronaviruses are a family of enveloped, single-stranded, positive-sense RNA viruses that are prevalent in bats and can affect many other species including humans. The name *corona* denotes the crown-like appearance of the surface projections of the virus under the electron microscope. They may cause respiratory, gastrointestinal, hepatic, and neurological diseases in various species [1]. They are grouped into four different genera which are alpha, beta, gamma, and delta coronaviruses. There are six types of coronaviruses that afflict humans and thus are called human coronaviruses (HCoV) which are HCoV-229E, HCoV-OC43, HCoV-NL63, HCoV-HKU1, SARS-CoV, and MERS-CoV (Table 1) [6]. Bats

TABLE 1: The human corona viruses (HCoV).

Virus	Year of discovery	Reservoir	Receptor	Cell type infected	Mode of transmission	Clinical presentation	Disease type	Severity and prognosis
OC43	1966	Bats	Receptor unknown, sialic acid and HLA class 1 involvement	Ciliated airway epithelial cells, macrophages in culture, and neuronal cells	Droplets	Coryza, cough, and fever	Upper respiratory infection, gastrointestinal infection, and pneumonia	Mild and harmless
229E	1967	Bats and camelids	APN	Nonciliated airway epithelial cells, human monocytes, and neuronal cells	Droplets	Coryza, cough, and fever	Upper respiratory infection, gastrointestinal infection, and pneumonia	Mild and harmless
NL63	2004	Bats	ACE2	Ciliated airway epithelial cells	Droplets	Fever, cough, sore throat, and rhinitis	Upper and lower respiratory infection, associated with croup in children	Mild and harmless
HKU1	2005	Bats	Unknown	Ciliated airway epithelial cells	Droplets	Rhinorrhea, fever, coughing, wheezing, and myalgia	Upper respiratory infection and pneumonia, enteric symptoms	Mild and harmless
SARS	2003	Bats, raccoon dogs, and civet cats	ACE2, role for DC-SIGN also known as CS209	Epithelial cells, ciliated cells, and type II pneumocytes	Droplets	Malaise, headache, chills, myalgia, fever, cough, and dyspnea	Lower respiratory infection, pneumonia, diffuse alveolar damage, and ARDS	Severe respiratory illness with high morbidity and mortality
MERS	2012	Bats and dromedary camels	DPP4 also known as CD26	Airway epithelial cells, renal epithelial cells, and dendritic cell	Droplets	Fever, cough, and breathing difficulties	Lower respiratory infection, pneumonia, ARDS, renal failure, and multiorgan failure	Severe respiratory illness with high morbidity and mortality

HLA: human leukocyte antigen, APN: aminopeptidase N, ACE2: angiotensin converting enzyme 2, DC-SIGN: dendritic cell-specific intercellular adhesion molecule-3-grabbing nonintegrin, CD209: cluster of differentiation 209, DPP4: dipeptidyl peptidase 4, CD26: cluster of differentiation 26, ARDS: acute respiratory distress syndrome.

are thought to be the natural reservoir of coronaviruses, and the viruses can spread to human through an intermediate reservoir. These viruses have been proven to have the ability to cross the species barrier to infect humans and other animals [7]. The human infection by coronaviruses has been mostly mild and harmless except in SARS-CoV and MERS-CoV where they cause severe morbidity and mortality. Among the human coronaviruses, HCoV-229E, HCoV-OC43, SARS-CoV, and more recently MERS-CoV were proven to be associated with neurological diseases [4, 5, 8].

MERS-CoV first appeared in September 2012 in Saudi Arabia in a 60-year-old male who died from respiratory and renal failure and multiorgan damage [1]. It is thought to have originated from bats and transferred to humans through dromedary camels as an intermediate host. Dromedary camels are part of the culture and economic resources for many businessmen and low-income citizens in Saudi Arabia. Although bats are found in large number in Africa, America, Asia, and Europe, they have been also found in small numbers scattered in caves and mountains in Saudi Arabia [9]. The disease in camels can be just as the common cold. However, it may lead to catastrophic effects in humans. In humans, the virus causes a lower respiratory tract disease and may progress to ARDS, multiorgan failure, and death in severe cases. The elderly and patients with multiple comorbidities appear to be more vulnerable and carry a bad prognosis [3]. The most affected country was Saudi Arabia with more than three-quarters of the confirmed cases in the world. There have been 1280 laboratory-confirmed cases in Saudi Arabia until the end of 2015 [10]. The mode of transmission is not understood thoroughly, but it is thought to transmit by lengthy close contact with an infected human or camel. The mean incubation period of MERS-CoV is five to six days, and it ranges from two to sixteen days [3]. To date, there is no effective treatment for MERS-CoV, and the cases are treated supportively depending on the patient's need [11]. There have been some endeavors to develop a vaccine, but to date there in no effective and approved vaccine for MERS-CoV [12].

Viruses, in general, may enter the brain and spinal cord through either hematogenous spread or retrograde neuronal dissemination. The hematogenous spread occurs through viremia (the presence and multiplication of a given virus in the blood stream). On the other hand, retrograde viral spread occurs when a given virus infects neuronal tissue in the periphery with subsequent spread to the CNS using transport mechanisms within the neurons to gain access to the affected vulnerable areas. Examples of the latter type include rabies and herpes simplex virus encephalitis [13]. Although studies have shown that some coronaviruses possess neurotropic and neuroinvasive properties in various hosts including humans, pigs, and rodents, MERS-CoV has never been isolated from neural tissues or fluids in affected human beings [8]. This could be due to the resistance of coronaviruses to culture by in vitro culture systems. In addition, routine viral culture services for coronaviruses is not available in most clinical laboratories and the process of isolation requires the use of labor-intensive embryonic organ cultures, which is time-consuming [14]. Some reports explained the mechanism by which coronaviruses reach the nervous system which is mainly through the hematogenous route where the virus can either remain dormant for a period before it can infect the endothelial cells of the blood-brain barrier or infect white blood cells that will become the reservoir for the dissemination to other sites [8]. This has never been proved by research. In addition, the blood-brain barrier has several protective characteristics to prevent viruses from entering the brain. In a recent communication by Joob and Wiwanitkit, they proposed that the size of MERS-CoV (150–320 nm) is an obstacle to enter through the 1 nm pore size within the blood-brain barrier [15]. From our point of view and through reviewing the neuroimaging studies, we did not find any meningeal enhancement in most of the cases which supports this theory. We are proposing a different theory which is the autoimmune theory with several involvements of the neural tissues and blood vessels through autoreactive T-cells recognizing both viral and myelin antigens as similar molecules. This immune response that participates in induction or exacerbation of neuropathologies occurs specifically

in genetically susceptible individuals [16]. This theory is predominant in explaining the neurological complications of other viruses such as the pandemic influenza A H1N1 pdm09 [17]. This has therapeutic implications which include the possible improvement with the early use of pulse steroid therapy and intravenous immunoglobulin before tissue damage occurs. Steroids and immunoglobulins have been reported previously in the literature in the treatment of SARS-CoV infected patients along with ribavirin. They were not proven to be effective or reduce the morbidity or mortality of the disease. In fact, four studies reported harm due to steroid therapy in terms of avascular necrosis and steroid-induced psychosis in SARS-CoV infected patients [18]. Steroids were also used empirically for the treatment of some MERS-CoV infected patients without proven benefit or positive effect observed [19]. However, we believe that using steroids in MERS-CoV infected cases that present with or develop neurological complications will be beneficial in reducing the mortality and helping with the disease course due to their known benefits in the treatment of neurological diseases. The lack of autopsy studies published in the literature on this topic may participate in keeping the explanation of neurological complications of coronaviruses unclear.

In our cases, none of the theories mentioned above are contributory since our patients presented with sequelae of systemic complications. The first case was explained by an intracerebral hemorrhage as a result of thrombocytopenia, disseminated intravascular coagulation, and platelet dysfunction. The second case was a case of critical illness polyneuropathy complicating a long ICU stay. He made a full recovery with supportive measures, immune modulating treatment, and physiotherapy. The three cases reported in the literature previously along with our cases are summarized in Table 2.

6. Conclusion

MERS-CoV infection is a serious disease that affects multiple organs and causes pulmonary, renal, hematological, and gastrointestinal complications. MERS-CoV has created an alarming anxiety in the health sector due to the number of confirmed cases and deaths, especially that there is no treatment available to counterattack this viral infection. Health authorities have released various guidelines to prevent transmission of the disease. Research and studies are ongoing to find the cure or, perhaps, ways to properly manage the case and minimize morbidity and mortality incidence of the disease. There have been some suggested mechanisms through which this virus affects the central nervous system, but the exact mechanism is not thoroughly understood. Autopsy studies are needed to further understand the mechanism.

Competing Interests

The authors declare that there is no conflict of interests.

TABLE 2: Patients with neurological complications of Middle East Respiratory Syndrome Coronavirus (MERS-CoV).

Patient	Age/sex	Presenting symptoms	Comorbidities	Diagnosis	Treatments	Outcome	Cause of death
Patient 1 [4]	74/M	Ataxia, vomiting, confusion, and fever	Diabetes, hypertension, and dyslipidemia	Acute disseminated encephalomyelitis (ADEM)	Broad-spectrum antibiotics, oseltamivir, bronchodilators, methylprednisolone, intravenous sedation, neuromuscular blockers, inhaled nitric oxide, vasopressors, renal replacement therapy, peginterferon alpha-2b and ribavirin	Death	Deep coma, poor overall condition, and worsening cardiovascular and respiratory status
Patient 2 [4]	57/M	Flu-like illness, fever, and a gangrenous toe	Diabetes, hypertension, and peripheral vascular disease	Bilateral anterior cerebral artery stroke	Broad-spectrum antibiotics	Death	Severe shock, acute kidney injury, and multiple cardiac arrests
Patient 3 [4]	45/M	Productive cough, dyspnea, rigors, fever, and diarrhea	Diabetes, hypertension, chronic kidney disease, and ischemic heart disease	Encephalitis	Broad-spectrum antibiotics, oseltamivir, renal replacement therapy, neuromuscular blockers, nitric oxide, vasopressors, peginterferon alpha-2b and ribavirin	Recovery	Not applicable
Patient 4	34/F	Fever, generalized bone pain, and fatigue	Diabetes mellitus	Intracerebral hemorrhage	Intravenous hydration, tazocin, azithromycin, mannitol, and dexamethasone	Death	Multiorgan failure and intracerebral hemorrhage with massive brain edema
Patient 5	28/M	Fever, generalized myalgia, dizziness, and productive cough	None	Critical illness polyneuropathy	Azithromycin, oseltamivir, antibiotics, intravenous immunoglobulins, and physiotherapy	Recovery	Not applicable

References

[1] A. M. Zaki, S. Van Boheemen, T. M. Bestebroer, A. D. M. E. Osterhaus, and R. A. M. Fouchier, "Isolation of a novel coronavirus from a man with pneumonia in Saudi Arabia," *The New England Journal of Medicine*, vol. 367, no. 19, pp. 1814–1820, 2012.

[2] World Health Organization, *Middle East Respiratory Syndrome Coronavirus (MERS-CoV)*, World Health Organization, Genève, Switzerland, 2016, http://www.who.int/emergencies/mers-cov/en/.

[3] I. M. Mackay and K. E. Arden, "MERS coronavirus: diagnostics, epidemiology and transmission," *Virology Journal*, vol. 12, no. 1, article 222, 2015.

[4] Y. M. Arabi, A. Harthi, J. Hussein et al., "Severe neurologic syndrome associated with Middle East respiratory syndrome corona virus (MERS-CoV)," *Infection*, vol. 43, no. 4, pp. 495–501, 2015.

[5] M. Saad, A. S. Omrani, K. Baig et al., "Clinical aspects and outcomes of 70 patients with Middle East respiratory syndrome coronavirus infection: a single-center experience in Saudi Arabia," *International Journal of Infectious Diseases*, vol. 29, pp. 301–306, 2014.

[6] L. E. Gralinski and R. S. Baric, "Molecular pathology of emerging coronavirus infections," *The Journal of Pathology*, vol. 235, no. 2, pp. 185–195, 2015.

[7] B. Hu, X. Ge, L. F. Wang, and Z. Shi, "Bat origin of human coronaviruses," *Virology Journal*, vol. 12, article 221, 2015.

[8] M. Desforges, A. Le Coupanec, É. Brison, M. Meessen-Pinard, and P. J. Talbot, "Neuroinvasive and neurotropic human respiratory coronaviruses: potential neurovirulent agents in humans," *Advances in Experimental Medicine and Biology*, vol. 807, pp. 75–96, 2014.

[9] Z. A. Memish, N. Mishra, K. J. Olival et al., "Middle East respiratory syndrome coronavirus in bats, Saudi Arabia," *Emerging Infectious Diseases*, vol. 19, no. 11, pp. 1819–1823, 2013.

[10] Saudi Ministry of Health, Command & Control Center, 2016, http://www.moh.gov.sa/en/ccc/pressreleases/pages/default.aspx.

[11] P. Sampathkumar, "Middle east respiratory syndrome: what clinicians need to know," *Mayo Clinic Proceedings*, vol. 89, no. 8, pp. 1153–1158, 2014.

[12] L. Du and S. Jiang, "Middle East respiratory syndrome: current status and future prospects for vaccine development," *Expert Opinion on Biological Therapy*, vol. 15, no. 11, pp. 1647–1651, 2015.

[13] S. H. Berth, P. L. Leopold, and G. Morfini, "Virus-induced neuronal dysfunction and degeneration," *Frontiers in Bioscience*, vol. 14, no. 14, pp. 5239–5259, 2009.

[14] D. S. Leland and C. C. Ginocchio, "Role of cell culture for virus detection in the age of technology," *Clinical Microbiology Reviews*, vol. 20, no. 1, pp. 49–78, 2007.

[15] B. Joob and V. Wiwanitkit, "Neurologic syndrome due to MERS: is there a possibility that the virus can cross the blood-brain barrier to cause a neurological problem?" *Annals of Tropical Medicine and Public Health*, vol. 8, no. 5, p. 231, 2015.

[16] P. J. Talbot, D. Arnold, and J. P. Antel, "Virus-induced autoimmune reactions in the CNS," *Current Topics in Microbiology and Immunology*, vol. 253, pp. 247–271, 2001.

[17] H. Algahtani, B. Shirah, S. Alkhashan, and R. Ahmad, "Neurological complications of novel influenza A (H1N1) pdm09 infection: report of two cases and a systematic review of the literature," *Journal of Neuroinfectious Diseases*, vol. 7, article 201, 2016.

[18] L. J. Stockman, R. Bellamy, and P. Garner, "SARS: systematic review of treatment effects," *PLoS Medicine*, vol. 3, no. 9, pp. 1525–1531, 2006.

[19] A. Zumla, D. S. Hui, and S. Perlman, "Middle East respiratory syndrome," *The Lancet*, vol. 386, no. 9997, pp. 995–1007, 2015.

10

A Horned Viper Bite Victim with PRES

Ahmed Mustafa Ibrahim, Tarek Talaat ElSefi, Maha Ghanem,
Akram Muhammad Fayed, and Nesreen Adel Shaban

Faculty of Medicine, Alexandria University, Alexandria, Egypt

Correspondence should be addressed to Ahmed Mustafa Ibrahim; amibrahim00@gmail.com

Academic Editor: Massimiliano Filosto

Neurological complications of snake bites have been well documented in the literature as neuromuscular paralysis and cerebrovascular complications; posterior reversible encephalopathy syndrome was rarely described. A 23-year-old lady presented near full term of her pregnancy with a horned snake *Cerastes cerastes* bite; after successful delivery she started complaining of altered mental status and visual disturbance with ulceration over the site of the snake bite. On admission, the patient had Glasgow Coma Score of 12, blood pressure 130/80 mmHg, temperature 38°C, sinus tachycardia at 120 beats per minute, severe dehydration, and reduction in visual acuity to "hand motion" in both eyes with poor light projection and sluggish pupillary reactions. CT brain was not conclusive; MRI revealed features of PRES. Treatment was mostly supportive within one week; the patient regained consciousness; visual disturbance, however, persisted. This patient as well as the few previously described cases highlights PRES as a possible complication of snake bites.

1. Background

The sand horned vipers (genus *Cerastes*) are the best identified and most abundant venomous snakes of the deserts of North Africa and the Middle East [1]. Various sequelae of human envenomation have been documented, with coagulopathy, hemolysis, and disseminated intravascular coagulopathy being the commonest findings [1, 2]. Both ischemic and hemorrhagic strokes, as well as acute renal failure and pancreatitis, have also been described [1, 3–7]. Many toxins have been identified from *Cerastes cerastes* venom. These include serine proteases and other thrombin-like enzymes (fibrinogenases) (IVa, Cerastocytin, Cerastotin, RP3 4, Afaâcytin, and Cerastase F-4), activators of platelet aggregation/agglutination (Cerastocytin, Cerastotin), inhibitors of platelet aggregation (IVa, Cerastatin, Cerastin), Factor X activators (calcium-dependent and calcium-independent serine proteases, Afaâcytin), a hemorrhagic protease (Cerastase F-4), and α/β fibrinogenase, which releases serotonin from platelets (Afaâcytin), and a phosphodiesterase exonuclease and a weakly toxic phospholipase A_2, which could contribute to local tissue damage. Obviously some of these toxins have opposite actions which suggest that the clinical picture of the snake bite would depend on the exact composition of the venom of the particular snake with large intraspecies variations [1].

Neurological complications of snake bites, primarily neuromuscular paralysis, hypopituitarism, and strokes, have also been recorded in the literature [8–10].

While intracranial hemorrhage in snake bite patients has been clearly attributed to the coexisting coagulopathy, the process by which ischemic strokes occur is still a matter of debate, with various mechanisms currently proposed such as endothelial injury, hypercoagulability, autoimmune vasculitis, thrombotic microangiopathy, and systemic hypotension [8, 9].

Posterior reversible encephalopathy syndrome (PRES) is a neurological disease whose pathophysiology is still not fully understood. Various theories have been put forward in an attempt to explain the mechanism by which PRES occurs, including endothelial injury and hypoperfusion [11, 12]. Only a handful of case reports have described the occurrence of PRES with snake bites as well as other animals' [13].

In this case report we describe the case of a young lady who presented to us with neurological symptoms following a horned sand viper bite that was later diagnosed as PRES.

2. Case Report

A previously healthy 23-year-old lady in her 37th week of pregnancy (G1P0A0) was bitten in her left leg by a snake that was later identified as the horned viper *Cerastes cerastes*. She developed pain and blisters at the site of the bite. A polyvalent antivenin was administered to the patient and she was transferred to a hospital in Tobruk, Libya. She presented to the hospital fully conscious. Her vital signs showed a blood pressure and heart rate of 110/70 mmHg and 130 beats per minute, respectively. Investigations were as follows: hemoglobin (Hb) 9.2 gm/dl, White Blood Cell (WBC) count 9.3×10^3, platelets (plt) 105×10^3, and INR 2.7. Fearing for fetal adverse events [14] and given that she was already at full term, pregnancy was terminated by caesarean section after fresh frozen plasma transfusion.

Over the following week, the patient started to become feverish and obtunded. Gradual loss of vision ensued. No seizures, headache, or paresis occurred. A brain CT scan was done but was unremarkable. Edema of the left leg worsened, with the ulcer at the bite site later on turning gangrenous. The patient had stable blood pressure throughout her stay in Libya with no evidence of preeclampsia. Urine analysis tested negative for proteinuria. The preliminary diagnosis was septic encephalopathy and the patient was transferred to our center, El-Ekbal Hospital, a private tertiary care facility in Alexandria, Egypt.

On admission, the patient was stuporous with a Glasgow Coma Score of 12 (E3M5V4). Vital signs were as follows: blood pressure 130/80 mmHg, temperature 38°C, respiratory rate 15 breaths per minute, and sinus tachycardia at 120 beats per minute which persisted even after adequate fever control and correction of anemia.

Neurological examination revealed a reduction in visual acuity to "hand motion" in both eyes with poor light projection and sluggish pupillary reactions.

On assessing the volume status, the patient was found to be severely dehydrated with an initial CVP reading of −3 and −2 cm H_2O. The C-section wound did not show any signs of infection; however her left leg displayed a gangrenous ulcer.

Her initial investigations were as follows: Hb 8.3 g/dL, WBC 8.1×10^3, Plt 63×10^3/uL, INR 1.1, Na^+ 142.6 mmol/L, K 3.21 mmol/L, Mg^{+2} 0.9 mg/dL, total bilirubin 0.7 mg/dL, creatinine 0.76 mg/dL, and urea 35.3 mg/dL. Urine analysis revealed a specific gravity of 1005, albumin: nil, urobilinogen: normal trace, pH 6.5, pus cells 2-3/HPF, RBCs 8–10/HPF, SGOT 11 U/L, SGPT 35 U/L, and total bilirubin 0.7 mg/dl.

A hypercoagulability panel was ordered. The patient tested positive for Factor V Leiden gene mutation and methylenetetrahydrofolate reductase (MTHFR) gene mutation and negative for protein C, protein S, antinuclear antibodies, and antiphospholipid antibodies.

Differential diagnosis of the altered sensorium was either a neurological complication of the snake bite or sepsis associated encephalopathy. Quantitative C-reactive protein and procalcitonin levels were 13.7 mg/L and 0.2 ng/mL, respectively, which correlated with mild-to-moderate localized bacterial infection rather than sepsis [19].

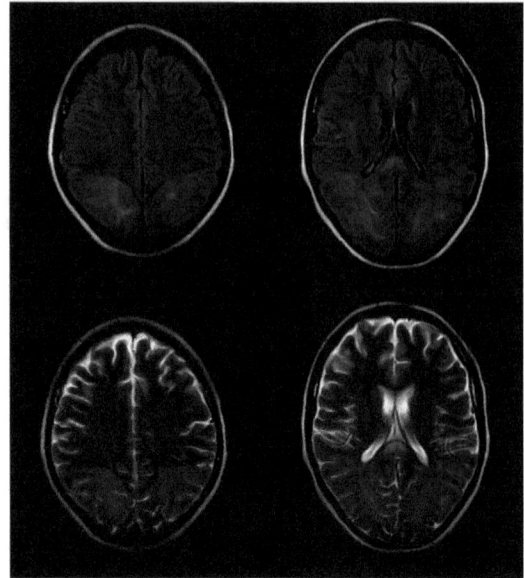

FIGURE 1: Bilateral symmetrical bright T2 and FLAIR white matter intensity involving the posterior parietal sections of both cerebral hemispheres, as well as the splenial segment of the corpus callosum.

A follow-up brain CT illustrated a very faint hypodense area in the posterior part of the parietal and occipital lobes. MRI revealed a bilateral symmetrical bright T2 and FLAIR white matter intensity involving the posterior parietal sections of both cerebral hemispheres, as well as the genu and splenial segments of the corpus callosum, with patchy diffusion restriction in the DW/ADC map series: features of PRES either with atypical findings of patchy diffusion restriction or complicated with ischemia. Magnetic resonance venography (MRV) was normal (Figures 1 and 2).

Doppler US of the left lower limb arterial system revealed a monophasic waveform in the posterior tibial and the dorsalis pedis arteries with good pulsatility and adequate peak systolic velocity, along with a hyperdynamic inflammatory pattern. Venous Doppler US showed superficial thrombophlebitis.

Treatment was mostly supportive: fluid and electrolyte replacement, antibiotics and debridement of the necrotic tissue, clopidogrel, folate, and vitamin B complex for MTHFR deficiency. Diltiazem was prescribed for inappropriate tachycardia and risperidone for agitation and blood transfusion for anemia.

Within one week of hospital stay the patient remained normotensive, her hyperthermia was rapidly controlled as well as the sinus tachycardia, and the patient regained consciousness and hemoglobin and platelet levels normalized. Blindness, however, persisted. She was discharged to home in Libya, no follow-up MRI was done, and the patient reported three months later still having visual impairment though her vision is improving.

3. Discussion

Snake venom contains a mixture of cytotoxic, hypotensive, neurotoxic, and anticoagulant substances and varies in composition according to the species of the snake [8].

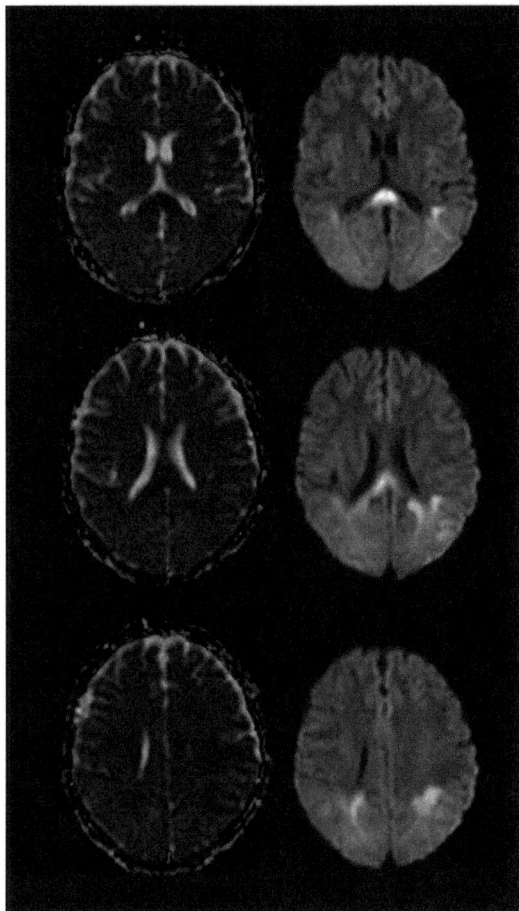

FIGURE 2: DW/ADC map series showing patchy diffusion restriction in posterior parietal sections as well as splenial segment of corpus callosum.

Neurotoxins are a major component of many venoms. These toxins cause paralysis by affecting the neuromuscular junction at presynaptic or postsynaptic levels. Presynaptic neurotoxins inhibit the release of acetylcholine from the presynaptic neuron. Postsynaptic neurotoxins are three-finger protein complexes, which have a curare-like action, causing a reversible blockage of acetylcholine receptors. Some venoms contain both types of neurotoxins, producing complex blockages of neuromuscular transmission [8]. This blockade presents as acute muscle weakness or, more dangerously, respiratory muscle failure which is potentially fatal [9].

Major neurological complications were described in cases of snake bites, most notably ischemic and hemorrhagic infarctions. These are most likely related to the components of the toxins that interfere with blood coagulation and cause bleeding or clotting [8]. While intracranial hemorrhages are related to pathology of hemostatic factors as decreased platelets or a severe consumptive coagulopathy, the mechanism underlying ischemia is still not established. Proposed mechanisms include hypercoagulability, endothelial damage, vasculitis, and hypotension. The presence of multiple cerebral infarctions in most of the cases supports the hypothesis that infarctions are most likely related to the prothrombotic effects

of the venom as well as endothelial damage [8], with the latter being the proposed mechanism by which PRES occurs in snake bite victims.

PRES is characterized by a variety of neurological symptoms including encephalopathy (50–80%), seizures (60–75%), headache (50%), visual disturbances (33%), focal neurological deficits (10–15%), and status epilepticus (5–15%) that is accompanied by a potentially reversible imaging pattern of subcortical vasogenic brain edema [11].

Two hypotheses were suggested to explain the pathogenesis of PRES: (1) hypertension exceeding the limits of autoregulation, causing breakthrough brain edema, and (2) hypertension leading to cerebral autoregulatory vasoconstriction, ischemia, and consequent brain edema [12].

Moderate-to-severe hypertension is encountered in about 70% of patients with PRES at presentation, and emergent hypertension treatment is associated with symptom improvement in many cases. Nevertheless, a significant number of PRES patients presented without hypertension, including the case we are discussing in this report. Data supporting hyperperfusion are scarce and the extent of brain edema does not correlate with the severity of hypertension [12]. The aforementioned findings delineate only two of the several problems affecting this theory.

Another theory proposed to explain PRES is the role of endothelial dysfunction. In the majority of patients who develop PRES; a complex underlying systemic inflammatory process is present as T-cell activation, inflammatory cytokine production, endothelial surface antigens activation, endothelial antibodies, immune system antigens, and VEGF elevation. Cytokines (TNF-a IL-1) upregulate endothelial surface antigens (P-selectin, E-selectin, ICAM-1, and VCAM-1) and increase leukocyte adherence (trafficking) leading to microvascular dysfunction. Enhanced systemic endothelial activation, leukocyte trafficking, and vasoconstriction, alone or in combination, will result in brain and systemic hypoperfusion [20].

Evidence of vasculopathy and cerebral hypoperfusion is present on current imaging studies and is likely reflected in the watershed appearance of the vasogenic edema that develops in PRES, which may support the theory of systemic inflammatory response leading to hypoperfusion [12, 20]. Other minor hypotheses put magnesium as part of the pathogenesis of PRES, either as a cause or as an aggravating factor. Noteworthy is that our patient had persistent hypomagnesemia [21].

PRES is associated with conditions as severe hypertension, blood pressure fluctuations, renal failure, eclampsia, preeclampsia, autoimmune disorders, and cytotoxic drugs. Few accounts described the occurrence of PRES in victims of animal bites [13] as scorpions [22], wasps [23], and snakes.

Four cases in the literature described the occurrence of PRES with snake bites (Table 1). The first case, described by Delgado and Del Brutto, was that of an 18-year-old man bitten by Bothrops asper. Two days after receiving the antivenin, he developed disturbance in the level of consciousness, respiratory distress, and coagulopathy; a brain CT with IV contrast revealed bilateral hypodensities that resolved upon resolution of the symptoms [15].

Table 1: A summary of the clinical presentation of five cases of PRES in patients with snake bites.

	Type of snake	Onset	Antivenin Received	Manifestations					Neurological symptoms			Reversibility
				Coagulopathy	Renal impairment	Respiratory failure	Hypertension	Seizures	Visual disturbance	DLC	Motor disorders	
Our patient	*Cerastescerastes*	Within a week	Yes, before symptoms	Yes	No	No	No	No	Yes	Yes	No	Partially
Delgado and Del Brutto [15]	*Bothropsasper*	2 days	Yes, before symptoms	Yes	No	Yes	No	Yes	No	Yes	No	Yes
Chaudhary et al. [16]	Not identified	30 min	Yes, after symptoms	Yes	No	No	No	No	No	Yes	Yes	Partially
Varalaxmi et al. [17]	Pit viper	2 days	No	No	Yes	No	No	No	Yes	Yes	No	Yes
Kaushik et al. [18]	*Bungaruscaeruleus*	hours	Yes, after symptoms	Not clear	Not clear	Yes	Yes	Yes	Yes	Yes	Yes	Yes

Chaudhary et al. illustrated the second case, being that of a 40-year-old woman bitten by an unknown species of snake. Unconsciousness and coagulopathy developed 30 minutes after the bite; MRI revealed signal intensity alteration in the caudate and lenticular nuclei as well as the thalami, along with involvement of the cortical rim suggestive of an asymmetrical leucoencephalopathy with the DW image excluding ischemia. Improvement of the general condition followed administration of the antivenin. Nonetheless, a parkinsonism-like state ensued which required long term treatment with a carbidopa-levodopa combination [16].

The third case was published in a letter by Varalaxmi et al. Following a bite by a pit viper, a 45-year-old man developed renal impairment. On the second day, the patient developed cortical blindness and headache. No antivenin was given. Brain MRI revealed cortical bilateral hyperintensity affecting the parietal, occipital, and subcortical white matter and a diagnosis of PRES was established. The neurological symptoms started to improve within 12 hours with complete resolution occurring 24 hours after the bite [17].

The fourth case, a 10-year-old boy bitten by an Indian Krait, was reported by Kaushik et al. The patient presented with respiratory distress, disturbed level of consciousness, sluggish light reflexes, uncontrolled hypertension, and autonomic disturbances. Improvement of the symptoms occurred 3 days after receiving the antivenin and the patient was discharged. Six days later, he presented with focal status epilepticus, uncontrolled hypertension, and visual disturbance. Brain MRI revealed hyperintensity on T2-FLAIR images in the parietooccipital subcortical white matter with a picture of PRES. His vision returned to normal within 2 days, and he was discharged on antiepileptic and antihypertensive medications. On follow-up, his blood pressure normalized and his antihypertensive medications were stopped. Repeated MRI studies revealed resolution of the findings [18].

What stands out in these cases as well as ours is that there was no hypertension in 4 of the 5 patients except Kaushik et al.'s [18]. Two of the cases had other clinical conditions that may explain the occurrence of PRES; the patient of Kaushik et al. [18] had uncontrolled hypertension and the patient of Varalaxmi et al. had renal impairment. Both conditions are known to be associated with PRES [11]. Our patient's symptoms developed in the early postpartum period. While eclampsia and preeclampsia are the most common conditions leading to PRES [24], our patient had neither hypertension nor proteinuria, which excludes preeclampsia as a cause of the disorder.

Two out of the five patients received antivenin prior to the development of the neurological symptoms. If the initial symptoms of the patient of Kaushik et al. [18] were not part of PRES, that would make them 3. Antivenin is known to have possible adverse neurological effects [8]. Four of the patients at one point or another received antivenin.

Although the exact mechanism of PRES is not clear in these cases, the temporal relation with the snake bites makes the association between the two very probable.

One of the remarkable features of the case we present here is the restricted diffusion pattern revealed in the MRI. Restricted diffusion is one of the atypical presentations of PRES. In a study by McKinney et al. it was the second most common atypical presentation of PRES [25]. It indicates the presence of cytotoxic edema rather than the vasogenic edema associated with PRES [26]. This finding was traditionally attributed to the development of ischemia on top of PRES and was regarded as a poor prognostic factor due to the irreversibility of the condition [26–28]. Other case reports and series suggest the contrary since reversible restricted diffusion was noted in cases of subarachnoid hemorrhage and transient ischemic attacks. Recent data suggests that the same may be true for PRES with patches of restricted diffusion [29–31]. In a study by Wagih et al., neither the extent of the lesion nor any imaging variable, such as the apparent diffusion coefficient (ADC), had statistically significant correlation with the reversibility of the disease [31], and other multicentric studies as the study done by Pande et al. also found that DWI, even with ADC maps, had limitations in predicting the course of PRES [32].

Despite resolution of most of our patient's symptoms, the persistence of vision loss for months after the bite may favor the possibility of irreversibility.

The relation between the patient's hypercoagulable state and PRES or the restricted diffusion pattern is unclear; scanty data are found in literature regarding the association between PRES and hypercoagulability [33], hypercoagulability may have been an added factor of endothelial injury in the patient.

Additional Points

Key Learning Points. (1) Due to the complexity of the structure of snake venom, all possible presentations must be anticipated no matter how rare they are. (2) The association between PRES and venomous animal bites may cast some light on the pathogenesis of the condition and thus requires further studying. (3) Most snake bite victims are inhabitants of remote and rural areas. A competent system for providing the essential primary care and referral must be established.

Conflicts of Interest

The authors declare that there are no conflicts of interest regarding the publication of this article.

Acknowledgments

The authors would like to thank Dr. Amira Harby, Dr. Emad Zakaria, Dr. Mustafa Ashmawy, and Dr. Islam Kotb, critical care specialists, Dr. Hani El-Boukhari, general surgery consultant, Dr. Ghada Ashmawy, neuropsychiatry consultant, and Dr. Ahmed Habiba, radiology specialist, for their effort with the patient.

References

[1] M. Schneemann, R. Cathomas, S. T. Laidlaw, A. M. El Nahas, R. D. G. Theakston, and D. A. Warrell, "Life-threatening envenoming by the Saharan horned viper (Cerastes cerastes) causing micro-angiopathic haemolysis, coagulopathy and acute renal

failure: clinical cases and review," *QJM*, vol. 97, no. 11, pp. 717–727, 2004.

[2] I. Berling and G. K. Isbister, "Hematologic effects and complications of snake envenoming," *Transfusion Medicine Reviews*, vol. 29, no. 2, pp. 82–89, 2015.

[3] D. Elkabbaj, K. Hassani, and R. El Jaoudi, "Acute renal failure following the Saharan horned viper (Cerastes cerastes) bite," *Arab Journal of Nephrology and Transplantation*, vol. 5, no. 3, pp. 159–161, 2012.

[4] J. Valenta, Z. Stach, and M. Svítek, "Acute pancreatitis after viperid snake cerastes cerastes envenoming: a case report," *Prague Medical Report*, vol. 111, no. 1, pp. 69–75, 2010.

[5] H. Rebahi, H. Nejmi, T. Abouelhassan, K. Hasni, and M.-A. Samkaoui, "Severe envenomation by cerastes cerastes viper: an unusual mechanism of acute ischemic stroke," *Journal of Stroke and Cerebrovascular Diseases*, vol. 23, no. 1, pp. 169–172, 2014.

[6] Y. Aissaoui, S. Hammi, K. Chkoura, I. Ennafaa, and M. Boughalem, "Association of ischemic and hemorrhagic cerebral stroke due to severe envenomation by the Sahara horned viper (Cerastes cerastes)," *Bulletin de la Societe de Pathologie Exotique*, vol. 106, no. 3, pp. 163–166, 2013.

[7] H. B. Ghezala and S. Snouda, "Hemorrhagic stroke following a fatal envenomation by a horned viper in Tunisia," *Pan African Medical Journal*, vol. 21, article 156, 2015.

[8] O. H. Del Brutto and V. J. Del Brutto, "Neurological complications of venomous snake bites: a review," *Acta Neurologica Scandinavica*, vol. 125, no. 6, pp. 363–372, 2012.

[9] U. K. Ranawaka, D. G. Lalloo, H. J. de Silva, and J. White, "Neurotoxicity in snakebite—the limits of our knowledge," *PLoS Neglected Tropical Diseases*, vol. 7, no. 10, Article ID e2302, 2013.

[10] S. Rajagopala, M. M. Thabah, K. K. Ariga, and M. Gopalakrishnan, "Acute hypopituitarism complicating Russell's viper envenomation: case series and systematic review," *QJM*, vol. 108, no. 9, pp. 719–728, 2015.

[11] J. E. Fugate and A. A. Rabinstein, "Posterior reversible encephalopathy syndrome: clinical and radiological manifestations, pathophysiology, and outstanding questions," *The Lancet Neurology*, vol. 14, no. 9, pp. 914–925, 2015.

[12] W. S. Bartynski, "Posterior reversible encephalopathy syndrome, Part 2: controversies surrounding pathophysiology of vasogenic edema," *American Journal of Neuroradiology*, vol. 29, no. 6, pp. 1043–1049, 2008.

[13] O. H. Del Brutto, "Reversible posterior leukoencephalopathy after venomous bites and stings," *NeuroToxicology*, vol. 39, article 10, 2013.

[14] R. L. Langley, "Snakebite during pregnancy: a literature review," *Wilderness and Environmental Medicine*, vol. 21, no. 1, pp. 54–60, 2010.

[15] M. E. Delgado and O. H. Del Brutto, "Reversible posterior leukoencephalopathy in a venomous snake (*Bothrops asper*) bite victim," *American Journal of Tropical Medicine and Hygiene*, vol. 86, no. 3, pp. 496–498, 2012.

[16] S. C. Chaudhary, K. K. Sawlani, H. S. Malhotra, and J. Singh, "Snake bite-induced leucoencephalopathy," *BMJ Case Reports*, vol. 2013, 2013.

[17] B. Varalaxmi, R. Ram, P. Sandeep, and V. Siva Kumar, "Posterior reversible encephalopathy syndrome in a patient of snake bite," *Journal of Postgraduate Medicine*, vol. 60, no. 1, pp. 89–90, 2014.

[18] J. S. Kaushik, B. Chakrabarty, S. Gulati et al., "Unusual late neurological complication in a child after an Indian krait bite," *Pediatric Neurology*, vol. 51, no. 1, pp. 130–132, 2014.

[19] U. Jongwutiwes, K. Suitharak, S. Tiengrim, and V. Thamlikitkul, "Serum procalcitonin in diagnosis of bacteremia," *Journal of the Medical Association of Thailand*, vol. 29, supplement 2, pp. S79–S87, 2009.

[20] A. Marra, M. Vargas, P. Striano, L. Del Guercio, P. Buonanno, and G. Servillo, "Posterior reversible encephalopathy syndrome: the endothelial hypotheses," *Medical Hypotheses*, vol. 82, no. 5, pp. 619–622, 2014.

[21] A. Chardain, V. Mesnage, S. Alamowitch et al., "Posterior reversible encephalopathy syndrome (PRES) and hypomagnesemia: a frequent association?" *Revue Neurologique*, vol. 172, no. 6-7, pp. 384–388, 2016.

[22] L. C. Porcello Marrone, B. F. Marrone, F. K. Neto et al., "Posterior reversible encephalopathy syndrome following a scorpion sting," *Journal of Neuroimaging*, vol. 23, no. 4, pp. 535–536, 2013.

[23] H. H. Loh and C. H. H. Tan, "Acute renal failure and posterior reversible encephalopathy syndrome following multiple wasp stings: a case report," *Medical Journal of Malaysia*, vol. 67, no. 1, pp. 133–135, 2012.

[24] M. Cozzolino, C. Bianchi, G. Mariani, L. Marchi, M. Fambrini, and F. Mecacci, "Therapy and differential diagnosis of posterior reversible encephalopathy syndrome (PRES) during pregnancy and postpartum," *Archives of Gynecology and Obstetrics*, vol. 292, no. 6, pp. 1217–1223, 2015.

[25] A. M. McKinney, J. Short, C. L. Truwit et al., "Posterior reversible encephalopathy syndrome: incidence of atypical regions of involvement and imaging findings," *American Journal of Roentgenology*, vol. 189, no. 4, pp. 904–912, 2007.

[26] W. S. Bartynski, "Posterior reversible encephalopathy syndrome, part 1: fundamental imaging and clinical features," *American Journal of Neuroradiology*, vol. 29, no. 6, pp. 1036–1042, 2008.

[27] S. Koch, A. Rabinstein, S. Falcone, and A. Forteza, "Diffusion-weighted imaging shows cytotoxic and vasogenic edema in eclampsia," *American Journal of Neuroradiology*, vol. 22, no. 6, pp. 1068–1070, 2001.

[28] R. Loureiro, C. C. Leite, S. Kahhale et al., "Diffusion imaging may predict reversible brain lesions in eclampsia and severe preeclampsia: initial experience," *American Journal of Obstetrics and Gynecology*, vol. 189, no. 5, pp. 1350–1355, 2003.

[29] A. Benziada-Boudour, E. Schmitt, S. Kremer et al., "Posterior reversible encephalopathy syndrome: a case of unusual diffusion-weighted MR images," *Journal of Neuroradiology*, vol. 36, no. 2, pp. 102–105, 2009.

[30] C. J. Stevens and M. K. S. Heran, "The many faces of posterior reversible encephalopathy syndrome," *British Journal of Radiology*, vol. 85, no. 1020, pp. 1566–1575, 2012.

[31] A. Wagih, L. Mohsen, M. M. Rayan, M. M. Hasan, and A. H. Al-Sherif, "Posterior reversible encephalopathy syndrome (PRES): restricted diffusion does not necessarily mean irreversibility," *Polish Journal of Radiology*, vol. 80, no. 1, pp. 210–216, 2015.

[32] A. R. Pande, K. Ando, R. Ishikura et al., "Clinicoradiological factors influencing the reversibility of posterior reversible encephalopathy syndrome: a multicenter study," *Radiation Medicine*, vol. 24, no. 10, pp. 659–668, 2006.

[33] Y. Yano, K. Kario, T. Fukunaga et al., "A case of reversible posterior leukoencephalopathy syndrome caused by transient hypercoagulable state induced by infection," *Hypertension Research*, vol. 28, no. 7, pp. 619–623, 2005.

11

Mercaptopurine Treatment in an Adult Man with Orbital and Intracranial Rosai-Dorfman Disease

Valentina Arnao, Marianna Riolo, Giovanni Savettieri, and Paolo Aridon

Dipartimento di Biomedicina Sperimentale e Neuroscienze Cliniche, Università degli Studi di Palermo, Palermo, Italy

Correspondence should be addressed to Paolo Aridon; paolo.aridon@unipa.it

Academic Editor: Samuel T. Gontkovsky

Background. Rosai-Dorfmann disease (RDD) is a rare, idiopathic non-Langerhans cell histiocytosis, affecting children and young adults, that commonly presents as painless, massive cervical lymphadenopathy with fever, weight loss, and polyclonal hypergammaglobulinemia. Cervical lymphadenopathy and extranodal involvement are the main presentations. On the contrary, ophthalmic involvement and localisation in the central nervous system are rare. *Case Report.* An old man was admitted to our hospital for first seizure. Brain imaging studies revealed on the left an extra-axial thickening of the dura mater with enhancement and perilesional oedema, infiltrating the sphenoorbital fissure and an isointense mass with enhancement in the orbital region with dislocation of the optic nerve. Pathological and immunohistochemistry examination of the bioptical specimen was consistent with a diagnosis of RDD. Treatment with levetiracetam and steroids was started obtaining only remission of seizures. Because of the patient refusal of the surgical debulking, therapy with mercaptopurine was started, stopping disease progression. *Conclusion.* So far, very few cases of extranodal RDD with multiple CNS lesions involving the orbital region have been described. Our case is significant because it is the first case in which the efficacy of mercaptopurine treatment has been documented in an adult patient with isolated ocular and intracranial RDD.

1. Introduction

Rosai-Dorfmann disease (RDD) is a rare idiopathic non-Langerhans cell histiocytosis, of unknown aetiology commonly presenting as painless, massive cervical lymphadenopathy with fever, weight loss, and polyclonal hypergammaglobulinemia. The disease mainly affects children and young adults [1, 2]. Over 90% of patients present with cervical lymphadenopathy. Extranodal involvement occurs in 40% of cases with anatomic distribution that include paranasal sinuses, respiratory tract, skin, nose, and bone. Ophthalmic involvement is seen in 10% of cases [3]. These include eyelid and orbital mass and rarely uveitis. Rosai-Dorfmann disease could mimic lymphoma, histiocytic and lacrimal gland tumours [3–7]. Localisation in the central nervous system (CNS) is rare (4% of cases) [8, 9]. Various treatments have been proposed, including steroid therapy, chemotherapeutic regimens, radiotherapy, surgery, and combinations of the above but optimal treatment has yet to be established.

2. Case Report

A 70-year-old man, with history of hypertension, presented an abrupt onset of tremor and jerking of his right arm and, after two days, he was admitted to our hospital for a critical sudden episode with secondary generalization with loss of consciousness, followed by amnesia about the event. For few months, he has been conscious of reduced vision and foreign body sensation in his left eye. He also complained of dizziness, clumsiness, and paraesthesia in his right arm especially while using little objects and playing the piano. His family history was positive for tumours. When he was five years old, his right eye was enucleated because of an eye infection and, since then, he carries a prosthetic eye. He had a moderate low vision (20/160) in his left eye. Neurological examination showed distal weakness in his right arm. Brain CT scan showed slight hyperdensity in the left frontoparietal region, suggesting a tumour. Brain and orbit MRI revealed in left frontoparietal-temporal region extra-axial thickening of the dura mater with enhancement and perilesional oedema, infiltrating the sphenoorbital fissure, and an isointense mass with enhancement in the orbital region with dislocation of the optic nerve, which was thought to be consistent with a meningioma (Figures 1(a) and 1(b)). EEG shows diffuse slowing with excessive delta and theta activity. Blood examination was normal, except for hyperlipidemia and mild elevation of erythrocyte sedimentation rate. The patient underwent surgery to perform cerebral biopsy. Histopathological evaluation of the surgical piece revealed a fibrotic tissue with a histiocytic reaction and a large number of histiocytes containing normal-appearing lymphocytes within their cytoplasm (emperipolesis). Immunohistochemistry was positive for S-100 protein and CD68 leucocyte antigens and negative for CD1a. According to published criteria, these findings were consistent with a diagnosis of Rosai-Dorfman disease. The patient refused the surgical debulking to salvage his vision. Treatment with levetiracetam (500 mg twice a day) and steroid (Dexamethasone 4 mg intravenously once a day) was started with remission of critical symptoms. MRI features showed a decreased of edema but no modification of the lesions previously reported.

Three months later, a therapy with mercaptopurine was started with a daily dosage of 2,5 mg/kg, and steroid treatment was stopped. One year later, MRI showed slight reduction of the parietal-temporal lesion (Figures 1(c) and 1(d)), and levetiracetam therapy was stopped. At his one-year follow-up appointment, the patient reported no seizure activity without further loss of vision. The third brain MRI, performed approximately two years after diagnosis, showed a further reduction of the parietal-temporal lesion and of the left intra-orbital mass that enhanced uniformly after gadolinium administration (Figures 1(e) and 1(f)).

3. Discussion

Sinus histiocytosis with massive lymphadenopathy was originally described by Rosai and Dorfman in 1969 [1]. This is a rare non-Langerhans histiocytosis of unknown aetiology that usually presents with painless bilateral cervical lymphadenopathy, fever, anemia, leukocytosis, an elevated erythrocyte sedimentation rate, and polyclonal hypergammaglobulinemia. The ophthalmic involvement of Rosai-Dorfman disease include eyelid, orbital, and lacrimal gland manifestations and uveitis. Orbital involvement is the most common of ophthalmic manifestations [3–6]. Recently, also a case of compressive neuropathy of the optic nerve (with consecutive gradual vision loss) due to a RDD mass in ethmoid and sphenoid sinus extending into suprasellar region and causing bone erosion has been described [7].

Involvement of the central nervous system is rare [8, 9] and it occurs generally in middle-aged men (mean 39,4 years) causing headaches, seizure, visual symptoms, and focal deficits [9–12]. Involvement of the spinal cord has also been described [13, 14]. The disease is frequently reported in leptomeninges and it typically presents as a meningioma-like, extra-parenchymal, dural-based mass, similar, on MRI, to meningioma histiocytosis X lymphoproliferative disorders,

plasma cell granulomas, and infectious disease [15, 16]. Nevertheless, there are also cases of isolated CNS presentation without dural involvement [17].

Histological and immunophenotypic assays are useful in establishing the diagnosis. In fact, RDD is characterized by abundant sheets of large and medium sized vacuolated histiocytes in a fibrous stroma, interspersed with foci of chronic inflammatory cells. In addition, the presence of emperipolesis is a hallmark of the disease, even if this may be less marked in intracranial disease [18]. In RDD, the histiocytes typically stain positive for S100 and CD68 and negative for CD1a [18–21]. These features with the absence of eosinophils and Birbeck's granules on electron microscopy make the differential diagnosis with CNS Langerhans Cell Histiocytosis (LCH) possible [18, 22, 23]. Another interesting differential diagnosis is Erdheim-Cester Disease (ECD), which is a rare non-Langerhans histiocytic disorder most commonly characterized by multifocal osteosclerotic lesions of the long bones. Neurologic involvement (mainly periorbital) is seen in 40 to 50 percent of cases. Biopsies of involved tissues are characterized by tissue infiltration by foamy (xanthomatous) histiocytes with interspersed inflammatory cells, multinucleate giant cells (Touton cells), and admixed or surrounding fibrosis. ECD cells express the histiocyte marker CD68, CD163, and Factor XIIIa but unlike Langerhans cell histiocytosis do not express CD1a or S100. Birbeck granules are absent (http://www.uptodate.com/).

In our case, the findings of emperipolesis, positivity for CD68 and S100 and negativity for CD1a were coherent with the diagnosis of RDD.

Most patients experience a course of spontaneous exacerbations and remissions [15]. However, if in 50% of systemic cases the disease will resolve spontaneously, a small percentage of patients (17%) will have asymptomatic persistent adenopathy and some will have residual symptoms for 5 to 10 years after onset [15]. Even if the course of intracranial lesions of RDD is generally considered to be benign, no spontaneous regression has been reported [1, 14]. Rarely intracranial RDD has an aggressive course [14].

Although a variety of treatments have been proposed [11, 13, 24], for the rare primary orbital and intracranial RDD only surgical resection, radical if possible, is considered the optimal treatment [25–27]. When this approach is not possible, according to the literature, roentgen therapy, chemotherapy, steroid therapy [11, 28], rituximab [29], interferon-alfa-2a [30], and immunosuppressive agents, such as azathioprine, methotrexate, and mercaptopurine [31–33], can be used.

Alqanatish et al. described a case of a 7-year-old child with concomitant LES and RDD, who was treated with rutiximab (500 mg/m^2/dose), with complete remission of the massive lymphadenopathy after 7 weeks of treatment [29]. Also high dose of interferon-alfa-2a, in particular, the pegylated form, has shown dramatic efficacy in cases of systemic RDD [30]. Nevertheless, it should be avoided because it could favour the occurrence of seizures [31]. Other options include immunosuppressive agents, such as azathioprine. Le Guenno et al. described a 57-year-old man with a history of diseases that involve the monocyte/macrophage system (Q fever and Crohn disease) who developed also RDD and was

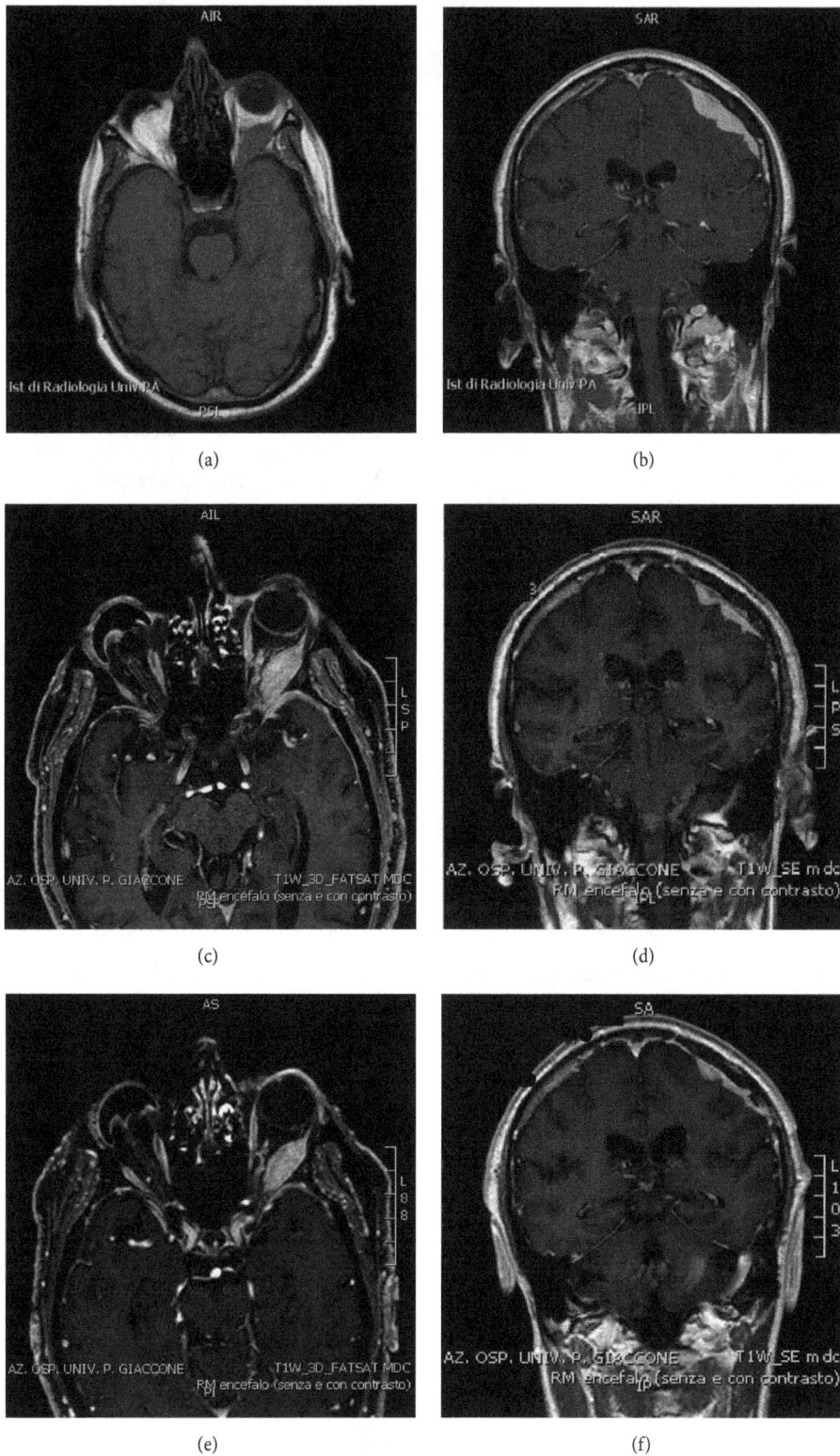

FIGURE 1: Axial (a, c, e) and coronal (b, d, f) enhanced T1 MR images reveal enhancing masses along the left frontoparietal-temporal region and the orbital region with dislocation of the optic nerve at onset (a, b) and in one-year (c, d) and two-year (e, f) follow-up, respectively.

successfully treated with azathioprine [32]. Moreover, two children showed a sustained response to a combination of methotrexate and mercaptopurine [33, 34]. Another two paediatric cases with nonintracranial involvement showed a good response to chemotherapy with vinblastine, prednisone, 6-mercaptopurine and methotrexate [35], and 2-chlorodeoxyadenosine (2-CdA, cladribine) [36].

Like a minority of patients with concurrent orbital and neurological manifestations as the sole extranodal site of involvement without synchronous nodal disease, surgery could have represented the best therapy for our patient; unfortunately, he refused this option. Therefore, considering the failure of conventional approach with steroid therapy, a treatment with mercaptopurine was started. This is a purine antagonist, which inhibits DNA and RNA synthesis acting as a false metabolite. The treatment caused a stabilization of the lesions and after 24 months, no adverse event has been reported including anemia, granulocytopenia, haemorrhage, lymphocytopenia, and leukopenia. Although spontaneous remissions are not uncommon and surgical resection appears to be the most efficacious approach, therapy with mercaptopurine in our patient led to stopping of the disease progression. To our knowledge, considering that the other reported cases are paediatric [33–36], this is the first reported case of an adult patient with isolated ocular and intracranial RDD in which the efficacy of mercaptopurine treatment has been documented. In this way, our case supports the use of purine antagonists and purine antimetabolite for an efficacious treatment of adult forms of RDD.

Competing Interests

The authors declare that there is no conflict of interests regarding the publication of this paper.

References

[1] J. Rosai and R. F. Dorfman, "Sinus histiocytosis with massive lymphadenopathy. A newly recognized benign clinicopathological entity," *Archives of Pathology*, vol. 87, no. 1, pp. 63–70, 1969.

[2] E. Foucar, J. Rosai, and R. Dorfman, "Sinus histiocytosis with massive lymphadenopathy (Rosai-Dorfman disease): review of the entity," *Seminars in Diagnostic Pathology*, vol. 7, no. 1, pp. 19–73, 1990.

[3] E. Foucar, J. Rosai, and R. F. Dorfman, "The ophthalmologic manifestations of sinus histiocytosis with massive lymphadenopathy," *American Journal of Ophthalmology*, vol. 87, no. 3, pp. 354–367, 1979.

[4] M. Lee-Wing, A. Oryschak, G. Attariwala, and M. Ashenhurst, "Rosai-Dorfman disease presenting as bilateral lacrimal gland enlargement," *American Journal of Ophthalmology*, vol. 131, no. 5, pp. 677–678, 2001.

[5] R. C. S. de Oliveira, M. Rigueiro, A. C. Vieira, D. De Freitas, and E. Sato, "Rosai-dorfman disease manifesting as an epibulbar ocular tumour," *Clinical and Experimental Ophthalmology*, vol. 39, no. 2, pp. 175–177, 2011.

[6] T. L. Vermeulen, T. W. Isaacs, D. Spagnolo, and B. Amanuel, "Rosai-Dorfman disease presenting as choroidal melanoma: a case report and review of the literature," *Graefe's Archive for Clinical and Experimental Ophthalmology*, vol. 251, no. 1, pp. 295–299, 2013.

[7] E. Shukla, A. Nicholson, A. Agrawal, and D. Rathod, "Extra nodal rosai–dorfman disease (Sinus Histiocytosis with Massive Lymphadenopathy) presenting as asymmetric bilateral optic atrophy," *Head and Neck Pathology*, vol. 10, no. 3, pp. 414–417, 2016.

[8] Md. Taufiq, A. Khair, F. Begum, S. Akhter, M. Shamim Farooq, and M. Kamal, "Isolated intracranial rosai-dorfman disease," *Case Reports in Neurological Medicine*, vol. 2016, Article ID 1972594, 4 pages, 2016.

[9] J. D. Sandoval-Sus, A. C. Sandoval-Leon, J. R. Chapman et al., "Rosai-dorfman disease of the central nervous system: report of 6 cases and review of the literature," *Medicine*, vol. 93, no. 3, pp. 165–175, 2014.

[10] A. O. Adeleye, G. Amir, S. Fraifeld, Y. Shoshan, F. Umansky, and S. Spektor, "Diagnosis and management of rosai-dorfman disease involving the central nervous system," *Neurological Research*, vol. 32, no. 6, pp. 572–578, 2010.

[11] C. M. McPherson, J. Brown, A. W. Kim, and F. DeMonte, "Regression of intracranial Rosai-Dorfman disease following corticosteroid therapy: case report," *Journal of Neurosurgery*, vol. 104, no. 5, pp. 840–844, 2006.

[12] M. B. Bhattacharjee, S. J. Wroe, B. N. Harding, and M. Powell, "Sinus histiocytosis with massive lymphadenopathy-isolated suprasellar involvement," *Journal of Neurology Neurosurgery and Psychiatry*, vol. 55, no. 2, pp. 156–158, 1992.

[13] D. P. Kidd, T. Revesz, and N. R. Miller, "Rosai-Dorfman disease presenting with widespread intracranial and spinal cord involvement," *Neurology*, vol. 67, no. 9, pp. 1551–1555, 2006.

[14] A. A. Ramos, M. A. Alvarez Vega, J. V. D. Alles, M. J. Antuña Garcia, and A. Meilán Martínez, "Multiple involvement of the central nervous system in Rosai-Dorfman disease," *Pediatric Neurology*, vol. 46, no. 1, pp. 54–56, 2012.

[15] A. Petzold, M. Thom, M. Powell, and G. T. Plant, "Relapsing intracranial rosai-dorfman disease," *Journal of Neurology Neurosurgery and Psychiatry*, vol. 71, no. 4, pp. 538–541, 2001.

[16] N. Ghosal, G. Murthy, K. Visvanathan, M. Sridhar, and A. S. Hegde, "Isolated intracranial Rosai Dorfman disease masquerading as meningioma: a case report," *Indian Journal of Pathology and Microbiology*, vol. 50, no. 2, pp. 382–384, 2007.

[17] C. S. Hong, R. M. Starke, M. A. Hays, J. W. Mandell, D. Schiff, and A. R. Asthagiri, "Redefining the prevalence of dural involvement in rosai-dorfman disease of the central nervous system," *World Neurosurgery*, vol. 90, pp. 702.e13–702.e20, 2016.

[18] R. N. Eisen, P. J. Buckley, and J. Rosai, "Immunophenotypic characterization of sinus histiocytosis with massive lymphadenopathy (Rosai-Dorfman disease)," *Seminars in Diagnostic Pathology*, vol. 7, no. 1, pp. 74–82, 1990.

[19] R. Kitai, J. Liena, A. Hirano, K. Ido, K. Sato, and T. Kubota, "Meningeal Rosai-Dorfman disease: report of three cases and literature review," *Brain Tumor Pathology*, vol. 18, no. 1, pp. 49–54, 2001.

[20] P. Lopez and M. L. Estes, "Immunohistochemical characterization of the histiocytes in sinus histiocytosis with massive lymphadenopathy: analysis of an extranodal case," *Human Pathology*, vol. 20, no. 7, pp. 711–715, 1989.

[21] M. Paulli, R. Rosso, S. Kindl et al., "Immunophenotypic characterization of the cell infiltrate in five cases of sinus histiocytosis with massive lymphadenopathy (Rosai-Dorfman disease)," *Human Pathology*, vol. 23, no. 6, pp. 647–654, 1992.

[22] M. Onciu, "Histiocytic proliferations in childhood," *American Journal of Clinical Pathology*, vol. 122, pp. S128–S136, 2004.

[23] W. H. McAlister, T. Herman, and L. P. Dehner, "Sinus histiocytosis with massive lymphadenopathy (Rosai-Dorfman disease)," *Pediatric Radiology*, vol. 20, no. 6, pp. 425–432, 1990.

[24] A. Pulsoni, G. Anghel, P. Falcucci et al., "Treatment of sinus histiocytosis with massive lymphadenopathy (Rosai-Dorfman disease): report of a case and literature review," *American Journal of Hematology*, vol. 69, no. 1, pp. 67–71, 2002.

[25] D. K. Resnick, B. L. Johnson, and T. J. Lovely, "Rosai-Dorfman disease presenting with multiple orbital and intracranial masses," *Acta Neuropathologica*, vol. 91, no. 5, pp. 554–557, 1996.

[26] A. J. Scumpia, J.-A. Frederic, A. J. Cohen, M. Bania, A. Hameed, and P. Q. Xiao, "Isolated intracranial Rosai-Dorfman disease with orbital extension," *Journal of Clinical Neuroscience*, vol. 16, no. 8, pp. 1108–1109, 2009.

[27] A. Hinduja, L. G. Aguilar, T. Steineke, D. Nochlin, and J. C. Landolfi, "Rosai-Dorfman disease manifesting as intracranial and intraorbital lesion," *Journal of Neuro-Oncology*, vol. 92, no. 1, pp. 117–120, 2009.

[28] S. S. Deodhare, L. C. Ang, and J. M. Bilbao, "Isolated intracranial involvement in Rosai-Dorfman disease: a report of two cases and review of the literature," *Archives of Pathology and Laboratory Medicine*, vol. 122, no. 2, pp. 161–165, 1998.

[29] J. T. Alqanatish, K. Houghton, M. Bond, C. Senger, and L. B. Tucker, "Rituximab treatment in a child with Rosai-Dorfman disease and systemic lupus erythematosus," *Journal of Rheumatology*, vol. 37, no. 8, pp. 1783–1784, 2010.

[30] G. Le Guenno, L. Galicier, C. Fieschi, V. Meignin, A. Chabrol, and E. Oksenhendler, "Dramatic efficiency of pegylated interferon in sinus histiocytosis with massive lymphadenopathy," *British Journal of Dermatology*, vol. 164, no. 1, pp. 213–215, 2011.

[31] F. Ahmed, I. M. Jacobson, J. L. Herrera et al., "Seizures during pegylated interferon and ribavirin therapy for chronic hepatitis C: observations from the WIN-R trial," *Journal of Clinical Gastroenterology*, vol. 45, no. 3, pp. 286–292, 2011.

[32] G. Le Guenno, L. Galicier, E. Uro-Coste, V. Petitcolin, V. Rieu, and M. Ruivard, "Successful treatment with azathioprine of relapsing Rosai-Dorfman disease of the central nervous system: case report," *Journal of Neurosurgery*, vol. 117, no. 3, pp. 486–489, 2012.

[33] G. Horneff, H. Jürgens, W. Hort, D. Karitzky, and U. Göbel, "Sinushistiocytosis with massive lymphadenopathy (Rosai-Dorfman disease): response to methotrexate and mercaptopurine," *Medical and Pediatric Oncology*, vol. 27, no. 3, pp. 187–192, 1996.

[34] Y. Jabali, V. Smrcka, and J. Pradna, "Rosai-Dorfman disease: successful long-term results by combination chemotherapy with prednisone, 6-mercaptopurine, methotrexate, and vinblastine: a case report," *International Journal of Surgical Pathology*, vol. 13, no. 3, pp. 285–289, 2005.

[35] S. Ambati, G. Chamyan, R. Restrepo et al., "Rosai-Dorfman disease following bone marrow transplantation for pre-B cell acute lymphoblastic leukemia," *Pediatric Blood and Cancer*, vol. 51, no. 3, pp. 433–435, 2008.

[36] M. Tasso, C. Esquembre, E. Blanco, C. Moscardó, M. Niveiro, and A. Payá, "Sinus histiocytosis with massive lymphadenopathy (Rosai-Dorfman disease) treated with 2-chlorodeoxyadenosine," *Pediatric Blood and Cancer*, vol. 47, no. 5, pp. 612–615, 2006.

12

Hemifacial Pain and Hemisensory Disturbance Referred from Occipital Neuralgia Caused by Pathological Vascular Contact of the Greater Occipital Nerve

Byung-chul Son[1,2] and Jin-gyu Choi[1]

[1]Department of Neurosurgery, Seoul St. Mary's Hospital College of Medicine, The Catholic University of Korea, Seoul, Republic of Korea
[2]Catholic Neuroscience Institute, College of Medicine, The Catholic University of Korea, Seoul, Republic of Korea

Correspondence should be addressed to Byung-chul Son; sbc@catholic.ac.kr

Academic Editor: Shahid Nimjee

Here we report a unique case of chronic occipital neuralgia caused by pathological vascular contact of the left greater occipital nerve. After 12 months of left-sided, unremitting occipital neuralgia, a hypesthesia and facial pain developed in the left hemiface. The decompression of the left greater occipital nerve from pathological contacts with the occipital artery resulted in immediate relief for hemifacial sensory change and facial pain, as well as chronic occipital neuralgia. Although referral of pain from the stimulation of occipital and cervical structures innervated by upper cervical nerves to the frontal head of V1 trigeminal distribution has been reported, the development of hemifacial sensory change associated with referred trigeminal pain from chronic occipital neuralgia is extremely rare. Chronic continuous and strong afferent input of occipital neuralgia caused by pathological vascular contact with the greater occipital nerve seemed to be associated with sensitization and hypersensitivity of the second-order neurons in the trigeminocervical complex, a population of neurons in the C2 dorsal horn characterized by receiving convergent input from dural and cervical structures.

1. Introduction

It is well known that patients with primary headaches often report pain not only involving the frontal head innervated by the first (ophthalmic) division of the trigeminal nerve, but also involving the occipital region innervated by the greater occipital nerve (GON), a branch of the C2 spinal root [1–3]. Likewise, stimulation of structures in the neck innervated by upper cervical roots in humans such as infratentorial dura mater, vessels, and tumors of the posterior fossa can lead to pain in the front of the head [4–7]. Trigeminocervical complex (TCC) is a population of neurons in the C2 dorsal horn characterized by receiving convergent input from dural and cervical structures [3]. These neurons show properties typical of dura-sensitive trigeminal neurons with a convergent input from the facial skin corresponding to the dermatome of the ophthalmic division of the trigeminal nerve [3, 8, 9]. This convergence of nociceptive afferents and sensitization of TCC neurons have clinical correlates such as hypersensitivity and the spread and referral of pain frequently seen in patients with primary headaches such as migraines.

Clinical evidence of referred pain in the frontal head with involvement of the TCC from cervical lesions has been reported in cases of posterior fossa tumors, stimulation of the infratentorial dura mater, direct stimulation of cervical roots, vertebral artery dissection, and stimulation of subcutaneous tissue innervated by the GON [3, 9]. However, the development of hemifacial sensory change associated with referred trigeminal pain from occipital neuralgia is extremely rare. We report a case of hemifacial sensory change associated with referred trigeminal pain from chronic occipital neuralgia. Furthermore, occipital neuralgia was found to be caused by

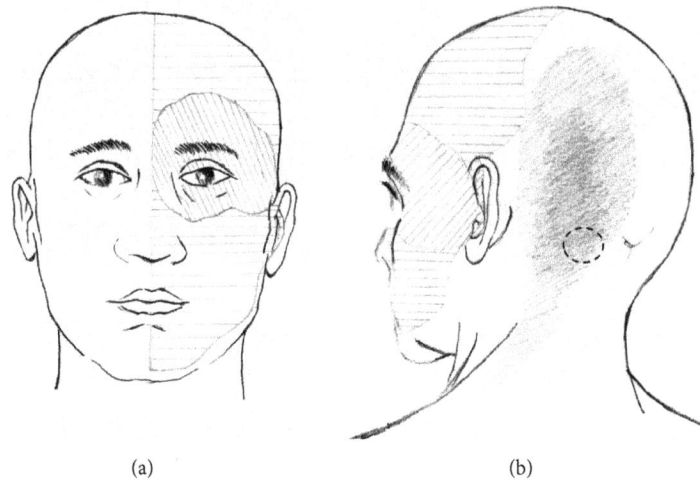

FIGURE 1: A schematic diagram demonstrating the distribution of occipital neuralgia and hemifacial sensory change with facial pain. (a) The grey areas over the left occipital area indicate the distribution of stabbing pain of occipital neuralgia. A tender point was present along the course of the greater occipital nerve. (b) The obliquely hatched area denotes regions of facial pain in addition to hypesthesia. The horizontally hatched area shows the distribution of hemifacial hypesthesia and paresthesia.

pathological vascular contact with the GON. Decompression of the GON immediately resulted in the disappearance of hemisensory deficit and hemifacial pain.

2. Case Presentation

A 53-year-old female with a 16-month history of chronic stabbing pain along the distribution of the left GON presented with a left-sided facial pain with 4 months of duration. A severe aching pain and tenderness over the left occipital area were associated during initial development of left occipital pain 16 months ago. There was no precipitating event before the onset of left occipital neuralgia. The onset was described as rather sudden. The pain was described as mainly stabbing and electric in nature with moderate severity (4–6/10 on numerical rating scale (NRS) ranging from 0 to 10). It was not aggravated with neck motion. Daily activity did not influence the continuous occipital pain. Her medical history was unremarkable, including diabetes and gout. Under the impression of occipital neuralgia, she had been treated with several nonsteroidal anti-inflammatory drugs, including tramadol (150 mg/day), carbamazepine (400 mg/day), and pregabalin (225 mg/day), with some degree of relief. Pain was so agonizing that treatment of repeated occipital nerve blocks on a regular schedule of a month for a year was given. The occipital nerve block over the tender point along the course of the GON was quite effective for the initial two injections. However, its effect lasted 3 hours thereafter.

Four months prior to presentation, an aching pain developed insidiously in the left orbit, cheek, temple, and left ear canal. Subsequently, paresthesia and numbness progressively developed in her left hemiface. Despite the development of left hemifacial pain and sensory disturbance, left occipital neuralgia was not aggravated. It remained present as it had been for the prior 16 months. Considering the chronic nature

of left occipital neuralgia with superimposed occurrence of hemifacial pain and sensory changes, she was referred to us for further evaluation of the trigeminal and occipital pain.

Upon examination, her left occipital pain was typically that of occipital neuralgia fulfilling the criteria of International Classification of Headache Disorders (ICHD) [10]. The stabbing occipital pain was present throughout the day with intermittent aggravation. It was present over the distribution of the left GON (Figure 1(a)). The tenderness which was severe at the onset was mild in our examination. Hemifacial pain was most severe in the left periorbital and temple. It was aching in nature. A moderate degree of hypesthesia to light touch, increased sensitivity to pinprick, and paresthesia were observed in her right face (V1, V2, and V3) (Figure 1(b)). However, no pain or hypesthesia was observed in the intraoral structures, including the buccal mucosa and the tongue. Corneal sensation was preserved. No allodynia was detected in the hypoesthetic left face. There was no tinnitus, visual disturbance, or lacrimation associated with the hemifacial pain. Repeated blocks with 1% lidocaine (3 mL) over the occipital tender point were effective for approximately 2 hours in relieving occipital neuralgia. However, the left-sided hemifacial pain and sensory disturbance were not influenced by the block.

Laboratory examinations were normal, including erythrocyte sedimentation rate and C-reactive protein, antinuclear antibody, and anti-DS-DNA. Cerebrospinal fluid examination was also normal. Pathological lesion to explain the left occipital and trigeminal pain was not observed in the enhanced MRI of the brain and cervical spine. Considering chronicity and medical intractability, exploration of the left GON was proposed. An approximately 8 cm sized hockey stick shaped incision and subcutaneous flap were elevated from the midline to identify the course of the GON. No entrapment of the GON was found in its course in the

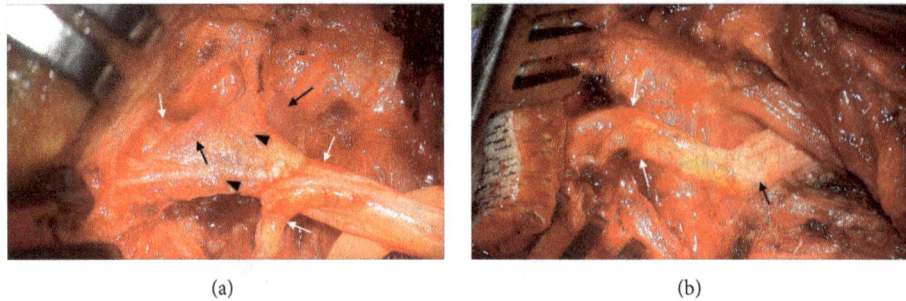

FIGURE 2: Intraoperative photographs during the decompression of the greater occipital nerve. (a) An intraoperative photograph showing adhesions of the greater occipital nerve *(white arrows)* with the connective tissue *(black arrow heads)* and occipital arteries *(black arrows)*. (b) An intraoperative photograph after decompression of the left greater occipital nerve. A reddish deformation is apparent in the compressed portion *(white arrows)* with pathological vascular contact compared to the normal proximal course *(black arrow)* of the greater occipital nerve.

trapezius or semispinalis capitis. Upon dissection along the distal course of the GON, a severe adhesion to the surrounding connective tissue and entrapment of the GON between tributaries of the occipital artery were encountered (Figure 2(a)). The occipital artery and veins were dissected and cut. The connective tissue adhesion around the GON was released to decompress the GON (Figure 2(b)). Immediately after the decompression of the GON, chronic stabbing pain of the occipital neuralgia and the left hemifacial pain as well as a sensory disturbance completely disappeared. Hypesthesia and paresthesia, aching hemifacial pain, and occipital neuralgia did not recur at 12 months of follow-up.

3. Discussion

3.1. Clinical Examples of V1 Trigeminal Pain Referred from Cervical Pathology. We present a rare case of neurological deficit in addition to typical referred pain to ipsilateral V1 trigeminal pain from chronic occipital neuralgia. It is extremely difficult to find a case in the literature describing the development of hemifacial hypesthesia associated with referred facial pain from cervical pathology. Of particular interest with regard to our case is the occurrence of cluster headaches, a rare form of primary headache marked by unilateral excruciating pain in association with autonomic features, associated with an ipsilateral vertebral artery aneurysm [11] and vertebral artery dissection [12]. The secondary cluster headache from a vertebral artery aneurysm was resolved when the aneurysm was clipped [11] or treated with sumatriptan (6 mg subcutaneously) [12]. These findings provided clinical affirmation of the existence of trigeminal/cervical convergence and hypersensitivity.

3.2. Trigeminocervical Complex as a Substrate of Convergence and Hypersensitivity. The upper cervical spinal roots can contribute to sensory innervation of cranial and cervical structures. Occipital and suboccipital structures such as vessels, the dura mater of the posterior fossa, deep paraspinal neck muscle, and zygapophyseal joints are recognized as sources of head and neck pain [1, 9, 13]. Nociceptive inflow

from these suboccipital structures is mediated by small-diameter afferent fibers in the upper cervical roots terminating from the C2 segment up to the medullary dorsal horn [9, 14, 15]. The major afferent contribution is mediated by the spinal root C2 peripherally represented by the GON [9, 16]. An anatomical overlap of the trigeminal and cervical afferents through the TCC from the level of the caudal trigeminal nucleus to at least the C2 segment has already been suggested [17]. Furthermore, an electrophysiological study [3] has described the convergence of dural afferents and cervical afferents in the GON on neurons in the TCC, with subsequent sensitization of dural input by stimulation of the GON, suggesting a neural mechanism of hypersensitivity, spread, and referral form structures of the upper cervical spine in the trigeminal domain [9].

Sensitization of the central nociceptive neurons in the TCC takes place in response to strong dural noxious inputs seen in secondary headache syndromes such as meningitis, subarachnoid hemorrhage, and experimental headaches [9]. Sensitization of these second-order neurons in the TCC could be explained by the following mechanisms: an increased afferent inflow from the periphery or central pain-modulatory influences can actively facilitate or disinhibit afferent inflow into the TCC. Occipital neuralgia in the case described herein caused by continuous vascular contact and compression could be a typical example of increased peripheral afferent inflow which resulted in the sensitization of central nociceptive neurons. The clinical correlates of this hypersensitivity include the development of spontaneous pain, hyperalgesia, and allodynia [18, 19]. In line with this, spontaneous pain and hyperalgesia to pinprick in addition to hemifacial hypesthesia were noted in the current case.

An occurrence of hemifacial hypesthesia not confined to V1 trigeminal distribution was observed in this case. This type of extension of a sensory deficit has been described in complex regional pain syndrome (CRPS) [20, 21]. Sensory deficit in patients with CRPS frequently extends past the painful area of the affected limb [20]. Increased frequency of mechanical allodynia and movement disorders in patients with hemisensory impairment or sensory deficits in the upper quadrant of the body may indicate central mechanisms. For example, functional alterations in the central processing of noxious stimuli are involved in the pathogenesis of an extension of the sensory deficit [20]. It is now well established that pain-modulating circuits in the brain stem such as the ventrolateral division of the periaqueductal grey (PAG), nucleus raphe magnus, and the rostroventral medulla are closely involved in the promotion of central sensitization and secondary hyperalgesia [10, 22]. The dynamic plasticity of descending pain-modulating pathways after peripheral nerve injury or continuous strong noxious inflow can lead to neuropathic pain and render the system vulnerable, resulting in pathological consequences [22].

3.3. Vascular Contact as a Cause of Occipital Neuralgia. While occipital neuralgia is mostly considered idiopathic, specific causes of occipital neuralgia should be excluded from individual cases [23–36]. The etiology in the present case is indeed the same as that reported by Cornely et al. [36], in which the GON was entrapped by pathological contact with the occipital artery. In their report, a 66-year-old woman with severe right-sided occipital neuralgia showed a severe tenderness over the trunk of the right GON with a strong pulsation of the occipital artery branch. We speculate that multiple and repeated injections of local anesthetics and steroids over the tender point during the past 16 months prior to presentation might have resulted in adhesion of connective tissues around the injection points around the pathological arterial contacts. Decompression and neurolysis with the removal of pathological arterial contacts led to immediate and complete relief of the referred hemifacial pain and chronic occipital neuralgia with immediate restoration of hemifacial sensory loss. Therefore, the contact between the GON and the occipital vessels was confirmed as the etiology of chronic occipital neuralgia with referred trigeminal pain and hemifacial sensory loss in this case.

4. Conclusion

An occurrence of hemifacial sensory disturbance associated with referred pain of trigeminal distribution from chronic occipital neuralgia due to pathological vascular contact of the greater occipital nerve is reported here. The present case may indicate that disturbance of sensory processing in higher central structures such as the thalamus may occur in addition to sensitization and hypersensitivity of the second-order neurons in the trigeminocervical complex, a population of neurons in C2 dorsal horn characterized by receiving convergent input from dural and cervical structures.

Competing Interests

The authors declare no conflict of interests regarding this manuscript and that this manuscript has not been previously published in whole or in part or submitted elsewhere for review.

References

[1] M. Anthony, "Headache and the greater occipital nerve," *Clinical Neurology and Neurosurgery*, vol. 94, no. 4, pp. 297–300, 1992.

[2] P. J. Goadsby, "The pathophysiology of headache," in *Wolff's Headache and Other Head Pain*, S. D. Silverstein, R. B. Lipton, and D. J. Dalessio, Eds., pp. 57–72, Oxford University Press, Oxford, UK, 7th edition, 2001.

[3] T. Bartsch and P. J. Goadsby, "Stimulation of the greater occipital nerve induces increased central excitability of dural afferent input," *Brain*, vol. 125, no. 7, pp. 1496–1509, 2002.

[4] H. G. Wolff, *Headache and Other Head Pain*, Oxford University Press, New York, NY, USA, 1948.

[5] B. S. Ray, "Experimental studies on headache," *Archives of Surgery*, vol. 41, no. 4, pp. 813–856, 1940.

[6] F. W. Kerr, "A mechanism to account for frontal headache in cases of posterior fossa tumours," *Journal of Neurosurgery*, vol. 18, pp. 605–609, 1961.

[7] E. J. Piovesan, P. A. Kowacs, C. E. Tatsui, M. C. Lange, L. C. Ribas, and L. C. Werneck, "Referred pain after painful stimulation of the greater occipital nerve in humans: evidence of convergence of cervical afferences on trigeminal nuclei," *Cephalalgia*, vol. 21, no. 2, pp. 107–109, 2001.

[8] P. J. Goadsby and K. L. Hoskin, "The distribution of trigeminovascular afferents in the nonhuman primate brain *Macaca nemestrina*: a c-fos immunocytochemical study," *Journal of Anatomy*, vol. 190, no. 3, pp. 367–375, 1997.

[9] T. Bartsch and P. J. Goadsby, "The trigeminocervical complex and migraine: current concepts and synthesis," *Current Pain and Headache Reports*, vol. 7, no. 5, pp. 371–376, 2003.

[10] Headache Classification Committee of the International Headache Society, "The International Classification of Headache Disorders, 3rd edition (beta version)," *Cephalalgia*, vol. 33, no. 9, pp. 629–808, 2013.

[11] P. West and D. Todman, "Chronic cluster headache associated with a vertebral artery aneurysm," *Headache*, vol. 31, no. 4, pp. 210–212, 1991.

[12] P. D. Cremer, G. M. Halmagyi, and P. J. Goadsby, "Secondary cluster headache responsive to sumatriptan," *Journal of Neurology, Neurosurgery & Psychiatry*, vol. 59, no. 6, pp. 633–634, 1995.

[13] N. Bogduk, "Cervicogenic headache: anatomic basis and pathophysiologic mechanisms," *Current Pain and Headache Reports*, vol. 5, no. 4, pp. 382–386, 2001.

[14] D. A. Bakker, F. J. R. Richmond, and V. C. Abrahams, "Central projections from cat suboccipital muscles: A Study Using Transganglionic Transport of Horseradish Peroxidase," *Journal of Comparative Neurology*, vol. 228, no. 3, pp. 409–421, 1984.

[15] P. J. Goadsby, Y. E. Knight, and K. L. Hoskin, "Stimulation of the greater occipital nerve increases metabolic activity in the trigeminal nucleus caudalis and cervical dorsal horn of the cat," *Pain*, vol. 73, no. 1, pp. 23–28, 1997.

[16] S. Scheurer, J. Gottschall, and V. Groh, "Afferent projections of the rat major occipital nerve studied by transganglionic tansport of HRP," *Anatomy and Embryology*, vol. 167, no. 3, pp. 425–438, 1983.

[17] F. W. L. Kerr, "Central relationships of trigeminal and cervical primary afferents in the spinal cord and medulla," *Brain Research*, vol. 43, no. 2, pp. 561–572, 1972.

[18] S. B. McMahon, G. R. Lewin, and P. D. Wall, "Central hyperexcitability triggered by noxious inputs," *Current Opinion in Neurobiology*, vol. 3, no. 4, pp. 602–610, 1993.

[19] M. Koltzenburg, "Neural mechanisms of cutaneous nociceptive pain," *Clinical Journal of Pain*, vol. 16, no. 3, pp. S131–S138, 2000.

[20] O. Rommel, M. Gehling, R. Dertwinkel et al., "Hemisensory impairment in patients with complex regional pain syndrome," *Pain*, vol. 80, no. 1-2, pp. 95–101, 1999.

[21] B. C. Son, M. C. Kim, D. E. Moon, and J. K. Kang, "Motor cortex stimulation in a patient with intractable complex regional pain syndrome Type II with hemibody involvement: case report," *Journal of Neurosurgery*, vol. 98, no. 1, pp. 175–179, 2003.

[22] K. Ren and R. Dubner, "Descending modulation in persistent pain: an update," *Pain*, vol. 100, no. 1-2, pp. 1–6, 2002.

[23] P. Vanelderen, A. Lataster, R. Levy, N. Mekhail, M. van Kleef, and J. van Zundert, "Occipital neuralgia," *Pain Practice*, vol. 10, no. 2, pp. 137–144, 2010.

[24] S. R. Hammond and G. Danta, "Occipital neuralgia," *Clinical and experimental neurology*, vol. 15, pp. 258–270, 1978.

[25] C. E. Poletti and W. H. Sweet, "Entrapment of the C2 root and ganglion by the atlanto-epistrophic ligament: clinical syndrome and surgical anatomy," *Neurosurgery*, vol. 27, no. 2, pp. 288–291, 1990.

[26] G. Ehni and B. Benner, "Occipital neuralgia and the C1-2 arthrosis syndrome," *Journal of Neurosurgery*, vol. 61, no. 5, pp. 961–965, 1984.

[27] P. Nikakis, G. Koutsis, C. Potagas, D. Mandellos, and C. Sfagos, "Occipital neuralgia as an isolated symptom of C2 myelitis," *Headache*, vol. 46, no. 8, pp. 1304–1306, 2006.

[28] G. Bruti, C. Mostardini, A. Pierallini, V. Villani, C. Modini, and R. Cerbo, "Neurovascular headache and occipital neuralgia secondary to bleeding of bulbocervical cavernoma," *Cephalalgia*, vol. 27, no. 9, pp. 1074–1079, 2007.

[29] P. Cerrato, M. Bergui, D. Imperiale et al., "Occipital neuralgia as isolated symptom of an upper cervical cavernous angioma," *Journal of Neurology*, vol. 249, no. 10, pp. 1464–1465, 2002.

[30] A. Hashiguchi, C. Mimata, H. Ichimura, and J.-I. Kuratsu, "Occipital neuralgia as a presenting symptom of cervicomedullary dural arteriovenous fistula," *Headache*, vol. 47, no. 7, pp. 1095–1097, 2007.

[31] I. Garza, "Craniocervical junction schwannoma mimicking occipital neuralgia," *Headache*, vol. 47, no. 8, pp. 1204–1205, 2007.

[32] R. R. Sharma, H. C. Parekh, S. Prabhu, N. T. Gurusinghe, and G. Bertolis, "Compression of the C-2 root by a rare anomalous ectatic vertebral artery: case report," *Journal of Neurosurgery*, vol. 78, no. 4, pp. 669–672, 1993.

[33] J. B. White, P. P. Atkinson, H. J. Cloft, and J. L. D. Atkinson, "Vascular compression as a potential cause of occipital neuralgia: a case report," *Cephalalgia*, vol. 28, no. 1, pp. 78–82, 2008.

[34] O. Gille, B. Lavignolle, and J.-M. Vital, "Surgical treatment of greater occipital neuralgia by neurolysis of the greater occipital nerve and sectioning of the inferior oblique muscle," *Spine*, vol. 29, no. 7, pp. 828–832, 2004.

[35] B.-C. Son, D.-R. Kim, and S.-W. Lee, "Intractable occipital neuralgia caused by an entrapment in the semispinalis capitis," *Journal of Korean Neurosurgical Society*, vol. 54, no. 3, pp. 268–271, 2013.

[36] C. Cornely, M. Fischer, G. Ingianni, and S. Isenmann, "Greater occipital nerve neuralgia caused by pathological arterial contact: treatment by surgical decompression," *Headache*, vol. 51, no. 4, pp. 609–612, 2011.

13

Impact of Methamphetamine Abuse: A Rare Case of Rapid Cerebral Aneurysm Growth

James Fowler,[1] **Brian Fiani** ⓘ**,**[1] **Syed A. Quadri** ⓘ**,**[1,2] **Vladimir Cortez,**[1]
Mudassir Frooqui,[2] **Atif Zafar** ⓘ**,**[2] **Fahad Shabbir Ahmed,**[3] **Asad Ikram,**[2]
Anirudh Ramachandran,[4] **and Javed Siddiqi**[1]

[1]*Department of Neurosurgery, Desert Regional Medical Center, Palm Springs, CA, USA*
[2]*Department of Neurology, University of New Mexico, Albuquerque, NM, USA*
[3]*Department of Pathology, Yale School of Medicine, New Haven, CT, USA*
[4]*College of Osteopathic Medicine of the Pacific, Western University of Health Sciences, Pomona, CA, USA*

Correspondence should be addressed to Brian Fiani; bfiani@outlook.com

Academic Editor: Isabella Laura Simone

Methamphetamine or "meth" is a sympathomimetic amine of the amphetamine-type substances (ATS) class with an extremely high potential for abuse. Illicitly abused neurostimulants like cocaine and meth predispose patients to the aneurysmal formation with reported rupture at a younger age and in much smaller sized aneurysms. However, very rapid growth of aneurysm within less than 2 weeks with methamphetamine abuse is very rarely observed or reported. In this report, we present a patient with repeated and recurrent meth abuse who demonstrated rapid growth of a pericallosal aneurysm over the period of less than two weeks. The pathophysiology of stroke related to meth and ATS abuse is multifactorial with hypertension, tachycardia, and vascular disease postulated as major mechanisms. The rapid growth of an aneurysm has a high risk of aneurysmal rupture and SAH, which is a neurosurgical emergency and therefore warrants careful consideration and close monitoring. This case confirms the dynamic temporal effects of methamphetamine use on intracranial vessels and this specific neurostimulants association to rapid aneurysmal formation. In light of vascular pathologies the possibility of drug-induced pseudoaneurysm should also be considered in young patients with history of meth abuse.

1. Introduction

Methamphetamine, commonly known as "meth", is a sympathomimetic amine of the amphetamine-type substances (ATS) class with an extremely high potential for abuse [1]. This abuse potential comes from side effects like euphoria, hallucination, central nervous system (CNS) stimulation, and anorexia. Excess use of meth has been implicated in the formation of renal and splanchnic artery aneurysms [2] and may cause myocardial infarction or stroke [3, 4]. Neurostimulants like cocaine and meth predispose patients to the aneurysmal formation with reported rupture at an earlier age and in much smaller sized aneurysms [4–7]

In this report, we present a patient with repeated and recurrent meth abuse who demonstrated rapid growth of a pericallosal aneurysm over the period of fewer than two weeks. Such rapid growth of aneurysm in the major intracranial vessels resulting from methamphetamine abuse is very rare. The pathophysiology of stroke form ATS Class substances is multifactorial but preexisting vascular disease, and meth-induced hypertension pays a major role [8]. The rapid growth of an aneurysm has a high risk of aneurysmal rupture and SAH, which is a neurosurgical emergency [3, 9]. Some underlying risk factors have been identified which can be helpful in recognizing susceptible individuals, which can benefit in clinical decision-making [10, 11].

2. Case

A 41-year-old Hispanic woman initially presented to the emergency room (ER) in 2012 with a severe excruciating headache for approximately 1 hour after the use of meth.

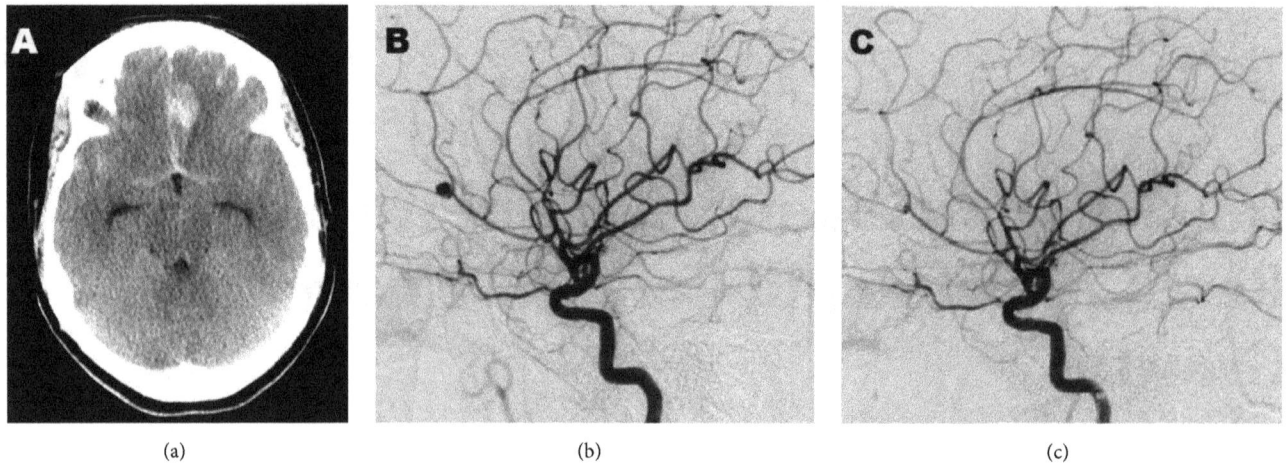

(a)   (b)   (c)

FIGURE 1: Imaging study upon patient's arrival at the hospital in 2012. (a) CT head without contrast showing diffuse subarachnoid hemorrhage that originated from an aneurysm identified by (b) Cerebral angiogram. (c) Cerebral angiogram imaging after coiling of an aneurysm.

Further history revealed patient had been an oral, snorting and intravenous user of meth. Her headache was also associated with nausea, vomiting, neck pain/stiffness, and photophobia. The patient had the following vitals: blood pressure 146/94 mmHg, heart rate 64 beats/min, respiratory rate 18 breath/min, and Temperature 36.5°C. The further patient assessment revealed a Hunt and Hess: grade I (+1) and Glasgow Coma Scale (GCS) of 15 with no focal deficits. Blood workup (hematological and blood chemistry) was within normal range. A head CT demonstrated left frontal intraparenchymal hemorrhage (IPH) measuring 1.2 × 2.6 cm with bilateral frontal and Sylvian fissure subarachnoid hemorrhage (Figure 1(a)) with hemorrhagic extension into the fourth ventricle; Fisher grade: IV. CT-A demonstrated a left distal anterior cerebral artery aneurysm measuring 3.7 × 3.4 mm pointing in a superior-medial direction. An EVD was placed for obstructive hydrocephalus. After coiling the ruptured aneurysm, postcoiling images were also obtained (Figure 1(c)). After procedure the patient was stable and without neurological deficit; her ICU stay was uneventful and eventually discharged home.

The patient was lost to follow-up and presented in the hospital emergency room after four years with complaints of acute onset headache similar to prior presentation with headache and vomiting identical to the symptoms she had in 2012. Follow-up history revealed she continued to struggle with meth abuse with last use around ten days before her presentation to the hospital. Her vitals on presentation were as follows: blood pressure 129/54 mmHg, heart rate 61 beats/min, respiratory rate 16 breath/min, and Temperature 37°C. The patient was assessed as Hunt and Hess grade II + 1 and a GCS of 15 with no focal deficits. There was a left medial frontal intracerebral hemorrhage adjacent to an aneurysm that was coiled previously on head CT (Figure 2(a)). A formal angiogram demonstrated rerupture with recannulation at the base of the previously coiled aneurysm. Additionally, three neoaneurysms that were found include a periophthalmic aneurysm of the right internal carotid artery,

approximately 5 mm, a fusiform dilation aneurysm at the pericallosal and callosomarginal bifurcation, and a basilar tip aneurysm, approximately 1.5-2 mm and 4 mm, respectively (Figures 2(b) and 2(c)) and were assessed as Fisher grade IV. She subsequently underwent a bifrontal craniotomy for clipping of her complex anterior cerebral branch aneurysm. Her postoperative course was uneventful, and the patient was eventually discharged home, GCS 15, and neurologically intact.

Five days after discharge in 2016, the patient again presented to the hospital as a transfer from an outside hospital, intubated, with a head CT demonstrating a 3.7 × 5.2 × 5 cm left frontal intracerebral hemorrhage (ICH) with extension into the bilateral lateral ventricles, third and fourth ventricles (Figure 3(a)). The patient was Hunt and Hess grade IV + 1, Fisher grade IV. Urine drug screen was positive for meth (records from another hospital). On arrival, her vitals were as follows: blood pressure 143/67 mmHg, heart rate 61 beats/min, respiratory rate 18 breath/min, and Temperature 37.4°C, and GCS was 11T with left-sided hemiparesis. Emergent left craniectomy was done for evacuation of the intraparenchymal hemorrhage and ventriculostomy tube placement. Postoperative formal angiogram, less than 3 weeks from her previous cerebral angiogram, showed that the previously identified fusiform dilations associated with the right pericallosal and callosomarginal bifurcation segment now had a small saccular component with a neck of 5 mm and a height of 7 mm (Figure 2(b)). The previous periophthalmic, basilar tip and left frontopolar aneurysms were identified and remained unchanged. She subsequently underwent angiography assisted coiling of the right pericallosal and callosomarginal bifurcation aneurysm (Figure 3(c)). Over the remainder of her hospital stay, she underwent revision of cranioplasty as well as angiogram for pipeline stent of the periophthalmic artery aneurysm. She was downgraded out of the ICU, ambulating with physical therapy with the assistance of a walker and subsequently discharged home.

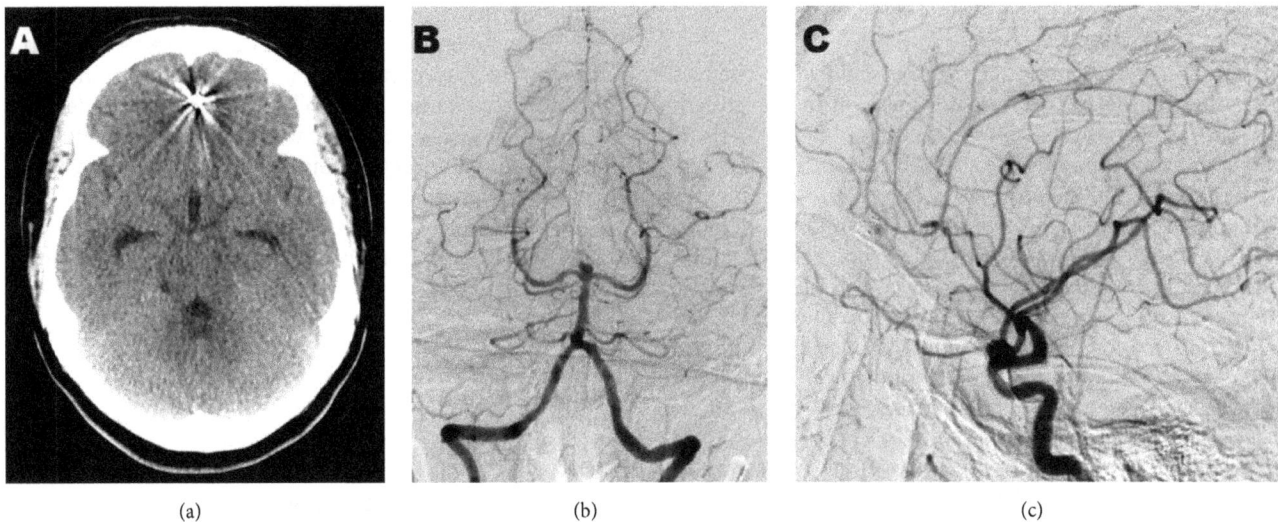

(a) (b) (c)

FIGURE 2: Imaging upon hospitalization in 2016. (a) CT head without contrast in 2016 showing intracerebral hemorrhage adjacent to the previously coiled aneurysm. (b and c) Cerebral angiogram of the anterior and posterior circulations showing the development of multiple new aneurysms.

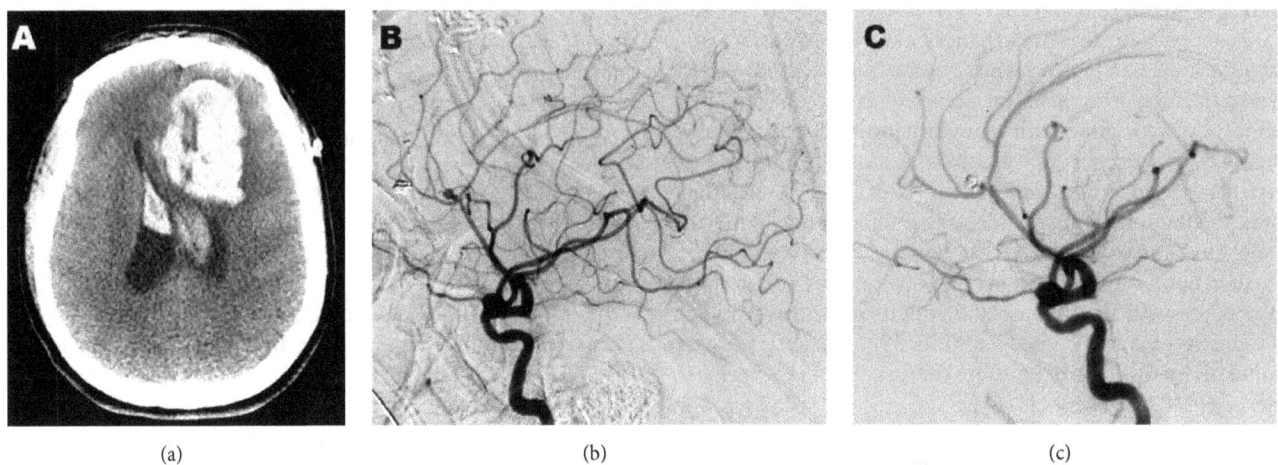

(a) (b) (c)

FIGURE 3: (a) 5 days after discharge in 2016: CT head shows large intracerebral hematoma. (b) A diagnostic cerebral angiogram less than 3 weeks from previous imaging demonstrating interval development of a saccular aneurysm at the callosomarginal and pericallosal bifurcation. (c) Cerebral angiogram postcoiling.

3. Discussion

Nontraumatic SAH is a neurosurgical emergency with a mortality rate as high as 45%, often secondary to aneurysm rupture [12–14]. Clinically, only two-thirds of all survivors regain functional independence, and nearly half of survivors have permanent cognitive deficits [15]. Among the risk factors for aneurysm rupture including location, morphology, family history, active smoking, and female sex, aneurysm growth is a consistent and significant finding [11, 16, 17]. Brinjijki et al. in a recent meta-analysis reported annual rupture rate in growing aneurysms versus a stable aneurysm as 3.1% and 0.1%, respectively [18]. Further, the greatest risk for aneurysm rupture is during rapid periods of growth and therefore such cases should be dealt with caution and close monitoring [19–21].

Amphetamine and its derivative, methamphetamine, are potent sympathomimetics and among the most common illicitly abused drugs. There is ample scientific data to suggest an association between meth abuse and large artery dissections and aneurysm formation over a period of time leading to rupture and SAH [22]. However, rapid growth of aneurysm, within weeks, and associated meth abuse is quite rare. Previously, Chen et al. was the only one to report the fast growth (within 2 weeks) of an aneurysm on a major intracranial vessel in a habitual amphetamine user [23]. Similarly, in our case where the patient struggling with chronic methamphetamine abuse, there was a very rapid aneurysm growth (within 3 weeks) leading to rupture and ICH. The etiology is hypothesized to be meth or cocaine-induced hypertension and tachycardia (sympathetic rush in the body) that leads to progression, evolution, and growth of intra- and extracranial aneurysms [24, 25].

Additionally vasculitis and other vasculopathic changes have also been postulated as major mechanisms for growth and subsequent rupture in meth abusers [4]. Meth is known to have numerous effects on the central nervous system, specifically the cerebral vasculature. Most prominently, pathological studies of cerebral vasculature have demonstrated necrosis of blood vessel walls with the destruction of the elastic and smooth muscle layer, without leukocytic infiltration of the blood vessel walls, commonly termed necrotizing angiitis or meth arteritis [3]. Chen et al. found much fibrotic adhesion and some fibrinoid necrotic material covering the aneurysm in their reported case [23]. Additionally, blood-brain barrier disruption [26], changes in cerebral perfusion [27], depletion of dopamine and serotonin [28], and cortical grey and white matter loss [29] have all been observed. These changes are seen in both binge and chronic users. Binge methamphetamine use is associated with compromised global and regional blood flow, likely representing severe and enduring neural toxicity of monoaminergic neurotransmitter systems in the brain, eventually producing a pattern of hypoperfusion [29].

Together with the CNS changes observed, transient and extreme increases in sympathetic output with blood pressure elevation can precipitate intracerebral hemorrhage either alone or in association with an underlying vascular pathology such as an aneurysm or vasculitis. A study comprising 30 patients by Ho et al. found all cases of SAH in a patient with methamphetamine abuse were aneurysmal with the majority of aneurysms located in the anterior circulation [30]. Further, numerous studies have demonstrated poor outcomes in patients with meth abuse and ruptured aneurysms when compared to age-matched controls [31, 32] and younger populations of illicit drug users are usually more prone to these devastating events [4, 6, 7].

In our opinion, this case corroborates the acute and chronic cerebrovascular repercussions associated with methamphetamine binge and abuse. In this case rapid growth of the aneurysm leads to rupture and intraparenchymal hemorrhage requiring emergent craniectomy and evacuation. Careful consideration should be given to the rapid development of aneurysms in this patient population as they are at higher risk of rupture. Meth use has been implicated in the growth and rupture of aneurysms, identifying opportunities for early intervention and potential benefit. It is necessary to identify this group of patients early because numerous studies have demonstrated poor outcomes in patients with meth abuse and ruptured aneurysms when compared to age-matched controls, making it imperative to prevent rupture when possible through endovascular or surgical interventions [31, 32]. Based on our experience, we anticipate vigilant monitoring of aneurysms and aggressive strategies treatment in patients with current or previous meth abuse.

4. Conclusion

This case highlights the risk of rapid aneurysm growth and rupture as well as the effects of meth on the CNS and cerebral vasculature that may contribute to the higher incidence of SAH in this patient population. The outcome after a ruptured aneurysm in this population is worse than age-matched controls, necessitating close follow-up, and a consideration for more aggressive treatment with endovascular embolization or open surgical clipping after aneurysms are found in patients with methamphetamine abuse. The possibility of a rapid drug-induced pseudoaneurysm should also be considered when faced with intracerebral or subarachnoid hemorrhage in young patients.

Abbreviations

SAH: Subarachnoid Hemorrhage
Meth: Methamphetamine
ATS: Amphetamine Like Substances
ER: Emergency Room
CNS: Central Nervous system
CT: Computed Tomography
CT-A: Computer Tomographic Angiography
GCS: Glasgow Coma Scale
EVD: Extraventricular Drain
ICU: Intensive Care Unit
ICA: Internal Carotid Artery
CNS: Central nervous system
ICH: Intracerebral hemorrhage.

Conflicts of Interest

The authors report no conflicts of interest concerning the materials or methods used in this study or the findings specified in this paper.

References

[1] K. E. Courtney and L. A. Ray, "Methamphetamine: An update on epidemiology, pharmacology, clinical phenomenology, and treatment literature," *Drug and Alcohol Dependence*, vol. 143, no. 1, pp. 11–21, 2014.

[2] L. C. Jang and S. S. Park, "Intensive long distance running as a possible cause of multiple splanchnic arterial aneurysms: a case report," *Vascular Specialist International*, vol. 32, no. 3, pp. 129–132, 2016.

[3] N. Miyazawa, I. Akiyama, and Z. Yamagata, "Risk factors for growth of unruptured intracranial aneurysms: follow-up study by serial 0.5-T magnetic resonance angiography," *Neurosurgery*, vol. 58, no. 6, pp. 1047–1052, 2006.

[4] J. A. Perez Jr., E. L. Arsura, and S. Strategos, "Methamphetamine-related stroke: Four cases," *The Journal of Emergency Medicine*, vol. 17, no. 3, pp. 469–471, 1999.

[5] A. Nanda, P. S. S. V. Vannemreddy, R. S. Polin, and B. K. Willis, "Intracranial aneurysms and cocaine abuse: Analysis of prognostic indicators," *Neurosurgery*, vol. 46, no. 5, pp. 1063–1069, 2000.

[6] M. M. El-Omar, K. Ray, and R. Geary, "Intracerebral haemorrhage in a young adult: Consider amphetamine abuse," *The British Journal of Clinical Practice*, vol. 50, no. 2, pp. 115-116, 1996.

[7] A. W. McEvoy, N. D. Kitchen, and D. G. T. Thomas, "Intracerebral haemorrhage and drug abuse in young adults," *British Journal of Neurosurgery*, vol. 14, no. 5, pp. 449–454, 2000.

[8] J. M. Lappin, S. Darke, and M. Farrell, "Stroke and methamphetamine use in young adults: a review," *Journal of Neurology, Neurosurgery and Psychiatry*, vol. 88, no. 12, pp. 1079–1091, 2017.

[9] L.-D. Jou and M. E. Mawad, "Growth rate and rupture rate of unruptured intracranial aneurysms: A population approach," *Biomedical Engineering Online*, vol. 8, article no. 11, 2009.

[10] R. Kleinloog, N. de Mul, B. H. Verweij, J. A. Post, G. J. E. Rinkel, and Y. M. Ruigrok, "Risk factors for intracranial aneurysm rupture: a systematic review," *Neurosurgery*, vol. 82, no. 4, pp. 431–440, 2018.

[11] S. Juvela, K. Poussa, H. Lehto, and M. Porras, "Natural history of unruptured intracranial aneurysms: a long-term follow-up study," *Stroke*, vol. 44, no. 9, pp. 2414–2421, 2013.

[12] A. A. Cohen-Gadol and B. N. Bohnstedt, "Recognition and evaluation of nontraumatic subarachnoid hemorrhage and ruptured cerebral aneurysm," *American Family Physician*, vol. 88, no. 7, pp. 451–456, 2013.

[13] S. A. Quadri, V. Ramakrishnan, O. Hariri, and M. A. Taqi, "Early Experience with the transform™ occlusion balloon catheter: a single-center study," *Interventional Neurology*, vol. 3, no. 3-4, pp. 174–183, 2015.

[14] M. Taqi, S. Quadri, A. Puri et al., "P-029 a prospective multicenter trial of transform™ occlusion balloon catheter (tobc): trial design and results," *Journal of NeuroInterventional Surgery*, vol. 7, p. A37, 2015.

[15] G. J. Rinkel and A. Algra, "Long-term outcomes of patients with aneurysmal subarachnoid haemorrhage," *The Lancet Neurology*, vol. 10, no. 4, pp. 349–356, 2011.

[16] G. Lanzino and R. D. Brown Jr., "Natural history of unruptured intracranial aneurysms," *Journal of Neurosurgery*, vol. 117, no. 1, pp. 50-51, 2012.

[17] M. A. Taqi, S. A. Quadri, A. S. Puri et al., "A prospective multicenter trial of the transform occlusion balloon catheter: trial design and results," *Interventional Neurology*, vol. 7, no. 1-2, pp. 53–64, 2018.

[18] W. Brinjikji, Y.-Q. Zhu, G. Lanzino et al., "Risk factors for growth of intracranial aneurysms: A systematic review and meta-analysis," *American Journal of Neuroradiology*, vol. 37, no. 4, pp. 615–620, 2016.

[19] C. Doenitz, K.-M. Schebesch, R. Zoephel, and A. Brawanski, "A mechanism for the rapid development of intracranial aneurysms: A case study," *Neurosurgery*, vol. 67, no. 5, pp. 1213–1221, 2010.

[20] V. Ramakrishnan, S. Quadri, A. Sodhi, V. Cortez, and M. Taqi, "E-064 safety and efficacy of balloon-assisted coiling of intracranial aneurysms: a single-center study," *Journal of NeuroInterventional Surgery*, vol. 6, no. Suppl 1, pp. A68.3–A69, 2014.

[21] S. Albano, B. Berman, G. Fischberg et al., "Retrospective analysis of ventriculitis in external ventricular drains," *Neurology Research International*, vol. 2018, Article ID 5179356, 9 pages, 2018.

[22] J. M. Lappin, S. Darke, and M. Farrell, "Stroke and methamphetamine use in young adults: a review," *Journal of Neurology, Neurosurgery & Psychiatry*, vol. 88, no. 12, pp. 1079–1091, 2017.

[23] H.-J. Chen, C.-L. Liang, K. Lu, and C.-C. Lui, "Rapidly growing internal carotid artery aneurysm after amphetamine abuse: Case report," *The American Journal of Forensic Medicine and Pathology*, vol. 24, no. 1, pp. 32–34, 2003.

[24] C. Fikar, "Methamphetamine and aortic dissection," *Journal of Cardiac Surgery*, vol. 23, no. 3, p. 282, 2008.

[25] E. Wako, D. LeDoux, L. Mitsumori, and G. S. Aldea, "The emerging epidemic of methamphetamine-induced aortic dissections," *Journal of Cardiac Surgery*, vol. 22, no. 5, pp. 390–393, 2007.

[26] N. A. Northrop, L. E. Halpin, and B. K. Yamamoto, "Peripheral ammonia and blood brain barrier structure and function after methamphetamine," *Neuropharmacology*, vol. 107, pp. 18–26, 2016.

[27] V. R. D. Kakhki, F. M. Sani, and B. Dadpour, "Abnormal cerebral blood flow in methamphetamine abusers assessed by brain perfusion single emission computed tomography," *Iranian Journal of Nuclear Medicine*, vol. 25, pp. 47–51, 2017.

[28] I. N. Krasnova, Z. Justinova, B. Ladenheim et al., "Methamphetamine self-administration is associated with persistent biochemical alterations in striatal and cortical dopaminergic terminals in the rat," *PLoS ONE*, vol. 5, no. 1, Article ID e8790, 2010.

[29] Y. A. Chung, B. S. Peterson, S. J. Yoon et al., "In vivo evidence for long-term CNS toxicity, associated with chronic binge use of methamphetamine," *Drug and Alcohol Dependence*, vol. 111, no. 1-2, pp. 155–160, 2010.

[30] E. L. Ho, S. A. Josephson, H. S. Lee, and W. S. Smith, "Cerebrovascular complications of methamphetamine abuse," *Neurocritical Care*, vol. 10, no. 3, pp. 295–305, 2009.

[31] K. Moon, F. C. Albuquerque, M. Mitkov et al., "Methamphetamine use is an independent predictor of poor outcome after aneurysmal subarachnoid hemorrhage," *Journal of NeuroInterventional Surgery*, vol. 7, no. 5, pp. 346–350, 2015.

[32] D. G. Zuloaga, J. Wang, S. Weber, G. P. Mark, S. J. Murphy, and J. Raber, "Chronic methamphetamine exposure prior to middle cerebral artery occlusion increases infarct volume and worsens cognitive injury in Male mice," *Metabolic Brain Disease*, vol. 31, no. 4, pp. 975–981, 2016.

14

A Case of Diffuse Leptomeningeal Glioneuronal Tumor Misdiagnosed as Chronic Tuberculous Meningitis without Brain Biopsy

Jung koo Lee,[1] Hak-cheol Ko (ID),[1] Jin-gyu Choi,[1] Youn Soo Lee,[2] and Byung-chul Son (ID)[1,3]

[1]Department of Neurosurgery, Seoul St. Mary's Hospital, College of Medicine, The Catholic University of Korea, Seoul, Republic of Korea
[2]Department of Hospital Pathology, Seoul St. Mary's Hospital, College of Medicine, The Catholic University of Korea, Seoul, Republic of Korea
[3]Catholic Neuroscience Institute, College of Medicine, The Catholic University of Korea, Seoul, Republic of Korea

Correspondence should be addressed to Byung-chul Son; sbc@catholic.ac.kr

Academic Editor: Chin-Chang Huang

Here we report a rare case of diffuse leptomeningeal glioneuronal tumor (DLGNT) in a 62-year-old male patient misdiagnosed as having tuberculous meningitis. Due to its rarity and radiologic findings of leptomeningeal enhancement in the basal cisterns on magnetic resonance imaging (MRI) similar to tuberculous meningitis, DLGNT in this patient was initially diagnosed as communicating hydrocephalus from tuberculous meningitis despite absence of laboratory findings of tuberculosis. The patient's symptoms and signs promptly improved after a ventriculoperitoneal shunting surgery followed by empirical treatment against tuberculosis. Five years later, mental confusion and ataxic gait developed in this patient again despite well-functioning ventriculoperitoneal shunt. Aggravation of leptomeningeal enhancement in the basal cisterns was noted in MRI. An additional course of antituberculosis medication with steroid was started without biopsy of the brain. Laboratory examinations for tuberculosis were negative again. After four months of improvement, his mental confusion, memory impairment, dysphasia, and ataxia gradually worsened. A repeated MRI of the brain showed further aggravation of leptomeningeal enhancement in the basal cisterns. Biopsy of the brain surface and leptomeninges revealed a very rare occurrence of DLGNT. His delayed diagnosis of DLGNT might be due to prevalence of tuberculosis in our country, similarity in MRI finding of prominent leptomeningeal enhancement in the basal cisterns, and extreme rarity of DLGNT in the elderly. DLGLT should be considered in differential diagnosis of medical conditions presenting as communicating hydrocephalus with prominent leptomeningeal enhancement. A timely histologic diagnosis through a leptomeningeal biopsy of the brain and spinal cord in case of unusual leptomeningeal enhancement with uncertain laboratory findings is essential because cytologic examination of the cerebrospinal fluid in DLGNT is known to be negative.

1. Introduction

Glioneuronal tumors are a group of primary brain neoplasms of relatively recent acquisition in the World Health Organization (WHO) classification of central nervous system (CNS) tumors [1]. In the literature, they have been described in a variety of similar terms, e.g., DLGNT or disseminated oligodendroglial-like leptomeningeal tumor of childhood [2, 3]. They mostly present as diffuse leptomeningeal diseases in children and adolescents. Their histologic characteristics include monomorphic clear cell glial morphology reminiscent of oligodendroglioma, although they often express synaptophysin in addition to OLIG2 and S-100 [2, 3]. The hallmark of neuroradiological appearance of diffuse leptomeningeal glioneuronal tumor (DLGNT) is prominent leptomeningeal enhancement with or without communicating hydrocephalus [1]. On T1 gadolinium-enhanced images, a thick and diffuse leptomeningeal enhancement on the surface of brain and basal cisterns similar to that described in tuberculous meningitis has been documented in all DLGNT patients [1].

We present an extremely rare occurrence of DLGNT in a 62-year-old male patient. Despite no evidence of tuberculous meningitis, consideration of typical MRI findings of leptomeningeal enhancement in basal cisterns associated with hydrocephalus and prevalence of tuberculosis led to a tentative diagnosis of tuberculous meningitis. A ventriculoperitoneal shunt and medical treatment for tuberculosis were performed without invasive brain biopsy. Indeed, the diagnosis of tuberculous meningitis is often difficult because its clinical features are not very specific. Detection of *Mycobacterium tuberculosis* in cerebrospinal fluid (CSF) by acid-fast staining, culture, or DNA analysis with polymerase chain reaction (PCR) has low sensitivity. The current case highlights the importance of histologic confirmation through brain biopsy for cases presenting leptomeningeal enhancement in the basal cistern in MRI with equivocal laboratory examinations to explain the etiology.

2. Case Presentation

A 62-year-old male patient presented with progressive worsening of mental function, dysphasia, and ataxic gait in the last six months. Five years prior to presentation (in August 2012), he was diagnosed with communicating hydrocephalus possibly caused by tuberculous meningoencephalitis because of mental confusion and gait disturbance. He underwent a ventriculoperitoneal shunt surgery in one hospital. His mental confusion and gait disturbance immediately improved following the ventriculoperitoneal shunt. Results of CSF study were negative for tuberculosis. However, a provisional diagnosis of communicating hydrocephalus caused by tuberculous meningitis was made based on MRI findings of leptomeningeal enhancement in the basal cisterns (Figures 1(a) and 1(b)). He had been treated with antituberculosis medication for the following six months after the shunting operation. After shunting and medical treatment, he returned to his work. He had been followed-up regularly every six months at that hospital. His physical and mental conditions were stable. He experienced no difficulty in work or daily activities.

Six months prior to the present presentation (December 2016), slurred speech and mental confusion with intermittent disorientation to time and place developed within several days. CSF analysis and MRI of the brain were performed. CSF analysis showed white blood cell (WBC) count of 9 cells/μL, red blood cell count of 33,000 cell/μL, protein level of 4228 mg/dL, lactic dehydrogenase (LDH) level of 224 mg/dL, and glucose level of 130 mg/dL. MRI of the brain showed multiple linear and nodular leptomeningeal enhancing lesions scattered in basal and left sylvian cisterns (Figure 1(c)). The extent of leptomeningeal enhancement in basal cisterns was markedly increased compared to that in MRI examination done in 2012. The size of the ventricle was small, indicating that shunt malfunction did not occur. There was no abnormal spike activity in his electroencephalography (EEG) except intermittent slow wave in his left frontocentral

area. Under an impression of aggravation of tuberculosis meningitis, he was referred to our hospital (January 2017).

The patient's consultation in the Department of Infectious Medicine was carried out for aggravation of tuberculous meningitis/encephalitis. The doctor in neurology thought that tuberculous meningitis aggravated again. For possibility of drug-resistant tuberculosis, four-drug regimen (isoniazid 75 mg, rifampicin 150 mg, pyrazinamide 400 mg, and ethambutol 300 mg; tubes tab 4 times a day for 2 months followed by isoniazide and rifampicin for 7 months) against tuberculosis was used. Beside antituberculosis medications, steroid was prescribed. The patient's mental confusion, dysphasia, and irritability progressively improved over the course of one month at the outpatient clinic. He returned to his usual life again. He was able to work in his previous job without apparent complications.

His mental confusion and dysphasia accompanying gait disturbance gradually developed again within four months (June 2017), leading to reevaluation of the brain by MRI. There was no fever or signs of meningeal irritation in neurologic evaluation. MRI of the brain surface revealed extensive progression of diffuse leptomeningeal enhancement in the basal and left sylvian cisterns (Figure 1(d)). No intraparenchymal enhancing lesion was noted. Hydrocephalic change was not shown either. CSF examination showed WBC count of 110 cells/μL (lymphocyte 70%, macrophage 7%, and neutrophils 3%), red blood cell count of 7200 cell/μL, protein level of 4272 mg/dL, and glucose level of 102 mg/dL. Levels of erythrocyte sedimentation rate (ESR) and C-reactive protein (CRP) were 4 mm/hr and 0.05 mg/dl, respectively. Levels of adenosine deaminase (ADA) and immunoglobulin G were 8.0 IU/L and 901 mg/dl, respectively. Results of CSF culture for toxoplasmosis, fungus, cryptococcus, and herpes simplex virus were all negative. Gram-staining revealed many WBC without microorganism. Polymerase chain reactions (PCR) of the CSF against *Mycobacterium tuberculosis*, herpes simplex virus, varicella zoster, enterovirus, and Epstein-Barr virus were all negative. Culture for acid-fast bacilli (AFB) did not show any growth until eight weeks after incubation. For possibility of leptomeningeal metastasis, biopsy of the brain, and leptomeninges was requested.

Biopsy of the brain surface and leptomeninges was performed on the left frontal cortex and sylvian fissure proceeded by a small frontotemporal craniotomy. Postoperative course was uneventful. Histologic diagnosis revealed DLGNT without intraparenchymal brain lesion (Figure 2(a)). Monotonous oligodendrocyte-like or neurocyte-like tumor cells with round nuclei and clear cytoplasm were found (Figure 2(b)). Mitosis, microvascular proliferation, and necrosis were not evident. Immunohistochemical stainings for Olig-2 and synaptophysin were positive (Figures 2(c) and 2(d)). Those for CD68, isocitrate dehydrogenase- (IDH-) 1, glial fibrillary acidic protein (GFAP), and neurofilament were negative. Ki67 proliferative index was low (5%). PCR for O^6-methylguanine-DNA-methyltransferase (MGMT) methylation was positive. However, 1p19q codeletion was not detected by interphase fluorescent in situ hybridization (FISH). Methenamine-silver and PAS staining for fungal organism,

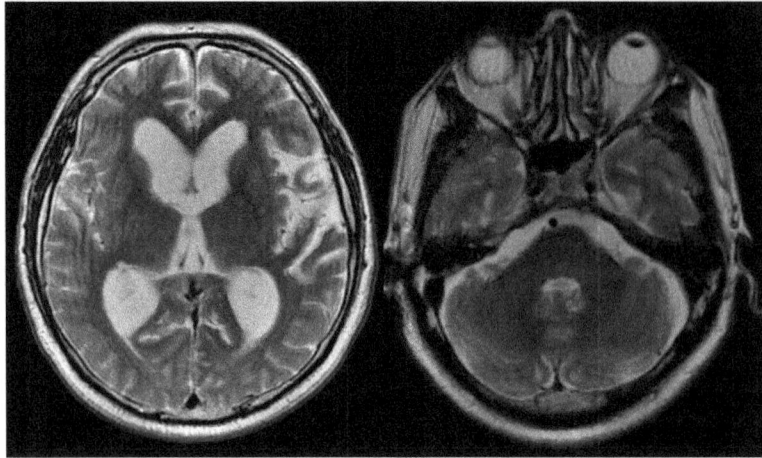

(a) A T2-weighted axial MRI image showing marked dilation of lateral and third ventricles indicating nonobstructive hydrocephalus

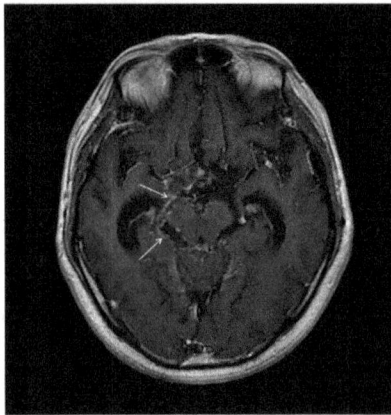

(b) A T1-weighted enhanced axial MRI image showing leptomeningeal enhancement (arrows) in the basal cisterns

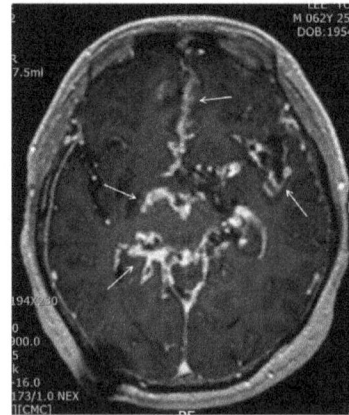

(c) Prominent leptomeningeal enhancement is noted in the basal, interhemispheric, and left sylvian cisterns in an enhanced T1-weighted axial MRI image at the time of recurrent mental confusion (January 2017). No intra-axial enhancing lesion is observed

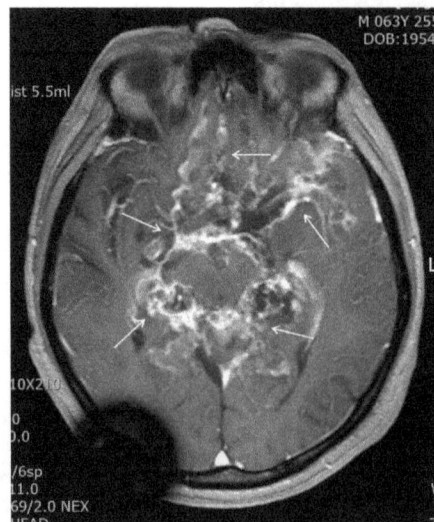

(d) Marked aggravation of leptomeningeal enhancement in the basal, interhemispheric, and left sylvian cisterns in an enhanced T1-weighted axial MRI image in August 2017

FIGURE 1: Continued.

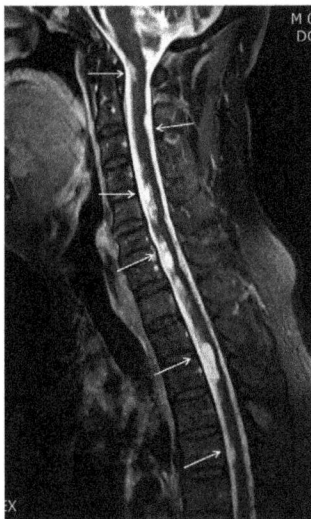

(e) Multiple leptomeningeal enhancing nodules along the whole spinal cord in a sagittal, fat suppressed, enhanced T1-weighted image. Indentation of the spinal cord is shown in some leptomeningeal nodules

FIGURE 1: Magnetic resonance imaging (MRI) findings of communicating hydrocephalus and leptomeningeal enhancement in the basal cistern at the time of initial manifestation of mental confusion (2012).

Ziehl-Neelsen staining, and PCR for *Mycobacterium tuberculosis* were all negative. After histologic diagnosis of DLGNT, MRI of the whole spine was subsequently performed in order to detect further leptomeningeal spread. MRI showed multiple leptomeningeal enhancing nodules displaying high signal intensity on T2-weighted images (Figure 1(e)), disseminating along the whole spinal cord without intramedullary lesion. With a final diagnosis of DLGNT by invasive brain biopsy, medical records and imaging results were thoroughly reviewed again. PCV (Procarbazine, CCNU, and Vincristine) chemotherapy and radiation therapy of the craniospinal axis were planned. The patient's condition gradually deteriorated with apparent worsening of severe memory impairment, disorientation, and gait ataxia.

3. Discussion

3.1. Leptomeningeal Enhancement and Tuberculous Meningitis. Contrast material enhancement for cross-sectional imaging has been used since the mid-1970s for computed tomography and the mid-1980s for MRI [4]. Knowledge of patterns of contrast enhancement has facilitated clinical and radiologic differential diagnosis. Extra-axial enhancement in the CNS may be classified as either pachymeningeal (dura mater, thick meninges) or leptomeningeal (pia and arachnoid, skinny meninges). Enhancement of the pia mater or enhancement extending into the subarachnoid spaces of the sulci and cisterns is leptomeningeal enhancement. It is also called "pial or pia-arachnoid enhancement". Leptomeningeal enhancement is usually associated with meningitis and meningoencephalitis that might be bacterial, viral,

or fungal. The primary mechanism of this enhancement is breakdown of the blood-brain barrier without angiogenesis. The subarachnoid space is infiltrated with inflammatory cells. The permeability in the meninges may increase due to bacterial glycoproteins released into the subarachnoid space [4]. Neoplasms may spread into the subarachnoid space and produce enhancement of the brain surface and subarachnoid space, a pathologic process often called "carcinomatous meningitis". Both primary tumors (medulloblastoma, ependymoma, glioblastoma, and oligodendroglioma) and secondary tumors (e.g., lymphoma and breast cancer) may spread through the subarachnoid space. Neoplastic leptomeningeal enhancement often produces thick, lumpy, or nodular enhancement, similar to fungal meningitis.

Tuberculosis has shown resurgence in nonendemic populations in recent years due to increased migration and endemic human immunodeficiency virus [5]. Although the thorax is most frequently involved, tuberculosis may involve any organ systems. Its involvement in the CNS is seen in approximately 5% of patients with tuberculosis [6]. CNS tuberculosis can manifest in a variety of forms, including tuberculous meningitis, tuberculomas, tuberculous abscesses, tuberculous cerebritis, and miliary tuberculosis. Among these, tuberculous meningitis is the most common manifestation of CNS involvement across all age groups [7]. It is usually due to hematogenous spread. However, it can be secondary to rupture of a Rich focus or direct extension from CSF infection [5–7]. Its typical radiographic finding is abnormal meningeal enhancement usually most pronounced in basal cisterns, although meningeal involvement at some degree within the sulci over the cerebral convexities and

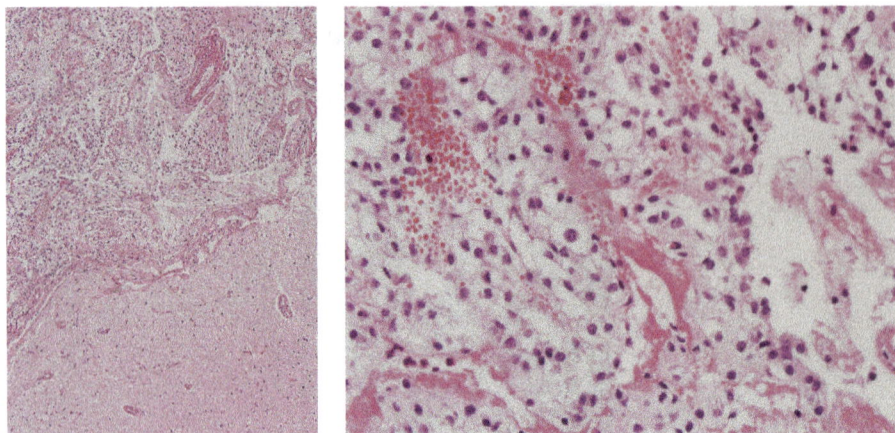

(a) Diffuse leptomeningeal dissemination of tumor cells without an intraparenchymal brain lesion (H & E, x 100)

(b) Monotonous oligodendrocyte-like or neurocyte-like tumor cells with round nuclei and clear cytoplasm (H & E, x 400)

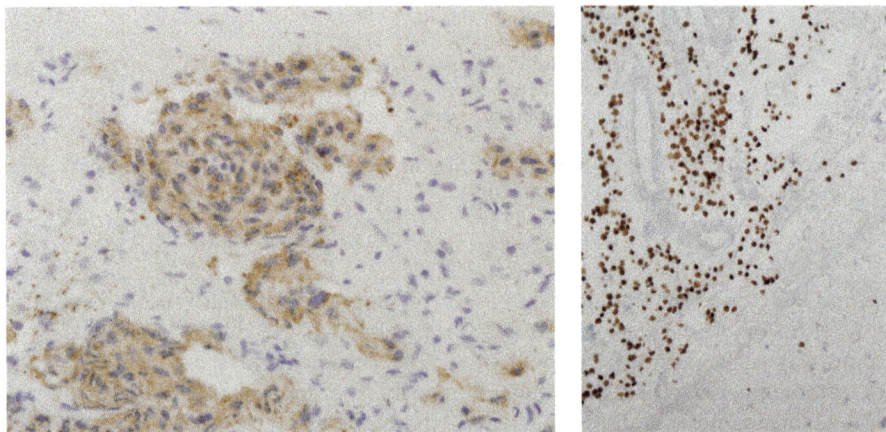

(c) Positive immunohistochemical staining for Olig-2 (x200)

(d) Immunohistochemical staining for synaptophysin is positive (x 400)

FIGURE 2: Histopathologic examination of disseminated leptomeningeal glioneuronal tumor.

in sylvian fissures is also seen in many cases [5–8]. Early diagnosis is important to reduce morbidity and mortality because delayed treatment is associated with severe morbidity. Unfortunately, history of infection or exposure to tuberculosis may or may not present in tuberculosis patients. Evidence of active tuberculosis is present in less than 50% of cases. Furthermore, clinical and radiologic features of tuberculosis may mimic those of many other diseases.

3.2. Delayed Diagnosis of DLGNT. The diagnosis of DLGLT was delayed in the current case. The patient initially presented with altered mentality with MRI findings of leptomeningeal enhancement of basal cisterns and communicating hydrocephalus. Characteristic basal meningeal inflammation resulting in leptomeningeal enhancement in basal cisterns is the most typical feature of gadolinium-enhanced MR imaging of tuberculous meningitis. The most common complication of tuberculous meningitis is communicating hydrocephalus caused by blockage of basal cisterns due to inflammatory exudates [4, 8]. In addition, tuberculosis is

still prevalent and multidrug-resistant tuberculosis is one of the major medical concerns in our country. Difficulty in establishing a diagnosis of tuberculous meningitis might have also contributed to the diagnostic error. A positive mycobacterial culture in the CSF remains the gold standard in the diagnosis of tuberculous meningitis. However, CSF acid-fast bacilli have been identified in less than 10% of cases. Mycobacteria culture positivity ranges from 50% to 75% after 8 weeks, an unacceptable length of time for the diagnosis of tuberculosis in making treatment decision [9, 10]. In the current case, real-time polymerase chain reaction (PCR) and mycobacterial cultures from sputum and CSF were negative. Despite absence of laboratory data supporting tuberculosis, the current case was treated with ventriculoperitoneal shunt and antituberculosis chemotherapy under clinical impression of tuberculous meningitis, complicated with hydrocephalus. In addition, radiological imaging study was not conducted to evaluate the efficacy of antituberculous treatment and resolution of leptomeningeal enhancement in the basal cisterns. According to medical standards, just clinical follow-up visits were scheduled and no control of clearance of the supposed tuberculous lesions was carried out.

Another reason for delayed diagnosis for this case might be an extreme rarity of DLGLT. Indeed, the patient did not show any past history or symptoms indicative of glial brain tumor. CSF cytology result was negative. Without an invasive brain biopsy including leptomeninges, it is hard to figure out such a rare DLGNT. The number of reported cases of DLGNT is less than 100 worldwide since the first report of the largest series of 36 patients by Rodrigues et al. in 2012 [2]. DLGNT has been mostly reported in children less than 10 years of age, although some of them have occurred in middle aged patients [1, 2, 11–17]. Prior to this report, there have been several case series and case reports published that might have the same entity. They were variably described as diffuse leptomeningeal glioneuronal tumor [1], superficially disseminated glioma in children [12], or diffuse leptomeningeal oligodendrogliomatosis [13–15]. These tumors including DLGNT are characterized radiologically by leptomeningeal enhancement on MRI usually involving basal cisterns and the spinal cord.

While various CNS tumors show diffuse leptomeningeal spread, Perilongo et al. [16] and Gardiman et al. [1] have reported a possibly novel entity of low-grade pediatric tumors with extensive leptomeningeal dissemination without a large solid component. It cannot be placed in the 2007 version of WHO classification of CNS tumors [18]. Histologically, these tumors are characterized as monomorphous oligoid tumor cells with round oval nuclei. Gardimann et al. [1] have suggested a "glioneuronal component" of these tumors and proposed a term of "diffuse leptomeningeal glioneuronal tumor". Although clinical presentation and course in patients with DLGNT are still largely unknown [17], most patients present an acute onset of signs and symptoms of raised intracranial pressure caused by communicating hydrocephalus necessitating extraventricular drainage or ventriculoperitoneal shunt [2, 17]. Most patients initially received antibiotic treatment for suspected meningeal infection and MRI showed typical findings of leptomeningeal enhancement, similar to reactive postinfectious changes. Extensive CSF examinations including virology, inflammation, and tumor markers (beta-HCG, AFF, and PLAP) are required.

If the CSF specimen is insufficient to confirm diagnosis, a prompt and open arachnoid biopsy is necessary to confirm the diagnosis. An aggressive behavior has been reported in 38% of cases. However, most tumors seem to show periods of stability or slow progress [2]. In the current case, an open leptomeningeal biopsy was requested for recurrence of mental confusion with MRI findings of extensive aggravation of leptomeningeal enhancement of the brain. MRI of the spinal cord was requested according to extensive leptomeningeal enhancement of basal cisterns and posterior fossa. Treatment and clinical outcomes of DLGNT are not defined yet [11]. It is known that up to a third of patients may die of DLGNT, although other outcomes are not well reported yet [11]. Chemotherapy and radiotherapy have been tried. However, their effects on the outcome of patients with DLGNT have not been firmly validated yet.

4. Conclusion

We report an extremely rare occurrence of DLGNT in an elderly patient. His diagnosis was delayed and he was misdiagnosed as having a communicating hydrocephalus caused by tuberculous meningitis. Diagnostic error seems to be caused by difficulty in establishing a diagnosis of tuberculous meningitis, prevalence of tuberculosis in Asian country, similarity in MRI finding of leptomeningeal enhancement in basal cisterns, and an extreme rarity of DLGNT in the elderly. Although invasive, a prompt open biopsy of leptomeninges of the brain and spinal cord should be performed in case of diagnostic uncertainty in patients with typical findings of extensive leptomeningeal enhancement in basal cisterns. DLGLT should be listed in differential diagnosis of diseases causing leptomeningeal enhancement.

Conflicts of Interest

The authors have no conflicts of interest regarding this manuscript to disclose.

References

[1] M. P. Gardiman, M. Fassan, E. Orvieto et al., "Diffuse leptomeningeal glioneuronal tumors: A new entity?" *Brain Pathology*, vol. 20, no. 2, pp. 361–366, 2010.

[2] F. J. Rodriguez, A. Perry, M. K. Rosenblum et al., "Disseminated oligodendroglial-like leptomeningeal tumor of childhood: a distinctive clinicopathologic entity," *Acta Neuropathologica*, vol. 124, no. 5, pp. 627–641, 2012.

[3] D. N. Louis, A. Perry, G. Reifenberger et al., "The 2016 World Health Organization Classification of Tumors of the Central Nervous System: a summary," *Acta Neuropathologica*, vol. 131, no. 6, pp. 803–820, 2016.

[4] J. G. Smirniotopoulos, F. M. Murphy, E. J. Rushing, J. H. Rees, and J. W. Schroeder, "Patterns of contrast enhancement in the brain and meninges," *RadioGraphics*, vol. 27, no. 2, pp. 525–551, 2007.

[5] J. Burrill, C. J. Williams, G. Bain, G. Conder, A. L. Hine, and R. R. Misra, "Tuberculosis: a radiologic review," *RadioGraphics*, vol. 27, no. 5, pp. 1255–1273, 2007.

[6] M. L. H. Whiteman, "Neuroimaging of central nervous system tuberculosis in HIV-infected patients," *Neuroimaging Clinics of North America*, vol. 7, no. 2, pp. 199–214, 1997.

[7] C. Morgado and N. Ruivo, "Imaging meningo-encephalic tuberculosis," *European Journal of Radiology*, vol. 55, no. 2, pp. 188–192, 2005.

[8] J. R. Jinkins, R. Gupta, and J. Rodriguez-Carbajal, "MR imaging of central nervous system tuberculosis," *Radiologic Clinics of North America*, vol. 33, no. 4, pp. 771–786, 1995.

[9] G. E. Thwaites, T. T. H. Chau, and J. J. Farrar, "Improving the Bacteriological Diagnosis of Tuberculous Meningitis," *Journal of Clinical Microbiology*, vol. 42, no. 1, pp. 378–379, 2004.

[10] D. Hillemann, E. Richter, and S. Rüsch-Gerdes, "Use of the BACTEC mycobacteria growth indicator tube 960 automated

system for recovery of mycobacteria from 9,558 extrapulmonary specimens, including urine samples," *Journal of Clinical Microbiology*, vol. 44, no. 11, pp. 4014–4017, 2006.

[11] A. J. Dodgshun, N. SantaCruz, J. Hwang et al., "Disseminated glioneuronal tumors occurring in childhood: treatment outcomes and BRAF alterations including V600E mutation," *Journal of Neuro-Oncology*, vol. 128, no. 2, pp. 293–302, 2016.

[12] D. P. Agamanolis, C. D. Katsetos, C. J. Klonk et al., "An unusual form of superficially disseminated glioma in children: Report of 3 cases," *Journal of Child Neurology*, vol. 27, no. 6, pp. 727–733, 2012.

[13] D. M. Armao, J. Stone, M. Castillo, K.-M. Mitchell, T. W. Bouldin, and K. Suzuki, "Diffuse leptomeningeal oligodendrogliomatosis: Radiologic/pathologic correlation," *American Journal of Neuroradiology*, vol. 21, no. 6, pp. 1122–1126, 2000.

[14] T. D. Bourne, J. W. Mandell, J. A. Matsumoto, J. A. Jane, and M. B. Lopes, "Primary disseminated leptomeningeal oligodendroglioma with 1p deletion," *Journal of Neurosurgery: Pediatrics*, vol. 105, no. 6, pp. 465–469, 2006.

[15] R. Chen, D. R. Macdonald, and D. A. Ramsay, "Primary diffuse leptomeningeal oligodendroglioma: Case report," *Journal of Neurosurgery*, vol. 83, no. 4, pp. 724–728, 1995.

[16] G. Perilongo, M. Gardiman, L. Bisaglia et al., "Spinal low-grade neoplasms with extensive leptomeningeal dissemination in children," *Child's Nervous System*, vol. 18, no. 9-10, pp. 505–512, 2002.

[17] M. Preuss, H. Christiansen, A. Merkenschlager et al., "Disseminated oligodendroglial cell-like leptomeningeal tumors: preliminary diagnostic and therapeutic results for a novel tumor entity," *Journal of Neuro-Oncology*, vol. 124, no. 1, pp. 65–74, 2015.

[18] D. N. Louis, H. Ohgaki, and O. D. Wiestler, "The 2007 WHO classification of tumours of the central nervous system," *Acta Neuropathologica*, vol. 114, no. 2, pp. 97–109, 2007.

15

Vasogenic Cerebral Edema following CT Myelogram with Nonionic Omnipaque 300

Sara Khodor ⓘ[1] **and Scott Blumenthal**[2]

[1]*University of South Florida, Tampa, FL, USA*
[2]*South Florida Neurology Associates, Boca Raton, FL, USA*

Correspondence should be addressed to Sara Khodor; skhodor@health.usf.edu

Academic Editor: Dennis J. Rivet

Computed Tomography (CT) with myelogram is a relatively safe procedure. It requires the use of nonionic contrast agents which, unlike ionic contrast agents, have been associated with low complication rates. We report a case of a 69-year-old female who developed diffuse bilateral cerebral edema following a lumber myelogram with the use of intrathecal nonionic contrast agent Omnipaque (Iohexol) 300. We were able to find one other reported case of cerebral edema following the use of intrathecal nonionic contrast agent in the literature.

1. Introduction

Vasogenic edema is the most common type of cerebral edema and develops as a result of breakdown of blood brain barrier and consequent albumin and fluid shift from the intravascular space and into the extravascular space. In turn, mass effect from vasogenic edema can cause reduced cerebral perfusion leading to ischemia and cytotoxic edema. Cerebral edema is not a well-known complication of intrathecal nonionic contrast material in CT myelograms. Intrathecal injection of nonionic contrast agents is known to be associated with adverse reactions related to pressure loss in the subarachnoid space and leakage at puncture site. These adverse reactions include headache, nausea, vomiting, and dizziness. Other reported complications of intrathecal nonionic contrast injections include aseptic meningoencephalitis, status epilepticus, and seizures.

2. Case Description

A 69-year-old Caucasian woman presents with confusion, headache, generalized weakness, ataxia, and increased agitation on the second day following a CT myelogram during which she received L2-L3 interspace lumbar puncture with fluoroscopic guided injection of 15 cc Omnipaque (Iohexol) 300, a nonionic water-soluble contrast material, in the prone position using a 20-gauge spinal needle. There were no complications during the procedure and after an adequate observation period the patient was discharged in a stable condition.

Her past medical history includes chronic back pain with spinal stenosis, diabetes, coronary artery disease, hyperlipidemia, colitis, gout, atrial fibrillation, and sick sinus syndrome. Her surgical history includes pacemaker placement, hysterectomy, and tonsillectomy. She has no known allergies. Her medication includes aspirin, allopurinol, amlodipine, colchicine, furosemide, gabapentin, metformin, pravastatin, metoprolol, pregabalin, and spironolactone.

On physical examination, the patient's vitals were stable. She was noted to be restless, agitated, and disoriented to place and had hyperactive deep tendon reflexes. She had no focal neurological deficits. Except for a mild elevation in WBC of 13.0, her laboratory values including CBC, CMP, urine analysis, and toxicity screen were all within normal limits.

A head CT revealed new supratentorial bilateral vasogenic edema with loss of all sulci and with poor differentiation of white and gray matter (Figure 1). There was no evidence of any compression of the quadrigeminal plate cistern or fourth

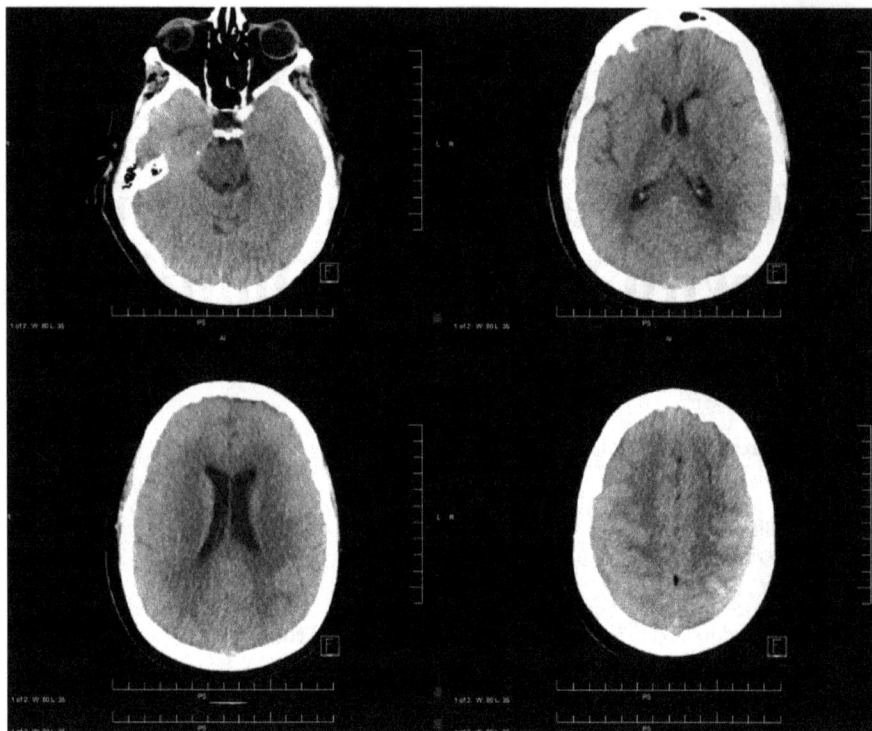

FIGURE 1: Supratentorial bilateral vasogenic edema with loss of all sulci and poor differentiation of white and gray matter.

ventricle on imaging. These findings were not visualized on previous imaging. Patient was admitted to the neurology intensive care unit (ICU) and was treated with mannitol, corticosteroids, and seizure prophylaxis. She was discharged in a stable condition after a 5-day admission with resolution of both clinical symptoms and radiographic findings of cerebral edema on head CT (Figure 2).

3. Discussion

3.1. Cerebral Edema. Cerebral edema is the accumulation of fluid in the brain as a response to cerebral injury such as trauma, infarction, hemorrhage, tumor, abscess, toxicity, and metabolism. Three types of cerebral edema include cytotoxic, vasogenic, and interstitial cerebral edema. Clinically there may be an overlap between the different types. Cytotoxic edema is the accumulation of fluid within glia, neurons, and endothelial cells most commonly due to hypoxia and usually starts within minutes of injury. Cytotoxic edema primarily affects the gray matter; however, ultimately white matter becomes involved as well [1]. Vasogenic edema, the most common type of cerebral edema, is secondary to the movement of albumin, other plasma proteins, and fluid from the intravascular space into the extravascular space. The breakdown of tight endothelial junction which compromises the blood brain barrier (BBB) facilitates this fluid shift [2]. This type of cerebral edema primarily affects the white matter [1]. Mass effect from vasogenic edema can cause reduced cerebral perfusion leading to ischemia and cytotoxic edema [2]. Interstitial

cerebral edema is seen in hydrocephalus with obstruction of CSF outflow causing an increase in intraventricular pressure and movement of fluid to the paraventricular space [1].

Clinical signs of cerebral edema will depend on the location of the edema if focal edema is with focal neurologic symptoms. However, with generalized edema, there may be symptoms of elevated intracranial pressure including central herniation with alteration in mental status, abnormalities in extraocular movement and pupil size, breathing pattern changes, elevation in blood pressure, bradycardia, extensor plantar response, etc. Neuroimaging is useful in identifying the location and the type of cerebral edema. Serial CT or MRI studies are important in monitoring the resolution of edema after therapeutic intervention. On CT, edema appears hypodense or hypoattenuated; whereas on T2 MRI or Flair pulse series it appears hyperintense.

3.2. CT Myelogram and Contrast Agents. CT myelogram is performed with the use of intrathecal contrast agent for an improved and enhanced visualization of spinal cord lesions. The first-generation contrast agents were ionic and were associated with high rates of intravascular adverse reactions due to their high osmolality. As a result, they have been replaced, for the most part except for gastrointestinal and urologic procedures, with nonionic second-generation water-soluble agents that are associated with fewer adverse reactions. Although rare, contrast-induced neurotoxicity has been well documented with intravascular use of nonionic low osmolar contrast material [3–7]. Kocabay et al. discuss

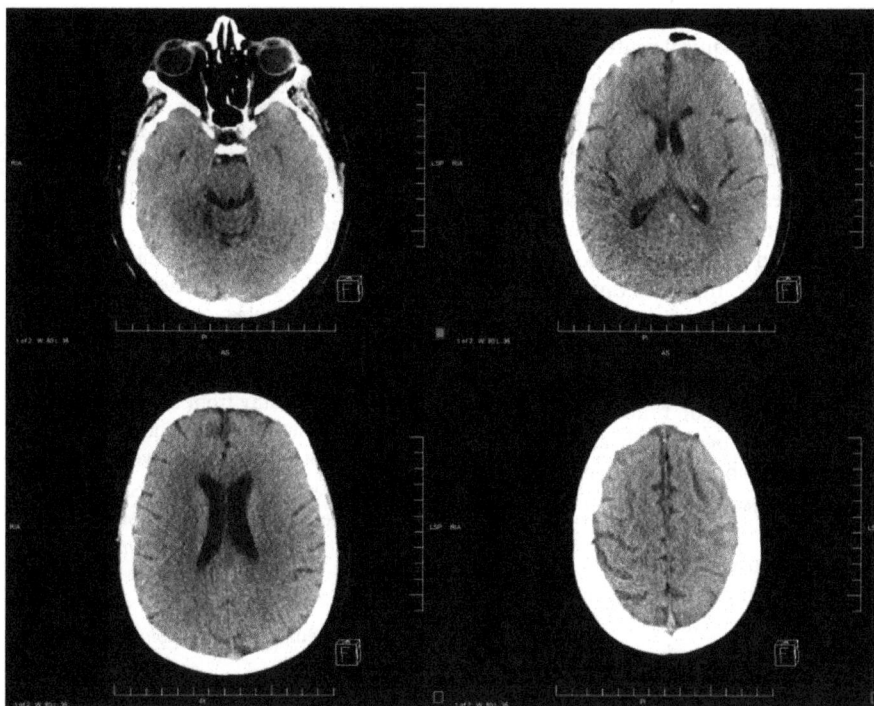

FIGURE 2: Improvement in vasogenic edema bilaterally with appreciation of sulci and improvement of white and gray matter differentiation.

contrast-induced encephalopathy, seizures, cortical blindness, and focal neurological deficits in their retrospective analysis of 9 patients with contrast-induced neurotoxicity after administration of Iopromide, a nonionic low osmolar contrast agent for coronary angiography [3]. They recognized that neurotoxicity may depend on doses, route of administration, and procedure and that the mechanism behind the pathophysiology is controversial and had been attributed to disruption of BBB [3].

As for intrathecal use in CT myelography, first-generation high osmolality contrast agents could not be used due to neurotoxicity. In 1974, this procedure was transformed with metrizamide and years later with iohexol, both nonionic contrast agents [8]. A newer agent iodixanol which is a iso-osmolar, nonionic dimer is preferable for procedures during which the central nervous system, cardiovascular, or renal system is exposed to insult [9]. However, due to its increased cost, it is reserved for known high risk patients.

The adverse reactions associated with intrathecal injections of nonionic contrast agents are headache, nausea, vomiting, or dizziness, which may largely be attributed to pressure loss in the subarachnoid space resulting from intracranial hypotension from leakage at the puncture site. However, several case reports have described complications such as aseptic meningoencephalitis [10], status epilepticus [11], and seizures [12], after intrathecal nonionic contrast injections. In a retrospective analysis, Klein et al. report a risk of seizures in nonepileptic individuals and risk of status epilepticus in patients with epilepsy who have received Iopamidol myelography [13]. Kelley et al. described a case of cerebral edema in a 50-year-old female patient who presented

with increased somnolence, headache, and visual changes a day following CT myelogram with Iopamidol [14]. Other reported cases have also described similar complications.

The pathophysiology for the development of neurotoxicity from intrathecal nonionic contrast injections is not well understood but has been linked to osmolarity disturbances [15], lipid solubility [16], or even direct toxicity [17] of these agents.

In our patient's case, she developed symptoms of cerebral edema manifested in altered mental status with reduced attention, agitation, and disorientation shortly after CT myelogram. Before the procedure, she was completely asymptomatic. This clinical presentation was supported with head CT findings of diffuse bilateral cerebral edema with absence of sulcal markings and poor differentiation of white and gray matter. We strongly suspect that the patient's presentation was a complication of the intrathecal use of nonionic Iohexol in CT myelogram.

3.3. Treatment and Management. General management of cerebral edema aims at optimizing cerebral perfusion, venous drainage, oxygenation, and minimizing cerebral metabolic demand [18]. Typical guidelines include maintenance of ICP < 20 mmHg and CPP 50 mmHg. There are various modalities which can be utilized to lower intracranial pressure and increase cerebral perfusion pressure. Elevating the head can decrease intracranial pressure (ICP) and usually recommended that the head is elevated at 30–60 degrees. Devices around the neck should be restricted as to not cause obstruction of venous outflow. Typically, patients are intubated for airway protection or to hyperventilate the patient to assist in lowering intracranial pressure. Mechanical ventilation should also be considered if the patient has hypoxia and hypercapnia as these conditions cause cerebral vasodilation and worsening edema. Controlled hyperventilation (PaCO2 25–30 mm Hg) can be used as a resuscitative measure for a short duration until more definitive therapies are instituted [18]. Other general measures including maintenance of intravascular volume with fluid management and vasopressors and adequate glycemic control are important for improved outcomes [18]. As for seizure prophylaxis, it is commonly used despite the lack of data proving its clinical benefit [18]. Specific measures such as corticosteroid therapy are used in selected patients; mostly those with vasogenic edema or brain neoplasm as it is thought to decrease capillary permeability of BBB [1]. Corticosteroids have not been shown to be effective in cytotoxic edema or stroke patients.

Medical management of cerebral edema may also entail the use of osmotic therapy, typically mannitol 20% or Hypertonic Saline. Mannitol acts as an immediate plasma expander by drawing fluid from extravascular to intravascular space, as a result improving cerebral blood flow which in turn causes cerebral vasoconstriction. Hypertonic saline acts as volume expander thus improving perfusion [19]. Loop diuretics are used sometimes in combination with osmotic agents to improve diuresis; however, their efficacy on cerebral edema is unknown and the risk of serious volume depletion may compromise cerebral perfusion. There is no strong data to support one osmotic agent over another.

In addition to the general management measures, our patient received mannitol. Close neuro exams were performed every 4 hours with gradual improvement. She was also treated with Keppra 500 oral BID for seizure prophylaxis in addition to dexamethasone 4 mg IV q6 h. Repeat CT scan showed resolution of edema (Figure 2). Patient was discharged after resolution of her symptoms and return to baseline in a stable condition after a 5-day admission to the neurology ICU.

4. Conclusion

Cerebral edema is not a well-known complication of intrathecal nonionic contrast material. We were only able to find one other similar case in the literature. Physicians should be aware of this rare complication after CT myelogram in order to implement early adequate therapeutic treatment to reduce patient's risk of mortality.

Conflicts of Interest

The authors declare that there are no conflicts of interest regarding the publication of this paper.

References

[1] S. K. Jha, "Cerebral edema and its management," *Medical Journal Armed Forces India*, vol. 59, no. 4, pp. 326–331, 2003.

[2] M. Ho, R. Rojas, and R. L. Eisenberg, "Cerebral edema," *AJR 2012*, vol. 199, pp. W258–W273, 2012.

[3] G. Kocabay, C. Y. Karabay, A. Kalayci et al., "Contrast-induced neurotoxicity after coronary angiography," *Herz*, vol. 39, no. 4, pp. 522–527, 2014.

[4] S. Law, K. Panichpisal, M. Demede et al., "Contrast-induced neurotoxicity following cardiac catheterization," *Case Reports in Medicine*, vol. 2012, Article ID 267860, 2012.

[5] J. Velden, P. Milz, F. Winkler, K. Seelos, and G. F. Hamann, "Nonionic contrast neurotoxicity after coronary angiography mimicking subarachnoid hemorrhage," *European Neurology*, vol. 49, no. 4, pp. 249–251, 2003.

[6] L. Guimaraens, E. Vivas, A. Fonnegra et al., "Transient encephalopathy from angiographic contrast: A rare complication in neurointerventional procedures," *CardioVascular and Interventional Radiology*, vol. 33, no. 2, pp. 383–388, 2010.

[7] R. Sawaya, R. Hammoud, S. Amaout, and S. Alam, "Contrast-Induced Encephalopathy following coronary angioplasty with iohexol," *The Southern Medical Journal*, vol. 100, no. 10, p. 1054, 2007.

[8] A. Torvik and P. Walday, "Neurotoxicity of water-soluble contrast media," *Acta Radiologica Supplements*, vol. 399, pp. 221–229, 1995.

[9] J. M. Widmark, "Imaging-related medications: a class overview," *Baylor University Medical Center Proceedings*, vol. 20, no. 4, pp. 408–417, 2017.

[10] J. Romesburg and M. Ragozzino, "Aseptic meningoencephalitis after iohexol CT myelography," *American Journal of Neuroradiology*, vol. 30, no. 5, pp. 1074-1075, 2009.

[11] H. Alimohammadi, A. Abdalvand, S. Safari, and A. Mazinanian, "Status epilepticus after myelography with iohexol (Omnipaque)," *The American Journal of Emergency Medicine*, vol. 30, no. 9, pp. e1–e3, 2012.

[12] S. Singh, C. Rajpal, S. Nannapeneni, and S. Venkatesh, "Iopamidol myelography-induced seizures," *MedGenMed : Medscape general medicine*, vol. 7, no. 2, p. 11, 2005.

[13] K. Klein, K. Shiratori, S. Knake et al., "Status epilepticus and seizures induced by iopamidol myelography," *Seizure*, vol. 13, no. 3, pp. 196–199, 2004.

[14] B. C. Kelley, S. Roh, P. L. Johnson, and P. M. Arnold, "Malignant cerebral edema following CT myelogram using isovuem 300 intrathecal nonionic water-soluble contrast," *Radiology Research and Practice*, vol. 2011, Article ID 212516, 2010.

[15] M. Donaghy, N. A. Fletcher, and G. D. Schott, "Encephalopathy after iohexol myelography," *The Lancet*, pp. 326–887, 1985.

[16] J. M. Caillé and M. Allard, "Neurotoxicity of hydrosoluble iodine contrast media," *Invest Radiol Suppl*, vol. 23, pp. S210–S212, 1988.

[17] T. Berod, O. Knebelmann, and F. Marjou, "Aseptic meningoencephalitis after iopamidol myelography," *Annals of Pharmacotherapy*, vol. 27, no. 9, p. 1140, 1993.

[18] A. Raslan and A. Bhardwaj, "Medical management of cerebral edema," *Neurosurgical Focus*, vol. 22, no. 5, p. E12, 2007.

[19] D. S. Mortimer and J. Jancik, "Administering hypertonic saline to patients with severe traumatic brain injury," *Journal of the American Association of Neuroscience Nurses*, vol. 38, no. 3, pp. 142–146, 2006.

16

A Case of Progressive Stroke on Posterior Circulation with Transient Bilateral Oculomotor Palsy

Chiaki Takahashi [ID]

Department of Neurosurgery, Takaoka City Hospital, 4-1, Takara-machi, Takaoka, Toyama, Japan

Correspondence should be addressed to Chiaki Takahashi; chiakit429@image.ocn.ne.jp

Academic Editor: Mehmet Turgut

Infarction located in the midbrain and pons presents various ophthalmic symptoms, because of the damage of the nuclei that control the movement of internal and external ocular and palpebral muscles. We experienced a case which presented with rare ocular symptoms and course. A 61-year-old man presented with left hemiparesis and dysarthria, bilateral ptosis, and bilateral impaired eyeball movement: right eyeball movement was totally impaired and left could only perform slight adduction. MRI showed fresh stroke in the right thalamus, cerebral crus, and posterior lobe and cuneate lesion on bilateral paramedian portion of the midbrain. MRA showed occlusion in the P1 area of the posterior cerebral artery (PCA). Transesophageal echocardiography (TEE) showed findings of a patent foramen ovale (PFO). These findings suggested cardioembolic stroke as a cause of PCA occlusion and we prescribed rivaroxaban. The patient's eyeball and eyelid movement, only on the left side, was improved imperfectly 2 weeks later. We thought that neurological findings and course of this case may have arisen from dysfunction of the oculomotor nucleus and oculomotor fascicles, and MLF results from the presence of the lesion in paramedian midbrain and pons.

1. Introduction

We sometimes encounter patients with cerebral infarction in whom the main lesion is located in the posterior circulation. In such patients, especially in a case where the lesion is in the midbrain, the severity and symptoms show great variety depending on the location and range. In particular, the vascular supply in the midbrain is much more complex than in the pons and medulla. The vasculature is supplied by branches of three arteries: the posterior cerebral artery (PCA) and the basilar and the superior cerebellar artery (SCA), depending on the level [1]. The eponymic symptoms which represent oculomotor paresis with the paramedian midbrain lesion have been named Claude syndrome [2] and Benedict syndrome [3], and these definitions are also complex. In addition, Nothnagel reported symptoms of ipsilateral or bilateral oculomotor paresis and contralateral cerebellar ataxia due to a lesion in ventral side of the midbrain including the superior colliculus [4]. We think the present case is a rare case that presented transient bilateral oculomotor paresis with ptosis and contralateral ataxia and hemiparesis. The clinical symptoms suggested Nothnagel syndrome; however, we were not able to explain some points.

2. Case Presentation

A 61-year-old man with no remarkable history had never had a regular medical examination. He has been smoking about forty cigarettes per day for more than forty years. On the morning of the day before admission, he found that he was not able to read a book as his vision became suddenly distorted. He had additionally noticed weakness in his left leg during the daytime but went to bed without going to the hospital. The next morning, his weakness grew worse and he visited our hospital in a wheelchair due to gait disturbance. At this first admission, his NIH Stroke Scale (NIHSS) score was 4 points: hemiparesis 2, sensory disturbance 1, and dysarthria 1. He complained of diplopia when he looked to the right, but we could not observe his ocular deviation. His head MRI-DWI showed a scattered fresh infarction including the right occipital lobe, cerebral crus, and thalamus, and MRA showed occlusion of the P2 area of the right PCA and left

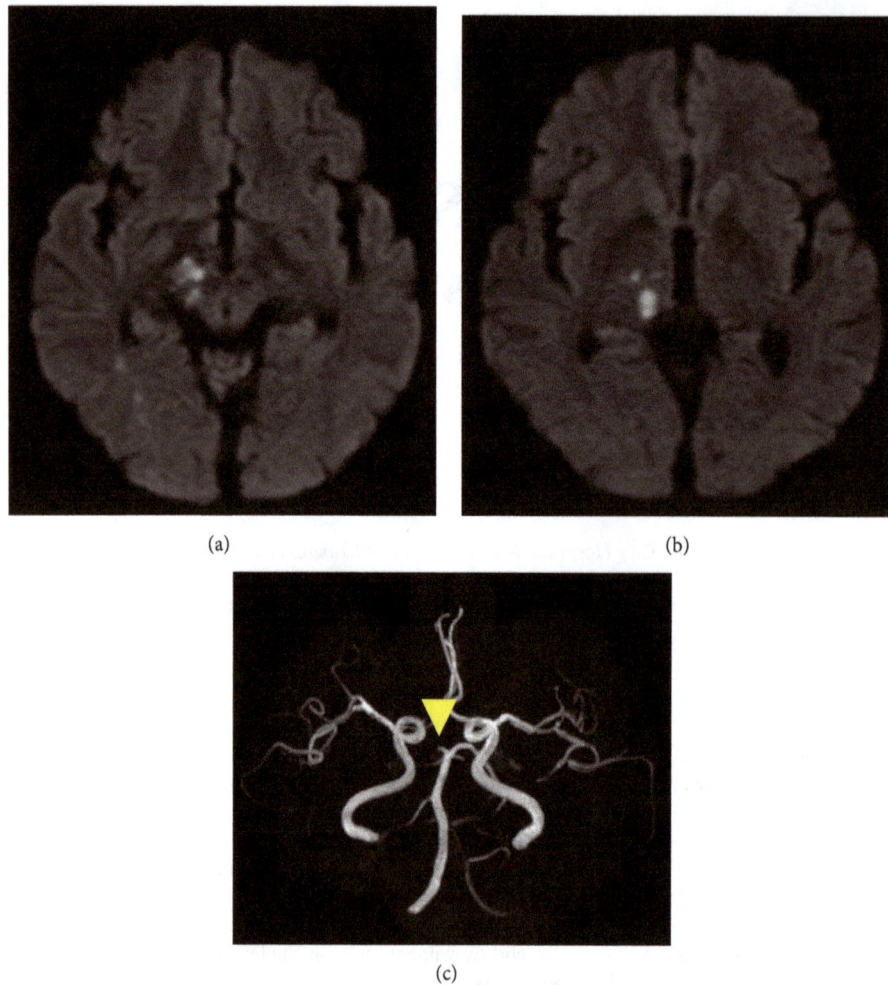

(a)

(b)

(c)

FIGURE 1: Head MRI performed about 24 hours after onset showed right occipital lobe, thalamus, cerebral crus, and midbrain fresh infarction (a, b). MRA showed right P2 (arrow head) and left SCA (superior cerebellar artery) occlusion (c).

SCA (Figure 1). Carotid ultrasound (CUS) showed findings of moderate arteriosclerosis, and plaque accumulation in the carotid bifurcation was not observed. He was admitted to our hospital. Electrocardiogram (ECG) and monitoring data showed no findings of arrhythmia. We speculated that the cause of this stroke might be atherosclerotic change at first. We decided to begin injection of argatroban hydrate and edaravone, and administered oral aspirin 100 mg.

Early the next morning, a drop in consciousness level and aggravation of left hemiparesis presented. Emergency MRI was performed and showed enlargement of the lesion in the thalamus and additional cuneate fresh stroke on the right paramedian portion of the midbrain and small spotty fresh stroke on the left paramedian portion. MRA showed the extension of the occlusion of the PCA to the P1 portion (Figure 2). At this point, we thought perforators branching from proximal part of PCA were occluded due to the progression of thrombosis in the PCA. We added cilostazol to avoid extra thrombosis. After half a day, his consciousness level began to improve, and we performed a

detailed neurological examination. At this time, we observed bilateral ptosis. He could not open his eyelids on his own and showed compensated contraction of the frontal muscle. His ocular position was median; right eyeball movement was totally impaired and left could only perform slight adduction with ocular nystagmus. The right and left pupil diameters were 6.0 mm and 5.0 mm. Light reflex was not observed on the right and was observed only slightly on the left.

During the course of treatment, transesophageal echocardiography (TEE) was performed to detect the cause of the stroke. It showed a patent foramen ovale (PFO) and noncompaction of the ventricular myocardium, which could have caused the stroke. According to the findings on TEE, we were convinced that the cause of the stroke was cardioembolic and changed his prescription from aspirin to rivaroxaban 20 mg.

His consciousness level improved gradually, and oculomotor paresis including ptosis only on the left side was also improved imperfectly 2 weeks later. Finally, disturbance of upward and downward abduction remained on the left side

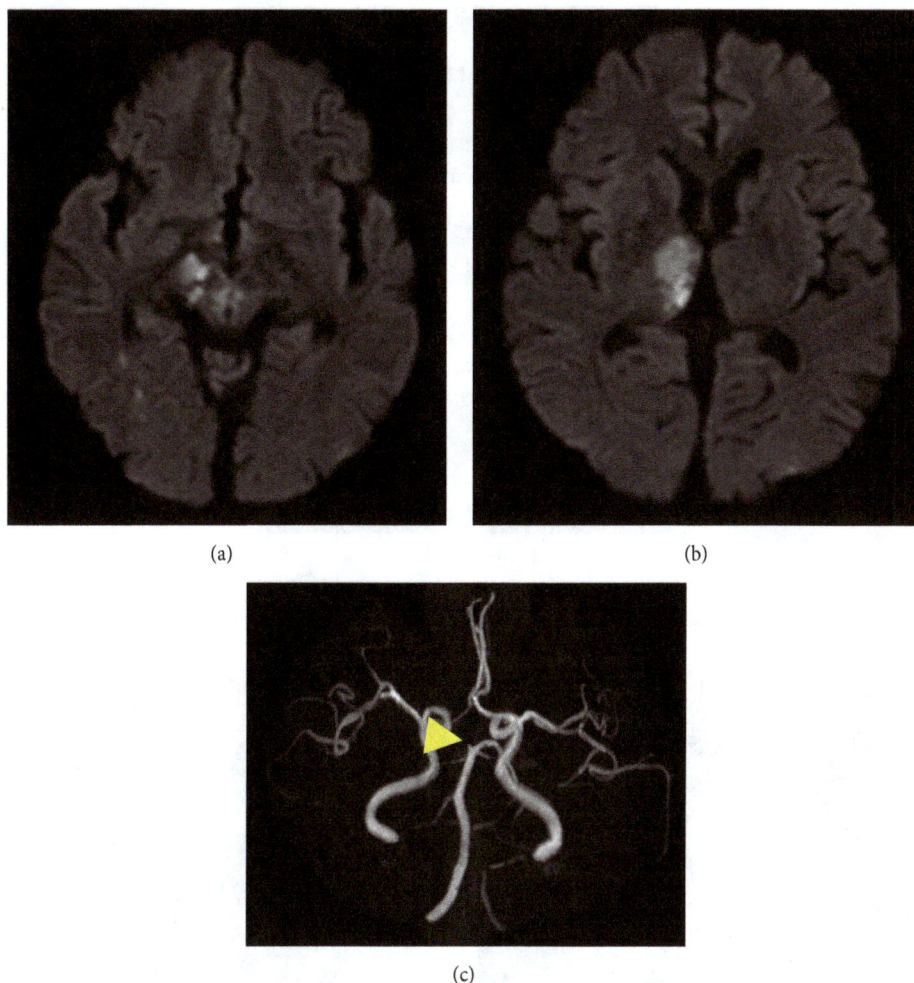

(a)

(b)

(c)

FIGURE 2: Head MRI performed after aggravation of neurological symptoms showed enlargement of infarction (a, b). MRA showed extension of occlusion (arrow head) to the P1 (c).

and severe oculomotor palsy also remained in the right side (Figure 3). He could not achieve ocular convergence and Bell phenomenon in both eyes.

In addition, with regard to the motor paresis, we observed complete hemiplegia in the left upper extremity in the flexed position and mild hemiparesis in the left lower extremity. With the improvement of his consciousness level, he started standing and walking training with physical therapists. Although his muscle strength on the left lower extremity was sufficient, he had difficulty with those types of training due to ataxia of bilateral body trunk and lower extremities and attentional deficit as a higher brain dysfunction. Ultimately, he acquired walking ability with a cane, but he risked losing his balance and falling down when he had a lapse of concentration. With regard to higher brain dysfunction, mild cognitive dysfunction and memory deficit were present. At 12 weeks after initial presentation, he could leave our hospital and go home in relatively good condition.

3. Discussion

At first, neurological deficits in this case due to the occlusion of the P2 area of the PCA were not severe; they later became

severe as a consequence of the enlargement of infarction due to the progressive thrombosis of the PCA and occlusion of the perforators branching from the P1 area. MRI showed a thalamic, cerebral crus and cuneate fresh stroke on the right paramedian portion of the midbrain and a very small spotty fresh stroke on the left paramedian portion. At first, we did not detect the left spotty infarction, but his clinical findings could not be explained; hence, we carefully reexamined his MRI referring to his apparent diffusion coefficient (ADC) map (Figure 4). The vasculature of the paramedian midbrain tegmentum was supplied by perforators branching like a fan from the P1 area up and down. These perforators are divided into 4 groups [5]. The first branch is called the thalamoperforating artery, and the second and third branches are the median mesencephalic arteries which supply the midbrain and the fourth branch is the superior pontine tegmental branch which supplies the pons [5]. Of these, the first and second branches bifurcate to the bilateral side with a probability of 10% [6]. In that case, the symptoms of the patient become potentially severe when the first or second branches are occluded by thrombus. It will bring the bilateral mesencephalic lesion. We detected the bilateral

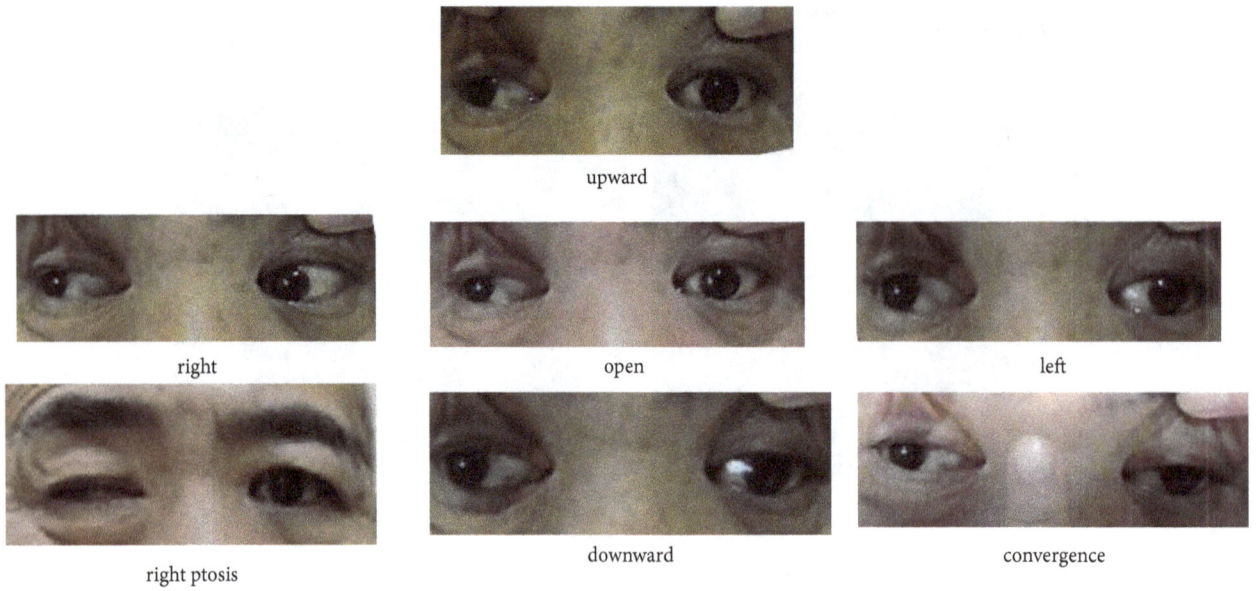

FIGURE 3: Findings of ptosis and oculomotor palsy one month after onset.

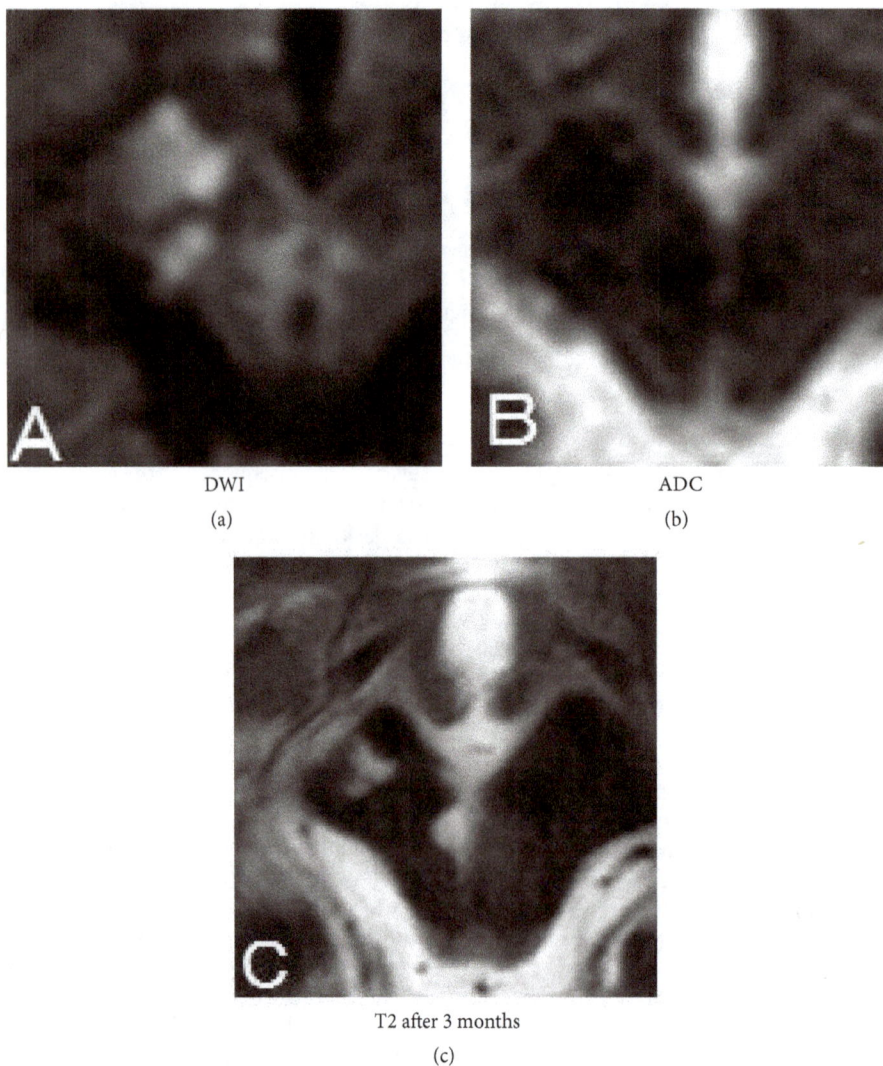

DWI

(a)

ADC

(b)

T2 after 3 months

(c)

FIGURE 4: Head MRI on midbrain performed after aggravation of neurological symptoms. ADC map indicates the left paramedian lesion as stroke (a, b). Bilateral paramedian lesions three months after onset (c).

mesencephalic lesions in our case and considered that the second branch might be occluded.

When the patient's condition showed abrupt change at first, we observed these neurological symptoms: (1) bilateral total ophthalmoplegia with bilateral ptosis (the left eye could only perform slight adduction with ocular nystagmus), (2) contralateral hemiparesis and ataxia, and (3) consciousness disturbance. One month later, his neurological symptoms had improved: (1) right oculomotor palsy with ptosis, (2) contralateral abducens palsy with ocular nystagmus, (3) disturbance of bilateral suprainfraduction, (4) contralateral hemiparesis and ataxia, and (5) cognitive dysfunction and attentional deficit.

We considered the mechanism of the change of the symptoms and the affected region. At first, we could posit that the bilateral oculomotor palsy affected his symptoms because of the existence of the distinctive symptoms, bilateral ptosis, pupillary abnormality, and so on, and the lesion on paramedian midbrain lesion in MRI.

The nucleus of the oculomotor nerve is placed in the midline region of the midbrain. It exists in complex with multiple independent subnuclei, controlling the superior, inferior, and medial rectus muscle, inferior oblique muscle, levator palpebrae superioris muscle, and sphincter pupillae, respectively. Of all others, the caudal central subnucleus (CCN), which controls the levator palpebrae superioris muscle, exists in the center area of the midbrain and dominates the bilateral elevation of the eyelids [7, 8] (Figure 5). The nerve fibers which arise from the oculomotor subnucleus form the oculomotor fascicles near the red nucleus and make a transition to the extramedullary oculomotor nerve [9, 10].

At first, we inferred from his MRI and clinical symptoms that his partial neurological findings were due to nuclear damage of the whole oculomotor complex including the CCN. At that time, the severity of bilateral ptosis was almost the same between right and left eyelid. In addition, his pupil showed bilateral mydriasis. We thought that these findings are not likely with the damage of the oculomotor fascicles. However, left ptosis and oculomotor palsy were improved one month later. As a damaged CCN cannot later show unilateral improvement of ptosis [10], we determined that the CCN was not damaged and that part of the fascicles was damaged bilaterally and then showed mild or incomplete improvement on the left side. Indeed, a case of oculomotor palsy without ptosis was reported as a result of the sparing of the CCN from the damage of stroke [10]. Besides, it is said that the subnuclei of the superior rectus muscle control the contralateral side [11]. In our case strong disturbance of the supra and infraduction of the bilateral side persisted one month later. We speculated about the two possibilities to be able to evoke it. At first, according to the figure of the oculomotor complex by Warwick (Figure 5), we thought that the subnuclei of the supra- and infraduction were damaged bilaterally due to the involvement of the dorsal side of the upper to lower oculomotor complex in the infarction lesion. We thought that the bilateral nerve fibers of the levator palpebrae superioris muscle were damaged in the oculomotor fascicles and that of the other external and internal muscles controlled by the oculomotor nerve were damaged supranuclearly.

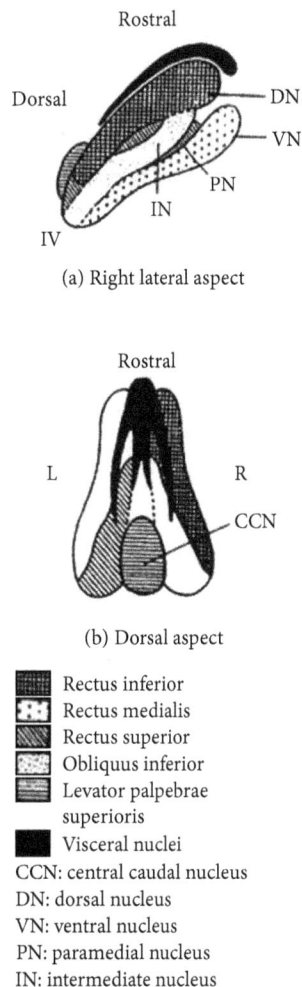

Rostral

Dorsal

DN
VN
PN
IN

IV

(a) Right lateral aspect

Rostral

L   R

CCN

(b) Dorsal aspect

Rectus inferior
Rectus medialis
Rectus superior
Obliquus inferior
Levator palpebrae superioris
Visceral nuclei

CCN: central caudal nucleus
DN: dorsal nucleus
VN: ventral nucleus
PN: paramedial nucleus
IN: intermediate nucleus

FIGURE 5: Structure of the oculomotor complex indicated by Warwick [7].

Secondly, ischemic lesion extended to the rostral interstitial nucleus of the medial longitudinal fascicles (riMLF) or interstitial nucleus of Cajal placed in rostral-medial side of the red nucleus might bring Parinaud's syndrome [12].

Then, we considered the behaviors which are impossible to explain only with the dysfunction around the level of the oculomotor nucleus.

The positions of the bilateral eyes were almost neutral at first and he could abduct only his left eyeball slightly with ocular nystagmus. One month later, his right eyeball was fixed completely to the abducted position and he could abduct his left eyeball incompletely with ocular nystagmus.

Granted that the stroke lesion in the upper pons which was impossible to detect by MRI existed, we considered several possibilities. One-and-a-half syndrome and medial longitudinal fascicles (MLF) syndrome are caused by the damage of paramedian area of the pons. The former does not fit into the behaviors of his eye movement, because he could adduct his left eye. Besides, we also considered WEBINO syndrome which is caused by the bilateral MLF syndrome. In such a case, we could observe the alternative exotropia when

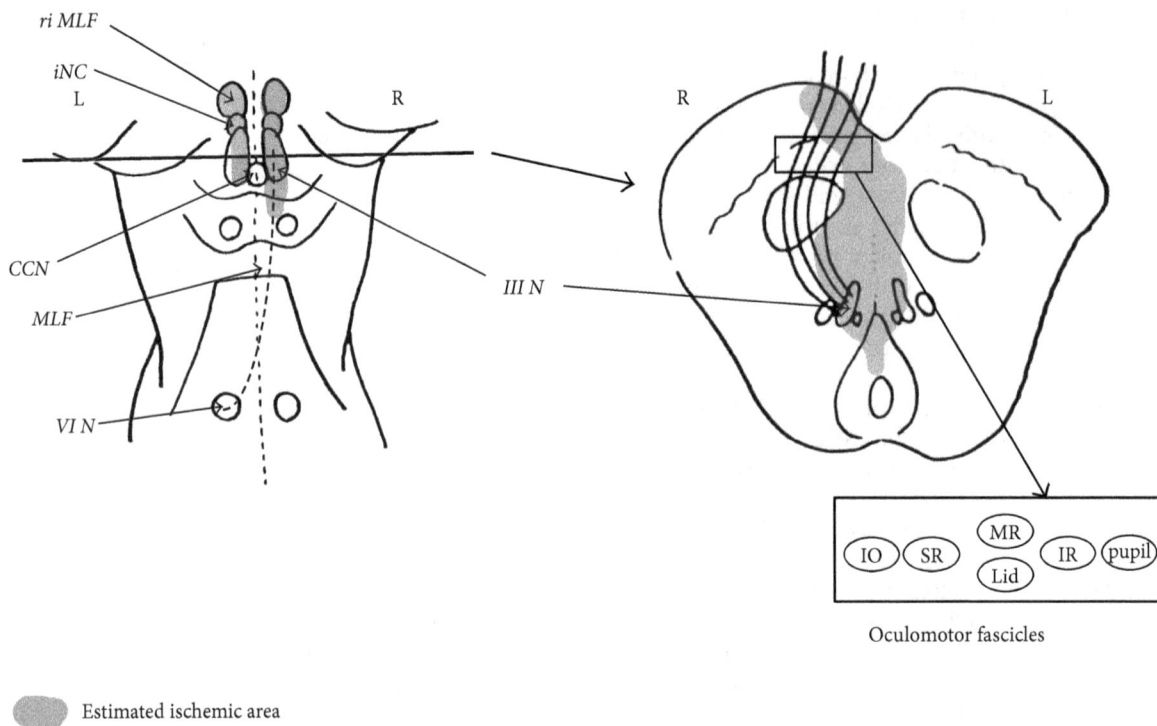

FIGURE 6: Picture in the left shows dorsal side of the midbrain and pons and in the right shows cross-sectional view of the midbrain along the line. Gray areas mark the ischemic area. riMLF: rostral interstitial nucleus of medial longitudinal fasciculus, iNC: interstitial nucleus of Cajal, CCN: caudal central subnucleus, MLF: medial longitudinal fasciculus, III N: oculomotor nucleus, VI N: abducens nucleus, IO: intraocular muscles, SR: superior rectus muscle, MR: medial rectus muscle, Lid: Levator palpebrae superioris muscle, IR: inferior rectus muscle, and pupil: sphincter pupillae muscles.

the patient holds fixation with a single eye. However his right eye always fixed into the abducted position regardless of the behavior of right eye; it also does not fit. Besides, it is reported that WEBINO syndrome due to pontine lesion often shows convergence impairment [13].

So, we speculated about it as follows.

At first, both bilateral oculomotor palsy which was stronger in the right eye and the right MLF syndrome existed, and then the left oculomotor palsy improved, and the right strong oculomotor palsy and the right MLF syndrome might remain finally. The left abducens palsy might be a movement of the intact side with nystagmus. Besides, his convergence palsy is explainable by coexisting dysfunction of the oculomotor nucleus.

We described the final estimated ischemic area in his brain stem (Figure 6). The figure in the left side shows the dorsal side of the brainstem and it describes ischemic area including the bilateral oculomotor nucleus without CCN and right MLF. The figure in the right side shows cross-sectional view of the midbrain along the line. It describes the ischemic part of the oculomotor fascicles pointed by the MRI image. Castro et al. reported these fascicles lines like the schema in the lower right side [14].

In addition, cognitive dysfunction and attentional deficit were presented and may have arisen from the inclusion of the thalamus [15]. Contralateral hemiparesis may have arisen from the stroke of the cerebral crus, and ataxia may have arisen from the thalamic stroke.

We obtained informed consent from the patient to use personal information and data including photographs of eyes, images of MRI, and health records.

Conflicts of Interest

The authors declare no conflicts of interest concerning this manuscript.

References

[1] E. Kumral, G. Bayulkem, A. Akyol, N. Yunten, H. Sirin, and A. Sagduyu, "Mesencephalic and associated posterior circulation infarcts," *Stroke*, vol. 33, no. 9, pp. 2224–2231, 2002.

[2] H. Claude, "Syndrome pedonculaire de la region du noyau rouge," *Revue Neurologique*, vol. 23, pp. 311–313, 1912.

[3] M. Benedikt, "Tremblement avec paralysie croisee du moteur oculaire commun," *Bulletin Medical (Paris)*, vol. 3, pp. 547-548, 1889.

[4] H. Nothnagel, "On the diagnosis of diseases of the corpora quadrigemina," *Brain*, vol. 12, no. 1-2, pp. 21–35, 1889.

[5] N. Goto, "Microanatomy of brainstem blood supply for clinical diagnosis," *Neurosurgeons*, vol. 5, pp. 127–138, 1985 (Japanese).

[6] A. Pedroza, M. Dujovny, J. I. Ausman et al., "Microvascular anatomy of the interpeduncular fossa," *Journal of Neurosurgery*, vol. 64, no. 3, pp. 484–493, 1986.

[7] R. Warwick, "Oculomotor organization," *Annals of the Royal College of Surgeons of England*, vol. 19, pp. 36–52, 1956.

[8] K. Ruchalski and G. M. Hathout, "A medley of midbrain maladies: a brief review of midbrain anatomy and syndromology for radiologists," *Radiology Research and Practice*, vol. 2012, Article ID 258524, 11 pages, 2012.

[9] N. Saeki, A. Yamaura, and K. Sunami, "Bilateral ptosis with pupil sparing because of a discrete midbrain lesion: magnetic resonance imaging evidence of topographic arrangement within the oculomotor nerve," *Journal of Neuro-Ophthalmology*, vol. 20, no. 2, pp. 130–134, 2000.

[10] J. Sargent, "Nuclear and infranuclear ocular motility disarders," in *Clinical Neuro-Ophthalmology*, N. R. Miller, P. S. Subramanian, and V. R. Patel, Eds., pp. 341–371, Wolters Kluwer, 2016.

[11] L. R. Caplan, "'Top of basilar' syndrome," *Neurology*, vol. 55, pp. 72–79, 1980.

[12] M. B. Bender, "Brain control of conjugate horjzontal and vertical eye movements: A survey of the stductural and functional correlates," *Brain*, vol. 103, no. 1, pp. 23–69, 1980.

[13] T. Yoshinaga, K. Nakamura, K. Kaneko, and A. Nakamura, "A case report of WEBINO syndrome with convergence impairment," *Journal of Neurology and Neurophysiology*, vol. 6, article 270, 2005.

[14] O. Castro, L. N. Johnson, and A. C. Mamourian, "Isolated inferior oblique paresis from brainstem infarction: perspective on oculomotor fascicular organization in the ventral midbrain tegmentum," *Archives of Neurology*, vol. 47, no. 2, pp. 235–237, 1990.

[15] R. P. Mills and P. D. Swanson, "Vertical oculomotor apraxia and memory loss," *Annals of Neurology*, vol. 4, no. 2, pp. 149–153, 1978.

17

A 66-Year-Old Woman with a Progressive, Longitudinally Extensive, Tract Specific, Myelopathy

Elizabeth O'Keefe,[1] Katherine E. Schwetye,[2] John Nazarian,[3]
Richard Perrin,[4] Robert E. Schmidt,[4] and Robert Bucelli[5]

[1]Department of Neurology, Division of Physical Medicine and Rehabilitation, Washington University School of Medicine,
  Campus Box 8518, 4444 Forest Park Blvd., St. Louis, MO 63108, USA
[2]Department of Pathology & Immunology, Division of Neuropathology, Saint Louis University School of Medicine,
  1402 South Grand Blvd., Saint Louis, MO 63104, USA
[3]Department of Radiology, Wake Radiology, 3949 Browning Place, Raleigh, NC 2760, USA
[4]Department of Pathology & Immunology, Division of Neuropathology, Washington University School of Medicine, Campus Box 8118,
  660 S. Euclid Ave., St. Louis, MO 63110, USA
[5]Department of Neurology, Divisions of Neuromuscular and General Neurology, Washington University School of Medicine,
  Campus Box 8111, 660 S. Euclid Ave., St. Louis, MO 63110, USA

Correspondence should be addressed to Robert Bucelli; bucellir@neuro.wustl.edu

Academic Editor: Peter Berlit

A 66-year-old woman presented with progressive lancinating pain and sensory deficits attributable to a myelopathy of unclear etiology. Spinal cord magnetic resonance imaging showed a longitudinally extensive T2-hyperintense lesion of the dorsal columns. Comprehensive serum, urine, and cerebrospinal fluid analyses failed to identify an etiology. Empiric intravenous methylprednisolone and intravenous immunoglobulin were of no benefit and serial screens for an occult malignancy were negative. She developed dysesthesias and allodynia affecting her entire body and lost the use of her arms and legs due to severe sensory ataxia that was steadily progressive from onset. She opted against additional aggressive medical management of her condition and passed away on hospice eleven months after symptom onset. Autopsy revealed findings most consistent with polyphasic spinal cord ischemia affecting the dorsal and lateral white matter tracts and, to a lesser extent, adjacent gray matter. The underlying etiology for the progressive vasculopathy remains unknown. Spinal cord ischemia affecting the posterior spinal cord is rare and to our knowledge this case represents the only instance of a progressive spinal cord tractopathy attributable to chronic spinal cord ischemia.

1. Introduction

Dorsal column myelopathies commonly present with a chief complaint of ataxia and incoordination. Exam findings include loss of proprioception (leading to sensory ataxia), vibration sense, two-point discrimination and light touch with preserved pain, and temperature sensation [1, 2]. The differential diagnosis includes infectious, inflammatory (including autoimmune, paraneoplastic, and demyelinating), metabolic, toxic, and vascular (e.g., dural arteriovenous

fistula) etiologies which may be seen as longitudinally extensive T2 hyperintensity localized to the dorsal columns on magnetic resonance imaging (MRI, see "Differential Diagnosis of Chronic Myelopathy") [2–11]. Although exceedingly rare, posterior cord syndromes can also be associated with an ischemic infarct of the spinal cord [5]. However, cases of dorsal spinal cord ischemia reported in the literature are associated with typical temporal features of a vascular disorder, including acute onset and monophasic course [5, 6].

Differential Diagnosis of Chronic Myelopathy

Inflammatory/Autoimmune

 (i) Vasculitis

 (ii) Neuro-Behcet's

 (iii) Sjögren's

 (iv) Neurosarcoidosis

 (v) Lupus

 (vi) Paraneoplastic (most common antibodies)

  (a) amphiphysin immunoglobulin G [IgG]

  (b) collapsin response-mediator protein 5 IgG

  (c) Purkinje-cell cytoplasmic autoantibody type 1, 2

  (d) antineuronal nuclear autoantibody (ANNA-1), and ANNA-3

 (vii) Neuromyelitis optica (NMO) and NMO spectrum disorders

  (a) Aquaporin-4 IgG

  (b) Myelin-oligodendrocyte glycoprotein (MOG) IgG (rare in adults)

  (c) Seronegative NMO (controversial entity)

 (viii) Multiple sclerosis

 (ix) Sarcoidosis

 (x) CLIPPERS (chronic lymphocytic inflammation with pontine perivascular enhancement responsive to steroids)

 (xi) Acute disseminated encephalomyelitis (ADEM) (rare in adults)

Vascular

 (i) Spinal cord infarction

 (ii) Arteriovenous malformations

 (iii) Diffuse atherosclerosis

 (iv) Dural arteriovenous fistula

Hereditary/Degenerative

 (i) Primary lateral sclerosis

 (ii) Hereditary spastic paraparesis

 (iii) Spinocerebellar ataxias

 (iv) Mitochondrial disorders

 (v) Adult polyglucosan body disease

Compressive/Structural

 (i) Tumor

 (ii) Atlantoaxial subluxation

 (iii) Syrinx

Metabolic

 (i) B12 deficiency

 (ii) Copper deficiency

 (iii) Vitamin E deficiency

Toxic

 (i) Radiation myelopathy

 (ii) Nitrous oxide

Infectious

 (i) Human immunodeficiency virus (HIV)

 (ii) Human T-lymphotropic virus (HTLV)-1

 (iii) Neurosyphilis

 (iv) Schistosomiasis

 (v) Brucellosis

Differential Diagnosis of a Dorsal Column Myelopathy

Metabolic

 (i) B12 deficiency

 (ii) Copper deficiency

Vascular

 (i) Posterior spinal artery infarction

 (ii) Vascular malformations

 (iii) AVFs

Infectious

 (i) Neurosyphilis

 (ii) HIV

See [1–6, 26–28].

We present the case of a woman with a predominantly progressive posterior cord syndrome of unclear etiology. Autopsy findings suggest that chronic, progressive microvasculopathy should be considered in the differential diagnosis of a dorsal column myelopathy when alternative, more common, etiologies have been ruled out.

2. Case Presentation

A 66-year-old woman presented with lancinating pain, allodynia, and numbness that steadily ascended from her feet to the level of her umbilicus over a three-month period. There was no clinical history to suggest an episodic or relapsing-remitting course. Her past medical history was significant for tobacco use, hypertension, poorly controlled type II diabetes mellitus, chronic kidney disease, chronic obstructive pulmonary disease, breast cancer (ductal carcinoma, otherwise unspecified; 13 years after mastectomy and reconstruction, not requiring chemotherapy), and a ruptured hepatic abscess (8 years after abdominal wall reconstruction). She had no known history of nitrous oxide exposure. Her

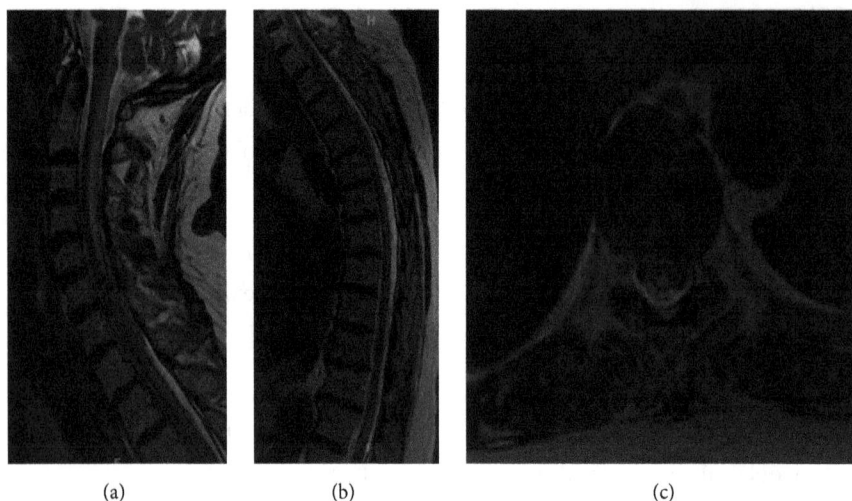

(a)   (b)   (c)

FIGURE 1: Sagittal T2-weighted MR images through the cervical (a) and thoracic (b) spine demonstrate diffuse, hyperintense signal in the posterior columns, extending nearly the entire length of the spinal cord. An axial T2W image at T9-T10 (c) demonstrates the cross-sectional extent of the signal abnormality.

neurologic examination showed normal mental status and cranial nerves and a normal motor exam when utilizing visual feedback to guide movement of the muscle groups being tested. She had no visual field deficits on bedside testing and there were no other clinical signs or symptoms of optic neuropathy. Joint position sense was severely impaired, with a corresponding severe sensory ataxia and impaired upper and lower extremity vibration sense (distal worse than proximal). Reflexes were symmetrically brisk (3+). Bilateral Babinski and Hoffman's signs were elicited.

MRI of the cervical and thoracic spine was obtained at the time of presentation and demonstrated mild, diffuse atrophy of the cord and a diffuse hyperintense signal on T2-weighted images within the dorsal columns, extending from the craniocervical junction to T12 (Figure 1). A low creatinine clearance precluded a contrast enhanced MRI of the spine and spinal angiography to evaluate for a dural arteriovenous fistula (AVF). MRI of the brain showed punctate T2 white matter hyperintensities, a finding felt to be most consistent with small vessel disease in this clinical context.

3. Clinical Discussion

The differential diagnosis for a dorsal column predominant "tractopathy" is broad and includes infectious, inflammatory/autoimmune/demyelinating, metabolic, toxic, and vascular (e.g., dural arteriovenous fistula or rarely ischemic infarction) etiologies (see *"Differential Diagnosis of Chronic Myelopathy"*). A lesion involving the dorsal columns symmetrically and extending over so many spinal levels with commensurate cord atrophy might suggest a metabolic process such as subacute combined degeneration from vitamin B12 deficiency or copper-deficiency myeloneuropathy. However, chronic sequelae from syphilis (tabes dorsalis) or HIV (vacuolar myelopathy) could have the same appearance. In contrast, homogenous extension over such a long spinal

segment, without contrast enhancement, would be unusual for a demyelinating disease, such as multiple sclerosis or neuromyelitis optica (NMO), or for a neoplasm. Although intravascular B cell lymphoma (IVBCL) can present with longitudinally extensive spinal cord lesions, this neoplasm would be expected to cause expansion of the cord and is rarely predominantly tract specific [13].

Paraneoplastic myelopathies, on the other hand, are commonly tract specific [8, 14–16]. Antineuronal nuclear antigen 1 (ANNA-1, also known as anti-Hu), antineuronal nuclear antigen 2 (ANNA-2), antineuronal antigen 3 (ANNA-3), antiamphiphysin, and anticollapsing response mediator protein 5 (CRMP-5) are among the most common antibodies identified in patients with paraneoplastic myelopathies [17]. However, antibodies directed against a number of other surface and intracellular antigens have also been reported [8, 18]. Paraneoplastic myelopathies have been reported in association with many forms of cancer, the most common being breast and lung cancer [17].

4. Diagnostic Evaluation and Management

An extensive evaluation for metabolic/toxic (vitamin B12 deficiency, copper deficiency, vitamin E deficiency, and heavy metals), infectious (bacterial (syphilis), viral (HIV, fungal, and tuberculosis)), and autoimmune etiologies (NMO, MS, and sarcoidosis) was nondiagnostic (Table 1). Neurosyphilis was excluded by the absence of pleocytosis on CSF analysis and a negative serum RPR and CSF VRDL. A purified-protein derivative skin test for tuberculosis was negative. A serum paraneoplastic autoantibody panel including anti-striated muscle, antiacetylcholine receptor (ganglionic neuronal), voltage-gated calcium channel P/Q type, anti-CRMP-5 IgG, antineuronal nuclear 1, 2, 3, anti-Purkinje cell cytoplasmic types 1 and 2 and TR, antiamphiphysin, antiglial nuclear, antineuronal voltage-gated potassium channel, and

TABLE 1: Relevant data.

Plasma/serum/urine		
Vitamin B12 (211–911 pg/mL)	524 pg/mL	
Methylmalonic acid (≤0.40 nmol/L)	0.31 nmol/L	
Homocysteine (5–15 μmol/L)	11.7 μmol/L	
Vitamin E (5.5–17.0 mg/L)	17.7 mg/L	
TSH (0.35–5.50 mcIU/mL)	1.07 mcIUnits/mL	
Free T4 (0.9–1.8 ng/dL)	1.12 ng/dL	
β2-Microglobulin (1.1–2.5 mg/L)	4.4 mg/L	
ANA, ANCA, anti-dsDNA, ENA	Negative	
24-hour urine heavy metals (mercury, lead, arsenic)	Negative	
24-hour urine zinc (300–600 mcg/24 h)	909 mcg/24 hr	
24-hour urine copper (15–60 mcg/24 h)	22 mcg/24 hr	
Serum paraneoplastic panel × 2*	0.03 and 0.04 nmol/L	
Negative except for calcium channel ab N-type (<0.03)		
Pathology		
CSF cytology	Negative	
Fine needle aspiration of right paratracheal lymph node	Negative	
Skin biopsy	Negative for lymphoma	
Quadriceps biopsy	Negative for lymphoma	
Microbiology		
HIV	Negative	
HTLV-1	Negative	
RPR	Negative	
Mycobacteria (AFB) culture and acid fast stain	Negative	
PPD	Negative	
Blood cultures	Negative	
Urine cultures	Negative	
Respiratory cultures from bronchoalveolar lavage	Negative	
CSF culture × 2	Negative	
Fungal culture of blood	Negative	
CSF	*Jun 14*	*Aug 14*
Glucose	113 mg/dL	120 mg/dL
Protein (15–45 mg/dl)	30 mg/dL	41 mg/dL
Nucleated cells (cells/μL)	0	0
Red blood cells	0	0
CSF IgG index (≤0.85)	0.6	0.62
CSF specific oligoclonal bands	0	0
CSF paraneoplastic panel*	Negative	
CSF cytology		

Electromyography (EMG)/ nerve conduction study

Length-dependent sensorimotor axonal polyneuropathy with small sural sensory nerve action potential amplitudes and EMG evidence of subacute and chronic neurogenic changes limited to a distal leg muscle.

TSH, thyroid stimulating hormone; HIV, human immunodeficiency virus; HTLV, human T-lymphotropic virus; RPR, rapid plasma reagin; ANA, anti-nuclear antibody; ANCA, anti-neutrophil cytoplasmic antibody; dsDNA, double-stranded DNA; ENA, extractable nuclear antigen.
*Paraneoplastic panel: antistriated muscle; antiacetylcholine receptor (ganglionic neuronal); anti-voltage-gated calcium channel binding P/Q type; CRMP-5 IgG; antineuronal nuclear 1, 2, 3; Purkinje cell cytoplasmic types 1 and 2 and TR; amphiphysin, antiglial nuclear; antineuronal voltage-gated potassium channel; and anti-GAD65 antibodies. CSF panel tested with indirect immunofluorescence assay and serum panel tested with indirect immunofluorescence assay and radioimmunoassay (RIA) [12].

anti-GAD65 antibodies, as well as serum aquaporin-4 IgG was performed by Mayo Clinic, Rochester, Minnesota [12]. This panel was borderline positive for N-type voltage-gated calcium channel (VGCC) antibodies at a titer of 0.03 nM on an initial sample and 0.04 nM on a repeat sample sent two months after her initial presentation. The patient underwent extensive screening for an occult malignancy, including a whole body positron emission tomography/computed tomography (PET/CT) scan, mammography, and colonoscopy, all of which were negative/nondiagnostic. PET scan did show FDG-avid lesions in lung parenchyma and paratracheal nodes which prompted biopsy of the paratracheal nodes which were negative for malignancy and showed no granulomatous disease. Electromyography and nerve conduction studies showed a mild, axonal, length-dependent sensorimotor polyneuropathy. A quadriceps biopsy performed to screen for IVBCL showed chronic neurogenic changes of increased fiber size variation, pyknotic nuclear clumps, and grouped atrophy with fiber type grouping. A skin biopsy also showed no evidence of intravascular B cell lymphoma. Empiric intravenous methylprednisolone (3 of 5 grams completed over 3 days, with the final two grams held due to significant hyperglycemia) and intravenous immunoglobulin (IVIg, 2 g/kg) were of no benefit. After discharge her disease continued to steadily progress and she was readmitted 3 weeks later with worsened upper limb sensory ataxia, rendering her unable to feed herself or live independently. Her allodynia and pain had similarly escalated and were no longer responsive to symptomatic therapies. Two additional IVIg (1 g/kg/month) treatments were of no benefit. Given her intractable pain, bedbound status with a hospitalization for pneumonia, and 100% dependency for all activities of daily living, she was placed on comfort care through home hospice. She passed away eleven months after onset of symptoms.

5. Neuropathologic Findings

Postmortem examination confirmed the cause of death as bilateral pneumonia with multiple flora and foreign material (consistent with aspiration) and found severe diffuse atherosclerosis within the aorta from the arch to the bifurcation, with evidence of ulceration. No neoplasm was detected. Gross examination of the spinal cord revealed atrophy and mild discoloration. Microscopic examination of the spinal cord showed a complex polyphasic myelopathy affecting dorsal and lateral white matter tracts and, to a lesser extent, adjacent gray matter. More specifically, the dorsal columns showed degeneration in a medial-to-lateral gradient, with evidence of acute, subacute, and chronic changes. The more acute/subacute changes included a neutrophilic infiltrate limited to the medial portions of the dorsal columns, appearing in association with acute/subacute necrosis, reactive/reparative vasculature, activated microglia, and numerous foamy macrophages (Figure 2). The chronic changes included loss of myelinated axons (Figures 3 and 4). Similar chronic changes were observed within the lateral corticospinal tracts, with extension into the ventrolateral white matter and adjacent gray matter (Figure 5). The superficial

white matter and ventral-most areas of white and gray matter were relatively spared.

Outside the areas of injury, blood vessels in the spinal cord showed only moderate arteriolosclerosis, without inflammation or thrombosis. Similar arteriolosclerosis was evident in the brain and meninges. The brainstem showed only very focal coarse vacuolation of the right spinothalamic tract and ventral spinocerebellar tract in the lateral medulla; other ascending and descending tracts were unremarkable. Sections of sampled dorsal root ganglia showed no evidence of nodules of Nageotte or of ganglion cell damage or loss. The feeding vessels of the vertebral and spinal arteries, which originate from the aorta, were not collected during prosection, so subsequent histopathologic examination of these vessels was not possible.

This pattern of spinal cord injury, involving the dorsal columns in a gradient of severity from medial (worst) to lateral (less severe) and also involving the dorsolateral white matter, correlated with the clinical history of ascending sensory symptoms. Coupled with damage to gray matter, this pattern also raised suspicion for chronic ischemia/infarction as an etiology for the patient's myelopathy.

6. Discussion

This case is unique and instructive for both the spatial (predominantly posterior columns on imaging with involvement of additional tracts on tissue analysis) and temporal (subacute-to-chronic and steadily progressive) pattern of myelopathy, presumed secondary to a polyphasic ischemic process. Typically, spinal cord infarction presents with an acute onset of deficits that vary based on the territories involved. Overall, nontraumatic spinal cord ischemia or infarction accounts for only ~1% of total strokes [17]. Usually, spinal cord ischemia/infarction results from hypoperfusion of the thoracolumbar spinal cord, which can occur in the settings of atherosclerotic disease of the aorta or vertebral arteries, dissecting aortic aneurysm, aortic surgical intervention, spinal trauma, or systemic hypotension [5]. Less common etiologies include vasculitis, cocaine abuse, presumed fibrocartilaginous embolism, decompression sickness, subclavian vein catheterization, sympathectomy, thoracoplasty, celiac plexus neurolysis, lumbar epidural anesthesia, intrathecal injection of lidocaine, dural arteriovenous fistula, intramedullary arteriovenous malformation, single radicular artery ligation, vertebral angiography, and renal artery embolization [5, 19]. Infarction of the posterior columns can be related to vertebral artery dissection and trauma of the spine or surgery. The histopathologic sequelae of ischemia are variable and depend on both the level and extent of vascular compromise. Autopsy findings in patients affected by spinal cord infarction often include preferential involvement of gray matter; however, in a large series, the most severe cases also showed white matter necrosis [18, 20]. Other reports describe involvement of both gray and white matter [21]. With respect to vascular territories, infarction localized predominantly to the region supplied by the posterior spinal arteries is very rare and the pathophysiology has not been clearly defined [17, 21]. Because the posterior columns have a consistent

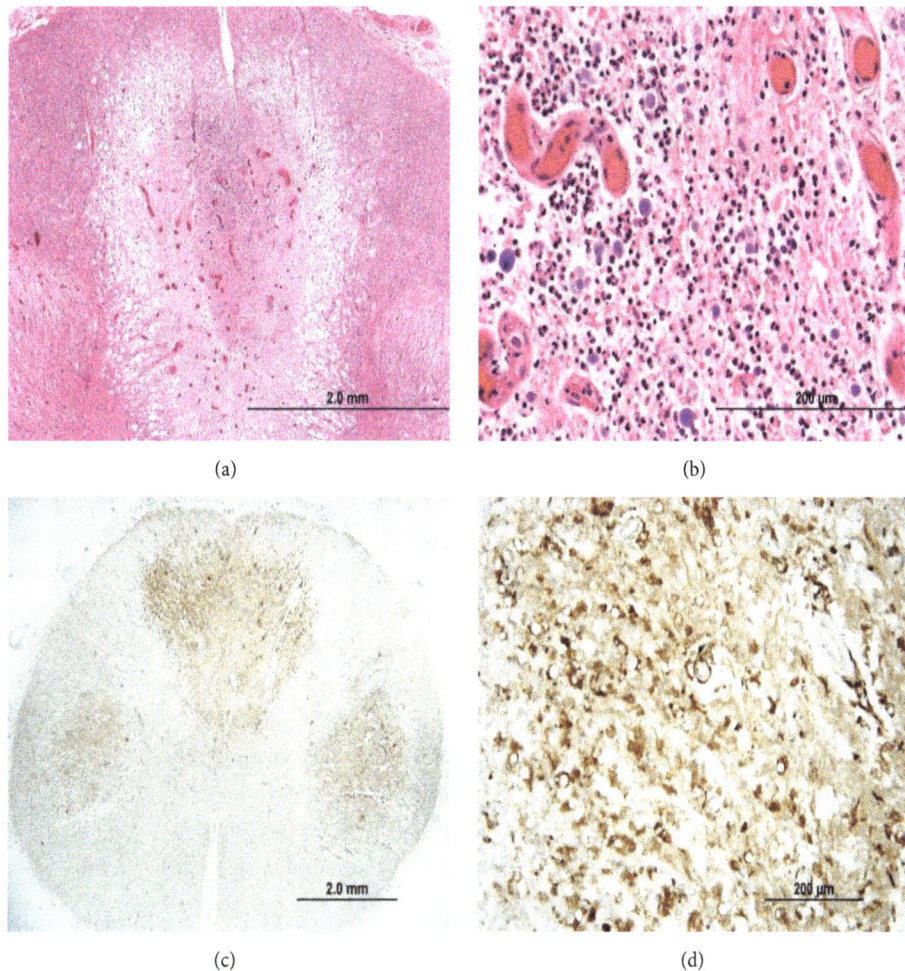

FIGURE 2: Acute and subacute ischemic changes in the spinal cord. (a, b) Intermediate-power and high-power photomicrographs of dorsal columns in a section with neutrophilic infiltrates and reactive vessels (original magnifications, ×40 and ×400, resp.; H-E stain); (c) low-power photomicrograph of spinal cord stained with antibody against CD68 to demonstrate foamy macrophages and microglia, primarily within dorsal columns and lateral white matter tracts (original magnification, ×20; CD68 immunostain); (d) higher-power photomicrograph of the dorsal columns showing CD68-positive macrophages and microglia (original magnification, ×200; CD68 immunostain).

blood supply from two posterior spinal arteries and the large number of anastomoses, it is hypothesized that this region is often spared [5, 6, 22]. However, in cases of hypoperfusion, a watershed effect may take precedence [17]. In the spinal cord, there is a dorsal watershed zone characterized by a capillary network where the penetrating branches of the anterior spinal artery meet the penetrating branches of the posterior spinal arteries and branches of the circumferential pial network [17]. This vascular anatomy may also contribute to the neurologic manifestations of chronic spinal cord ischemia in the setting of arteriovenous malformations and AVFs.

Signs and symptoms of spinal cord ischemia may vary in intensity and evolve over a few days before deficits become fixed. This patient presented with a subacute-to-chronic history of pain and severe sensory ataxia, and MRI findings supported localization to the posterior cord; accordingly, our initial differential diagnosis focused on common causes of this form of myelopathy. This patient did not fit the typical case of spinal cord infarction as she had no acute inciting

event and it is uncommon for spinal cord infarction to preferentially involve the dorsal columns [5, 6, 17, 22, 23]. Furthermore, these acute inciting events have a much stronger association with anterior, rather than posterior, spinal cord infarctions in the literature [17]. A spinal angiogram (to evaluate for a dural AVF) was not possible in the setting of the patient's low creatinine clearance.

The underlying etiology of this patient's apparent polyphasic spinal cord infarction remains unclear. The lack of an inflammatory CSF profile, nodular contrast enhancing lesions in the spine (typical of sarcoidosis), nondiagnostic paratracheal lymph node biopsy guided by results of a full body PET scan, and lack of pathologic features of noncaseating granulomas on complete autopsy, all argued against neurosarcoidosis. The patient's serum anti-aquaporin-4 IgG was negative and other than radiologic evidence of a longitudinally extensive lesion of the dorsal columns there were no clinical features suggestive of NMO or NMOSD. Radiological and postmortem examinations identified severe

(a)   (b)

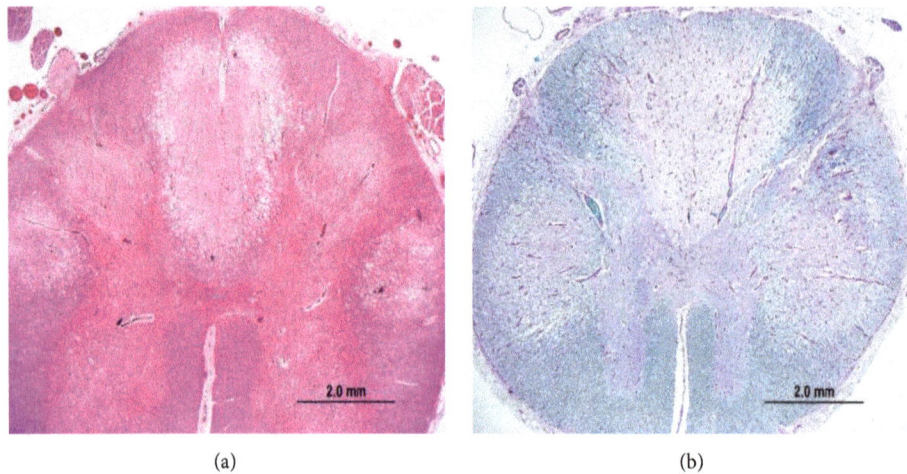

FIGURE 3: Histologic sections of spinal cord demonstrate extensive white matter pathology. (a) Low-power photomicrograph of spinal cord with dorsal column and lateral white matter degeneration (original magnification, ×20; hematoxylin-eosin [H-E] stain); (b) low-power photomicrograph of spinal cord stained with Luxol fast blue-periodic acid Schiff (LFB-PAS) histochemistry to demonstrate loss of myelinated axons (original magnification, ×20; LFB-PAS stain).

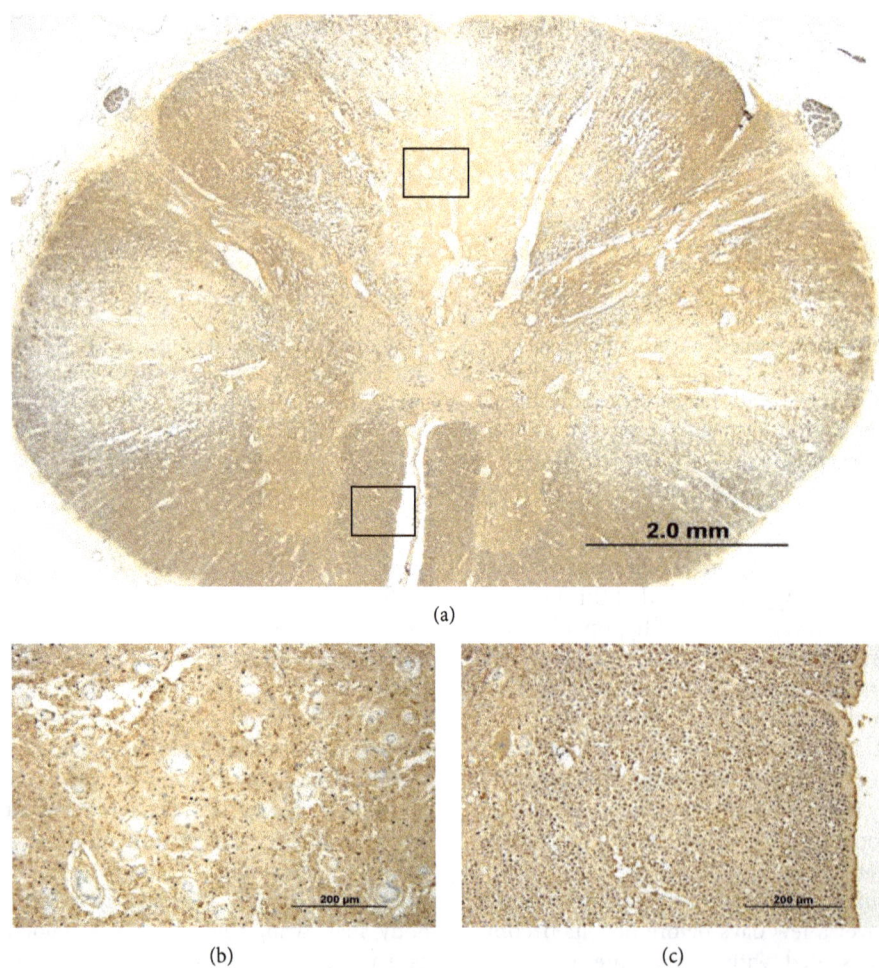

(a)

(b)   (c)

FIGURE 4: Spinal cord stained immunohistochemically with antibody to neurofilament (NF) demonstrates regional axonal loss; (a) low-power photomicrograph demonstrates areas of axonal loss most pronounced in the dorsal (upper boxed area) and lateral white matter tracts, in contrast to ventral spinal cord (lower boxed area) (original magnification, ×20; NF immunostain); (b, c) higher-power photomicrographs of boxed areas to demonstrate axonal loss in dorsal columns ((b) upper boxed area from (a)) with relative axonal preservation in ventral area ((c) lower boxed area from (a)) (original magnifications, ×200; NF immunostain).

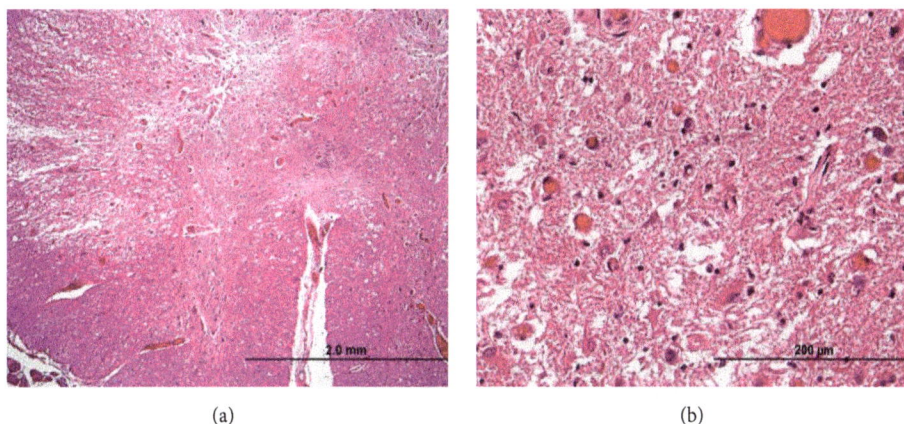

(a)   (b)

FIGURE 5: Gray matter damage. (a) Lower-power photomicrograph of gray matter adjacent to ventrolateral tracts (original magnification, ×40; H-E stain); (b) higher-power photomicrograph of adjacent gray matter with neuronal loss and gliosis (original magnification, ×400; H-E stain).

atherosclerosis in the aorta and visceral blood vessels, but there was no definitive evidence of thrombosis or vasculitis to explain the more acute changes. Given the symmetric, tract specific changes on imaging, symmetric clinical deficits, and the progressive course, a paraneoplastic myelopathy remains possible, despite the lack of an identified occult malignancy at autopsy or on PET/CT scan. Although VGCC autoantibodies have been reported in cases of paraneoplastic myelopathy they are not specific to this disorder; and, given the low titers, this finding has unclear clinical significance [14, 16]. Nonetheless, given the many factors suggestive of a paraneoplastic etiology and the possibility of an unidentified antibody-mediated disorder, the patient underwent extensive screening for an occult malignancy, including a whole body positron emission tomography/computed tomography (PET/CT) scan, mammography, and colonoscopy. PET/CT scans certainly improve the likelihood of identifying an occult malignancy in suspected paraneoplastic disorders but are not 100% sensitive and in this case serial PET scans did not identify a malignancy [24, 25]. The unusual findings of ischemia/infarction suggest that if this were paraneoplastic in nature, it would be associated with a novel form of a paraneoplastic microvasculopathy [14]. The pathologic features of paraneoplastic myelopathies are not well characterized, precluding a comparison of our findings to others reported in the literature.

7. Conclusion

Chronic, progressive microvasculopathy should be considered in the differential diagnosis of a progressive myelopathy with imaging evidence of a dorsal column tractopathy when alternative, more common, etiologies have been ruled out. Given the strong suspicion for an occult malignancy in our case and the strong clinical resemblance to previously reported cases of paraneoplastic dorsal column myelopathy, we propose that an immune mediated microvasculopathy be considered in the list of potential pathophysiologic mechanisms for paraneoplastic myelopathies. To our knowledge, no

comparable cases exist in the literature and additional cases are necessary to further test this hypothesis, emphasizing the importance of postmortem examinations in this unfortunate patient population.

Competing Interests

The authors declare that there is no conflict of interests regarding the publication of this paper.

References

[1] K. W. I. B. R. C. J. V. G. Lindsay, *Neurology and Neurosurgery Illustrated*, Churchill Livingstone, 5th edition, 1991.

[2] A. Jacob and B. G. Weinshenker, "An approach to the diagnosis of acute transverse myelitis," *Seminars in Neurology*, vol. 28, no. 1, pp. 105–120, 2008.

[3] N. Kumar, "Metabolic and toxic myelopathies," *Seminars in Neurology*, vol. 32, no. 2, pp. 123–136, 2012.

[4] C. K. Petito, B. A. Navia, E.-S. Cho, B. D. Jordan, D. C. George, and R. W. Price, "Vacuolar myelopathy pathologically resembling subacute combined degeneration in patients with the acquired immunodeficiency syndrome," *The New England Journal of Medicine*, vol. 312, no. 14, pp. 874–879, 1985.

[5] S. Weidauer, M. Nichtweiß, E. Hattingen, and J. Berkefeld, "Spinal cord ischemia: aetiology, clinical syndromes and imaging features," *Neuroradiology*, vol. 57, no. 3, pp. 241–257, 2015.

[6] J. Novy, A. Carruzzo, P. Maeder, and J. Bogousslavsky, "Spinal cord ischemia: clinical and imaging patterns, pathogenesis, and outcomes in 27 patients," *Archives of Neurology*, vol. 63, no. 8, pp. 1113–1120, 2006.

[7] J. R. Berger and A. Sabet, "Infectious myelopathies," *Seminars in Neurology*, vol. 22, no. 2, pp. 133–141, 2002.

[8] E. P. Flanagan and B. M. Keegan, "Paraneoplastic myelopathy," *Neurologic Clinics*, vol. 31, no. 1, pp. 307–318, 2013.

[9] D. M. Wingerchuk, V. A. Lennon, C. F. Lucchinetti, S. J. Pittock, and B. G. Weinshenker, "The spectrum of neuromyelitis optica," *The Lancet Neurology*, vol. 6, no. 9, pp. 805–815, 2007.

[10] O. Andersen, "Myelitis," *Current Opinion in Neurology*, vol. 13, no. 3, pp. 311–316, 2000.

[11] L. P. Caragine Jr., V. V. Halbach, P. P. Ng, and C. F. Dowd, "Vascular myelopathies-vascular malformations of the spinal cord: presentation and endovascular surgical management," *Seminars in Neurology*, vol. 22, no. 2, pp. 123–132, 2002.

[12] Mayo Medical Laboratories, *Paraneoplastic Autoantibody Evaluation, Serum*, 2016, http://www.mayomedicallaboratories .com/test-catalog/Overview/83380.

[13] Y. Hidekazu, I. Keisuke, H. Masashi et al., "A case of acute progressive myelopathy due to intravascular large B cell lymphoma diagnosed with only random skin biopsy," *Clinical Neurology*, vol. 55, no. 2, pp. 115–118, 2015.

[14] E. P. Flanagan, A. McKeon, V. A. Lennon et al., "Paraneoplastic isolated myelopathy: clinical course and neuroimaging clues," *Neurology*, vol. 76, no. 24, pp. 2089–2095, 2011.

[15] Y. Jiao, W. Zhang, X. Li et al., "Longitudinally extensive spinal cord lesion: etiology and imaging features," *Zhonghua Yi Xue Za Zhi*, vol. 94, no. 41, pp. 3229–3233, 2014.

[16] E. P. Flanagan, V. A. Lennon, and S. J. Pittock, "Autoimmune myelopathies," *Continuum (Minneap Minn)*, vol. 17, no. 4, pp. 776–799, 2011.

[17] A. H. Ropper, M. A. Samuels, and J. P. Klein, "Diseases of the spinal cord," in *Adams & Victor's Principle's of Neurology*, A. H. Ropper, M. A. Samuels, and J. P. Klein, Eds., vol. 44, chapter 44, 10th edition, 2014.

[18] K. Ishizawa, T. Komori, T. Shimada et al., "Hemodynamic infarction of the spinal cord: involvement of the gray matter plus the border-zone between the central and peripheral arteries," *Spinal Cord*, vol. 43, no. 5, pp. 306–310, 2005.

[19] M. N. Rubin and A. A. Rabinstein, "Vascular diseases of the spinal cord," *Neurologic Clinics*, vol. 31, no. 1, pp. 153–181, 2013.

[20] N. Duggal and B. Lach, "Selective vulnerability of the lumbosacral spinal cord after cardiac arrest and hypotension," *Stroke*, vol. 33, no. 1, pp. 116–121, 2002.

[21] H. K. Wolf, D. C. Anthony, and G. N. Fuller, "Arterial border zone necrosis of the spinal cord," *Clinical Neuropathology*, vol. 9, no. 2, pp. 60–65, 1990.

[22] M. F. Shamji, D. E. Maziak, F. M. Shamji, R. J. Ginsberg, and R. Pon, "Circulation of the spinal cord: an important consideration for thoracic surgeons," *Annals of Thoracic Surgery*, vol. 76, no. 1, pp. 315–321, 2003.

[23] W. P. Cheshire, C. C. Santos, E. W. Massey, and J. F. Howard Jr., "Spinal cord infarction: etiology and outcome," *Neurology*, vol. 47, no. 2, pp. 321–330, 1996.

[24] A. McKeon, M. Apiwattanakul, D. H. Lachance et al., "Positron emission tomography-computed tomography in paraneoplastic neurologic disorders: systematic analysis and review," *Archives of Neurology*, vol. 67, no. 3, pp. 322–329, 2010.

[25] R. R. Patel, R. M. Subramaniam, J. N. Mandrekar, J. E. Hammack, V. J. Lowe, and J. R. Jett, "Occult malignancy in patients with suspected paraneoplastic neurologic syndromes: value of positron emission tomography in diagnosis," *Mayo Clinic Proceedings*, vol. 83, no. 8, pp. 917–922, 2008.

[26] L. Pandit, "Neuromyelitis optica spectrum disorders: an update," *Annals of Indian Academy of Neurology*, vol. 18, supplement 1, pp. S11–S15, 2015.

[27] D. M. Wingerchuk, B. Banwell, J. L. Bennett et al., "International consensus diagnostic criteria for neuromyelitis optica spectrum disorders," *Neurology*, vol. 85, no. 2, pp. 177–189, 2015.

[28] W. O. Tobin, B. G. Weinshenker, and C. F. Lucchinetti, "Longitudinally extensive transverse myelitis," *Current Opinion in Neurology*, vol. 27, no. 3, pp. 279–289, 2014.

18

Nonvisualization of the Internal Carotid Artery on Computed Tomography Angiography

Sonal Saran, Rengarajan Rajagopal, Pushpinder S. Khera, and Neeraj Mehta

Department of Radiology, AIIMS Jodhpur, Jodhpur 342005, India

Correspondence should be addressed to Sonal Saran; sonalsaranmalik@gmail.com

Academic Editor: Jorge C. Kattah

Nonvisualization of the internal carotid artery (ICA) on cross-sectional imaging studies can be due to congenital (dysgenesis of the ICA) or acquired (complete occlusion of ICA) causes. We report two cases, one with absent carotid canal on bone window setting of computed tomography (CT) suggestive of congenital cause and the other with normal carotid canal, suggesting acquired cause. Development of aortic arches with six pathways of collateral circulation in brain is also discussed.

1. Introduction

Nonvisualization of the internal carotid artery (ICA) on cross-sectional imaging studies can be due to dysgenesis of the ICA or due to complete occlusion. In both the cases the clinical possibility ranges from that of an asymptomatic patient to one having transient ischemic attack (TIA) and fatal stroke [1].

The aorta develops at around 21st day of embryonic life. Primitive aorta consists of ventral and dorsal segments that are continuous through the first aortic arch. The two ventral aortae fuse to form the aortic sac. The dorsal aortae fuse to form the midline descending aorta. Six paired aortic arches (brachial arch arteries) develop between the ventral and dorsal aortae (Figure 1).

(i) First Arch. It contributes to the formation of the maxillary and external carotid arteries.

(ii) Second Arch. It contributes to the formation of the stapedial arteries.

(iii) Third Arch (Also Known as Carotid Arch). Proximal segments of the third pair form the common carotid arteries. The distal portions contribute to the formation of the internal carotid arteries along with segments of the dorsal aortae. The ECA arises as a sprout from the CCA (i.e., the third aortic arch) and also receives contribution from the first and second aortic arches.

(iv) Fourth Arch. The left fourth arch forms the aortic arch. The proximal right subclavian artery is formed from the right fourth arch whereas the distal right subclavian artery is derived from a portion of the right dorsal aorta and the right seventh intersegmental artery.

(v) Fifth Arch. It forms the rudimentary vessels that regress early.

(vi) Sixth Arch. The left sixth arch contributes to the formation of the main and left pulmonary arteries and ductus arteriosus. The right sixth arch contributes to the formation of the right pulmonary artery.

Initially, the aortic arches are connected to the dorsal aorta. As development progresses, the connection of the first and second arches to the dorsal aorta regresses and they contribute to the formation of the ECA. Persistence of the connection with the dorsal aorta may present as transcranial ECA-ICA anastomosis. Through this anastomosis

Dorsal aorta
Ventral aorta
Right subclavian artery
Internal carotid artery
External carotid artery
Common carotid artery
Arch of aorta
Ductus arteriosus
Pulmonary artery bifurcation

1 2 3 4 5 6

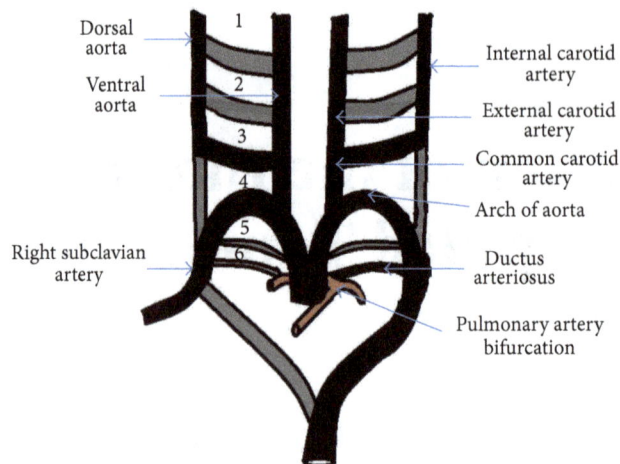

FIGURE 1: Development of aortic arches is depicted. Numbers one to six represent the aortic arches.

the internal maxillary artery and middle meningeal arteries can supply the distal ICA in cases of hypoplasia of the ICA (known as rete mirabile in the region of the cavernous sinus) [2].

Two longitudinal vascular plexuses dorsal to the third and fourth arches form the basilar artery during the 5th week of intrauterine development. Multiple primitive vessels connect the developing basilar artery and the ICA. All of these vessels involute except for the most cranial one, which persists as the posterior communicating artery [2].

2. Case Presentation

We hereby present two cases, which presented to our hospital with symptoms of TIA and, on evaluation with computed tomography angiography (CTA) of carotid vessels, diagnosis of nonvisualization of the ICA was made.

2.1. Case One. A 64-year-old male, hypertensive for 20 years (on medication), presented with transient right-sided weakness and numbness. The patient underwent CTA imaging of the carotid vessels and circle of Willis, which showed absent ICA on left side and collateral flow to the left hemisphere through the circle of Willis. Absence of the left carotid canal was also discovered at bone window setting of computed tomography (CT), which confirmed the congenital nature of the nonvisualization of left ICA. Maximum intensity projection (MIP) reconstruction revealed that the left middle cerebral artery was fed through a dilated left anterior cerebral artery supplied by the anterior communicating artery (Figure 2).

There was no associated vascular malformation or any transcranial ECA-ICA anastomosis or any embryonic persistent artery. The patient's symptoms resolved spontaneously and were attributed to either transient ischemic attacks or migraine headaches. No thromboembolic source was identified.

2.2. Case Two. A 59-year-old male, hypertensive for 5 years (on medication), presented with transient left-sided weakness and numbness. The patient underwent CTA imaging of the carotid vessels and circle of Willis, which showed nonvisualization of ICA on right side and collateral flow to the right hemisphere through the circle of Willis. Right carotid canal was normal at CTA, which confirmed the acquired nature of the nonvisualization of right ICA. A diagnosis of complete occlusion of the right ICA along its whole course was made (Figure 3).

3. Discussion

Our first case was diagnosed as agenesis of the left ICA with absent left carotid canal assessed on bone window setting of CT. Dysgenesis of the ICA includes agenesis, aplasia, and hypoplasia. Complete failure of development of the ICA leads to agenesis whereas hypoplasia refers to a very small caliber ICA after the development started and the term aplasia is used when only vestiges of the ICA are present [3]. Dysgenesis of ICA is a rare congenital anomaly, occurring in less than 0.01% of the population. The left ICA is reported to be affected three times more than the right one as in our case. Most of the patients with dysgenesis of the ICA are asymptomatic. In this setting, the most common type of collateral flow is through the circle of Willis. Secondly, collateral flow can be provided via persistent embryonic vessels or from transcranial collaterals arising from the external carotid artery system [4].

Agenesis of the ICA occurs before 24 mm stage of the embryonic growth [5].

Lie reported the first case of agenesis of the ICA and defined agenesis as the total absence of the entire length of the artery. According to Lie, there are six pathways (types A to F) of collateral circulation associated with agenesis of the ICA. In type A, there is unilateral absence of the ICA with collateral circulation to the ipsilateral anterior cerebral artery and middle cerebral artery through anterior communicating

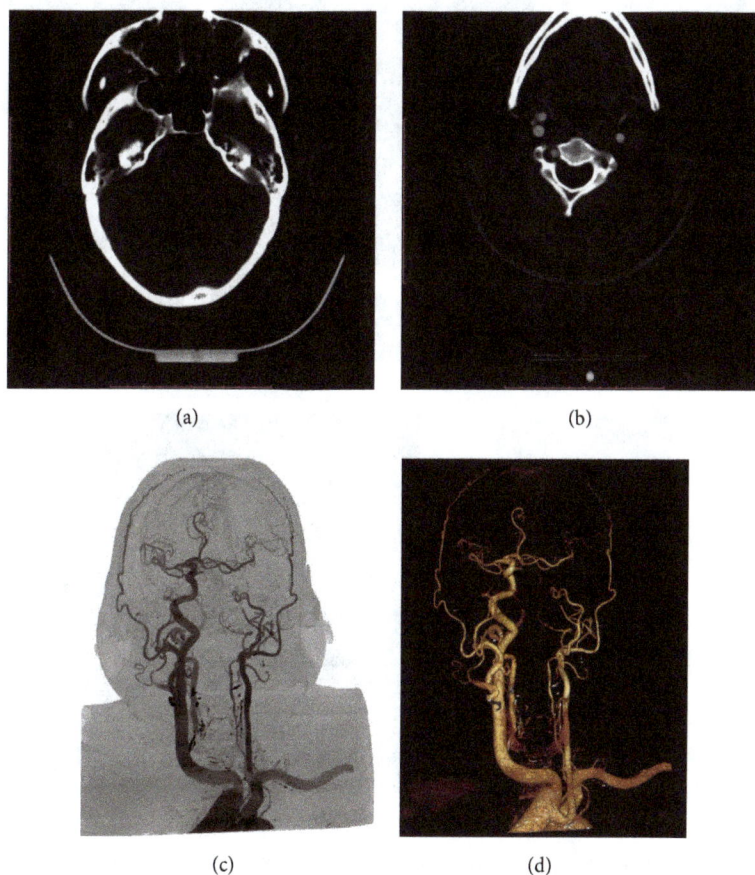

FIGURE 2: (a) Computed tomographic angiography axial image of the patient shows nonvisualization of the left internal carotid artery with absence of left carotid canal. (b) Computed tomographic angiography axial image of the patient at caudal level shows nonvisualization of the left internal carotid artery. Normal internal and external carotid arteries are seen on the contralateral side. (c) Digital subtraction angiographic image reconstructed by the volumetric rendering techniques shows absent left internal carotid artery with left middle cerebral artery being supplied by the collateral circulation through the anterior cerebral artery and anterior communicating arteries. (d) Three-dimensional reconstruction by the volumetric rendering techniques shows absent left internal carotid artery with left middle cerebral artery being supplied by the collateral circulation through the anterior cerebral artery and anterior communicating arteries.

artery and hypertrophic posterior communicating artery, respectively. Unilateral absence of ICA with collateral flow to the ipsilateral anterior cerebral artery and middle cerebral artery across a patent anterior communicating artery comes under type B as in our cases. In type C, bilateral ICA agenesis is associated with patent anastomoses between carotid and vertebra-basilar system. Unilateral agenesis of the cervical portions of the ICA with collateral from an intercavernous communication from the cavernous segment of contralateral ICA comes under type D. In types E and F, there is bilateral ICA hypoplasia with bilateral posterior communicating arteries supplying the middle cerebral arteries in type E and the hypoplastic ICA getting flow from bilateral rete mirabile in type F. Retia mirabilia are transcranial anastomoses between the branches of ICA and external carotid artery system [2].

Congenital absence of ICA is often associated with intracerebral aneurysm formation. The carotid canals in petrous bone form secondary to the presence of the embryonic ICA.

Absence or hypoplasia of embryonic ICA leads to hypoplasia of the carotid canal. Absence of carotid canal on a computed tomography scan should suggest a congenital ICA abnormality and suggest an extensive search for associated intracranial vascular malformations [6].

In patients with agenesis of the ICA, cross-sectional imaging techniques are currently the modality of choice [7]. Our second case was diagnosed as complete occlusion of right ICA along its whole course with absolutely normal right carotid canal.

Dysgenesis of the ICA should be differentiated from complete occlusion especially when unilateral. Complete occlusion of the ICA is more likely due to severe atherosclerosis, chronic dissection, or fibromuscular dysplasias [8].

In patients with occlusion of the ICA, postocclusive diminished arterial pressure causes collaterals to develop via the circle of Willis which is important to prevent stroke. The anterior communicating artery and the posterior communicating artery are the collateral channels through which

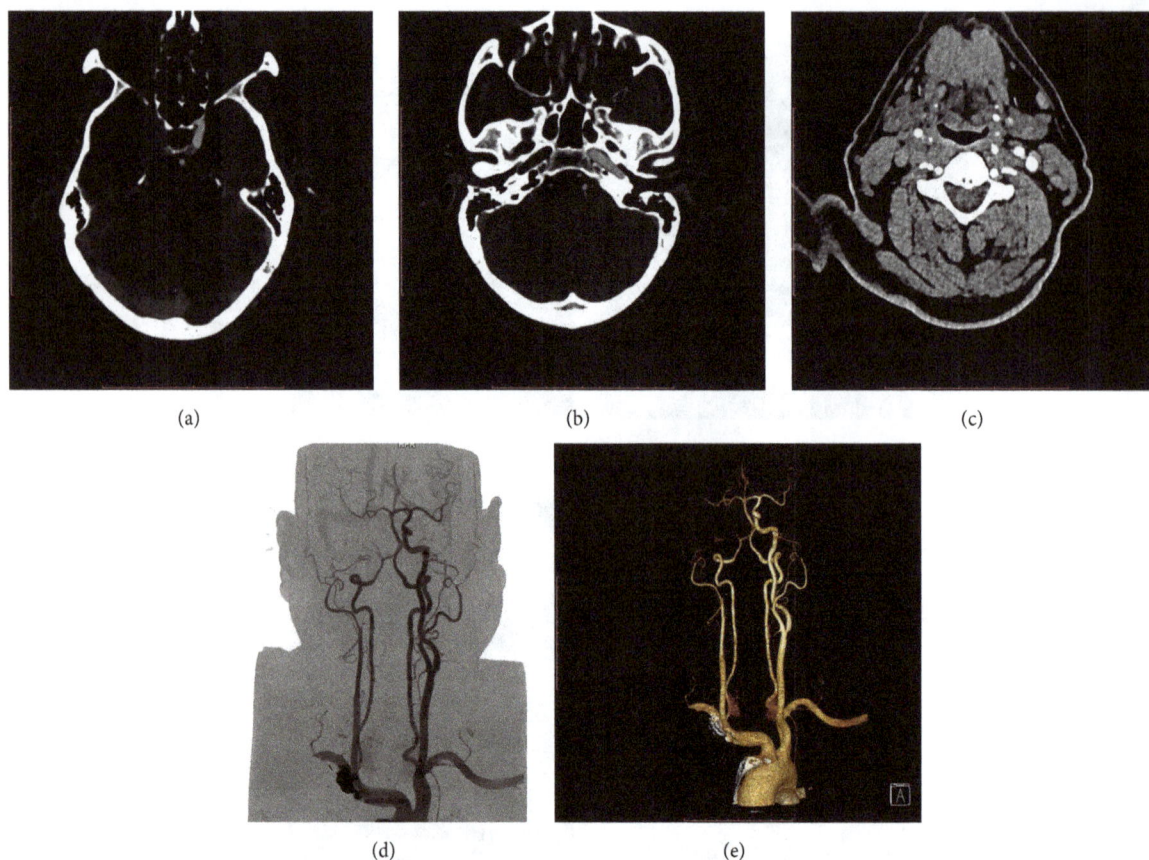

FIGURE 3: (a) Computed tomographic angiography axial image of the patient shows nonvisualization of the right internal carotid artery. (b) Computed tomographic angiography axial image of the patient shows nonvisualization of the right internal carotid artery with normal right carotid canal. (c) Computed tomographic angiography axial image of the patient at caudal level shows nonvisualization of the right internal carotid artery. Normal internal and external carotid arteries are seen on contralateral side. (d) Digital subtraction angiographic image reconstructed by the volumetric rendering techniques shows absent right internal carotid artery with right middle cerebral artery being supplied by the collateral circulation through the anterior cerebral artery and anterior communicating arteries. (e) Three-dimensional reconstruction by the volumetric rendering techniques shows absent right internal carotid artery with right middle cerebral artery being supplied by the collateral circulation through the anterior cerebral artery and anterior communicating arteries.

the circle of Willis can supply blood flow to the affected side of the brain. When collateral compensation mechanisms fall short, low-flow infarcts in border zone areas of the brain may develop [9].

Cote et al. evaluated forty-seven patients with ICA occlusion who were asymptomatic or had only mild neurological deficit and prospectively followed them up for an average of 34.4 months. During that period of time, they found that 51% of patients experienced TIAs in the territory of the occluded artery and 23.5% of patients suffered a cerebral infarction [10].

4. Conclusion

Agenesis of ICA is mostly asymptomatic, being identified only incidentally. The finding of absent carotid canal on routine CT should suggest the diagnosis. It is important in the management of cerebrovascular accidents as the single ICA supplies both the cerebral hemispheres. ICA dysgenesis has to be distinguished from acquired stenosis as the management of the two conditions is different.

Competing Interests

The authors declare that there is no conflict of interests regarding the publication of this paper.

Authors' Contributions

All persons listed as authors in the paper have made substantial contribution in the production of this paper.

References

[1] M. Fisher, "Occlusion of the carotid arteries: further experiences," *AMA Archives of Neurology and Psychiatry*, vol. 72, no. 2, pp. 187–204, 1954.

[2] T. A. Lie, "Amsterdam: excerpta medica," in *Congenital Anomalies of the Carotid Arteries*, pp. 35–51, 1968.

[3] S. Ito, H. Miyazaki, N. Iino, Y. Shiokawa, and I. Saito, "Unilateral agenesis and hypoplasia of the internal carotid artery: a report of three cases," *Neuroradiology*, vol. 47, no. 5, pp. 311–315, 2005.

[4] L. Paşaoğlu, U. Toprak, B. Akdal, G. Yagiz, D. Acar, and F. Gurel, "Unilateral hypoplasia of the internal carotid artery," *International Journal of Medical and Pharmaceutical Case Reports*, vol. 3, no. 5, pp. 132–137, 2015.

[5] P. C. Janicki, J. P. Limbacher, and F. C. Guinto Jr., "Agenesis of the internal carotid artery with a primitive transsellar communicating artery," *American Journal of Roentgenology*, vol. 132, no. 1, pp. 130–132, 1979.

[6] D. J. Quint, R. Silbergleit, and W. C. Young, "Absence of the carotid canals at skull base CT," *Radiology*, vol. 182, no. 2, pp. 477–481, 1992.

[7] O. Kiritsi, G. Noussios, K. Tsitas, and D. Lappas, "Unilateral agenesis of the internal carotid artery presented as transient ischaemic attack: a case report," *Surgical and Radiologic Anatomy*, vol. 34, no. 5, pp. 475–477, 2012.

[8] C. A. Given II, F. Huang-Hellinger, M. D. Baker, N. B. Chepuri, and P. Pearse Morris, "Congenital absence of the internal carotid artery: case reports and review of the collateral circulation," *American Journal of Neuroradiology*, vol. 22, no. 10, pp. 1953–1959, 2001.

[9] C. P. Derdeyn, A. Khosla, T. O. Videen et al., "Severe hemodynamic impairment and border zone—region infarction," *Radiology*, vol. 220, no. 1, pp. 195–201, 2001.

[10] R. Cote, H. J. M. Barnett, and D. W. Taylor, "Internal carotid occlusion: a prospective study," *Stroke*, vol. 14, no. 6, pp. 898–902, 1983.

19

Reversible Akinetic Mutism after Aneurysmal Subarachnoid Haemorrhage in the Territory of the Anterior Cerebral Artery without Permanent Ischaemic Damage to Anterior Cingulate Gyri

François-Xavier Sibille,[1] Philippe Hantson,[1] Thierry Duprez,[2] Vincent van Pesch,[3] and Simone Giglioli[1]

[1]*Department of Intensive Care, Université Catholique de Louvain, Cliniques St-Luc, 1200 Brussels, Belgium*
[2]*Department of Neuroradiology, Université Catholique de Louvain, Cliniques St-Luc, 1200 Brussels, Belgium*
[3]*Laboratory of Neurophysiology, Université Catholique de Louvain, Cliniques St-Luc, 1200 Brussels, Belgium*

Correspondence should be addressed to Philippe Hantson; philippe.hantson@uclouvain.be

Academic Editor: Mehmet Turgut

We report on two cases of transient akinetic mutism after massive subarachnoid haemorrhage due to the rupture of an intracranial aneurysm of the anterior cerebral artery (ACA). In the two cases, vasospasm could not be demonstrated by imaging studies throughout the clinical course. Both patients shared common radiological features: a hydrocephalus due to haemorrhagic contamination of the ventricular system and a mass effect of a subpial hematoma on the borders of the corpus callosum. Patients were also investigated using auditory event-related evoked potentials at acute stage. In contrast to previous observations of akinetic mutism, P300 wave could not be recorded. Both patients had good recovery and we hypothesized that this unexpectedly favourable outcome was due to the absence of permanent structural damage to the ACA territory, with only transient dysfunction due to a reversible mass effect on cingulate gyri.

1. Introduction

In contrast to the high incidence of subarachnoid haemorrhage (SAH) due the rupture of an intracranial aneurysm (RIA) of the anterior cerebral artery (ACA), akinetic mutism complicating vasospasm-related bilateral stroke within anterior cingulate gyri and supplementary motor area (SMA) remains uncommon [1–3]. We describe two cases of akinetic mutism occurring in the course of massive SAH from RIA in the ACA territory in whom diffusion-weighted MR imaging (DW-MRI) failed to reveal ischaemic damage to the cingulate gyri. Both patients experienced a rapid recovery. We speculate that mass effect synergistically due to oedematous changes, hydrocephalus, and subpial hematoma impinging on the corpus callosum may have led to reversible dysfunction of the cingulate gyri in the absence of permanent

ischaemic damage. Both patients were also investigated at the acute phase using event-related auditory evoked potentials.

2. Case 1 Presentation

A 61-year-old woman with a heavy medical history of arterial hypertension, sarcoidosis, hypothyroidism, and bilateral optic nerve atrophy was referred to the Emergency Department for severe headache, vomiting, and alteration of consciousness. Her Glasgow Coma Score on admission was 15/15 but the patient had a slurry speech and exhibited choreic movements of the upper limbs. The admission brain computed tomography (CT scanner) revealed a Fisher grade 4 SAH with initially mild intraventricular bleeding uncomplicated by hydrocephalus. Angiographic examination confirmed the presence of a saccular aneurysm at the junction

(a)   (b)   (c)

(d)

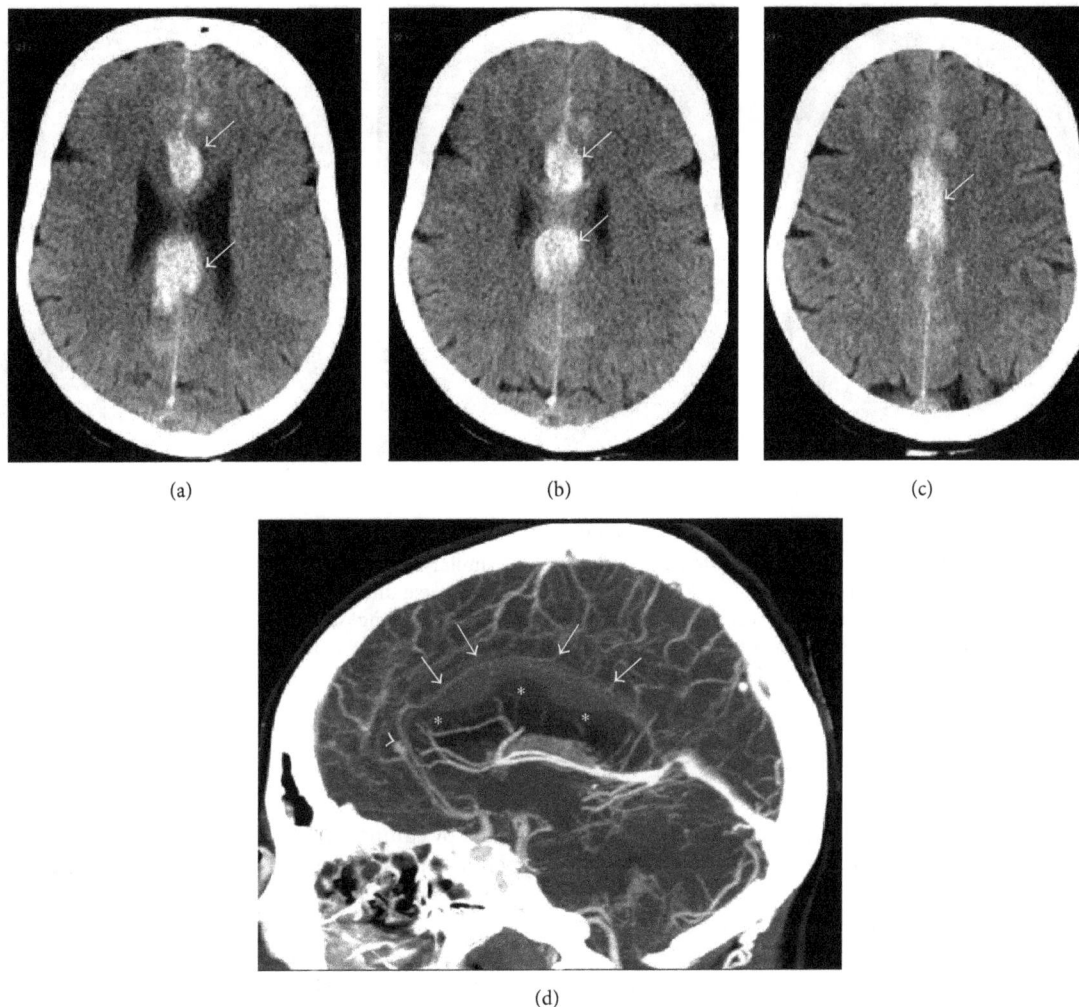

FIGURE 1: Admission brain CT scanner work-up of patient 1. (a–c) Serial unenhanced axial transverse views through the level of the corpus callosum showing massive hyperintense subpial hematoma at the cranial border of the corpus together (white arrows) with a mild SAH at the lateral borders of the frontal and parietal lobes, mainly on the left side. (d) Contrast-enhanced mid-sagittal reformatted Maximum Intensity Proton (MIP) view showing severe polylobulated impingement of the subpial hematoma (white arrows) on the corpus callosum (asterisks) and the causative microaneurysm on the left ACA (arrowhead). Note artifactual lowering of the apparent density of the hematoma because of changes in image scaling (window/level) after contrast agent injection.

of the left pericallosal and callosomarginal arteries, which was successfully treated by coiling. The neurological status worsened a few hours after the procedure and an early follow-up brain CT scanner was performed with increased hydrocephalus and the *de novo* constitution of a subpial hematoma collected at the upper border of the corpus callosum (Figure 1). Extubation was possible soon after surgery for intraventricular drainage. The neurological examination showed spontaneous eye opening and some spontaneous movements of the upper and lower limbs with a mild left hemiparesia. When stimulated, the patient remained completely mutic but demonstrated some orientating reactions toward the source of intense verbal and/or auditory stimulation. A brain magnetic resonance imaging (MRI) performed on day 6 failed to reveal vasospasm or ischaemic injury in both ACA territories (Figures 2(a)-2(b)). In contrast, there

was a significant impingement by the mass effect of the subpial hematoma on the superior border of the corpus callosum. Expectedly, major haemorrhagic contamination of the whole ventricular system was still present.

Event-related evoked potentials were recorded on days 13 and 28, using an auditory oddball paradigm (at least two independent acquisitions of 100 stimuli, consisting of an 85 dBHL binaural tone burst at 500 Hz for the frequent stimulus and 750 Hz for the rare stimulus, with a standard/deviant ratio of 85/15 and an interstimulus interval of 0,8 Hz). Exogenous activities were normal (N100: 85 ms; P200: 120 ms). In contrast, no endogenous activities were obtained.

The patient was discharged from the Intensive Care Unit on day 11 with persisting mutism and some uncontrolled movements in the right hemibody and left hemiparesia.

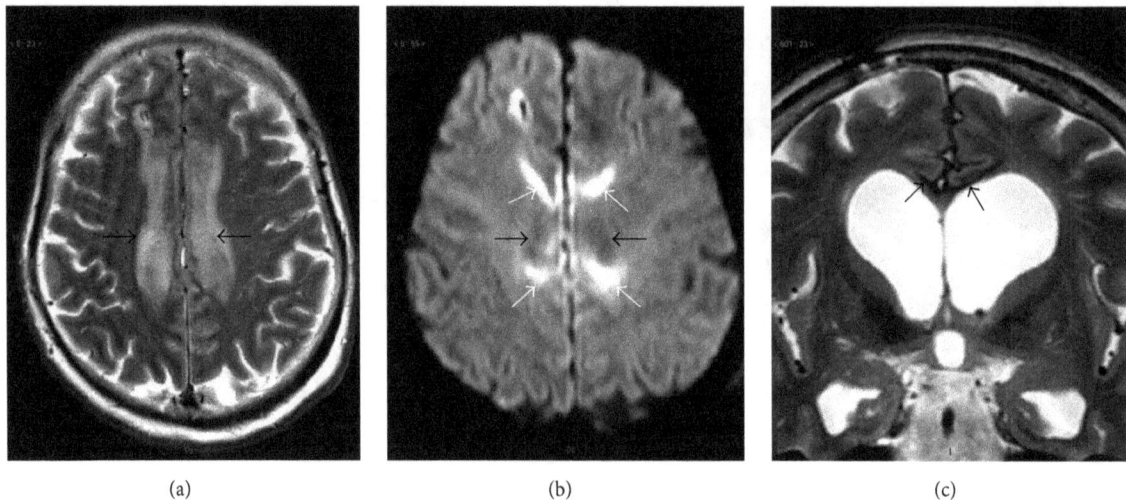

(a)   (b)   (c)

FIGURE 2: MRI work-up (a-b) at acute phase and delayed (7 months) MRI follow-up examination (c) of patient 1. (a) Axial transverse T2-weighted fast-spin echo (FSE) view through cingulate gyri demonstrating similar findings as in previous patient: oedema-related strong hypersignal intensity within them on both sides (black arrows). (b) Axial transverse diffusion-weighted (b factor = 1000 s/mm^2) view in similar slice location (black arrows) failed to reveal hypersignal intensity, thereby excluding ischaemic cytotoxic damage. Only false positive artifacts due to adjacent hematoma were seen (white arrows). (c) Coronal T2-weighted FSE MR view at chronic phase (7 months) showed intrinsic textural integrity of the cingulate gyri. Meningeal hemosiderosis surrounding cingulate gyri featured by pial strong hyposignal intensity was present (arrows).

Levodopa (125 mg orally t.i.d) had been initiated from day 7 but was stopped at the time of her transfer to the rehabilitation clinic on day 27. At this moment, the patient was still mutic and unable to produce spontaneous movements. Mutism almost resolved after 6 weeks. At 6-month follow-up, the patient had a fluid speech with minor episodes of dysarthria. The recovery of neurocognitive functions was very satisfactory, with a mild fatigability impairing attention demanding tasks. Memory was well preserved. Slower improvement was noted regarding motor recovery. After 6 months, the patient was able to walk with some help and could return home to follow an outpatient rehabilitation program. At 7-month follow-up, brain MRI was repeated and documented the integrity of cingulate gyri (Figure 2(c)). At 12-month follow-up, some postural instability persisted but language had completely recovered.

3. Case 2 Presentation

A 56-year-old woman was found unconscious at home and transferred to the Emergency Department with a Glasgow Coma Score of 5/15 (E2V1 M2). The admission brain CT scanner revealed the presence of a Fisher grade 4 subarachnoid haemorrhage. Secondary hypertensive hydrocephalus was present together with a subpial dissecting hematoma at the posterior part of the corpus callosum (Figure 3). Angiographic examination confirmed the presence of a saccular microaneurysm arising at the junction of the right pericallosal and callosomarginal arteries. An external ventricular drain was immediately placed and her neurological status improved subsequently. The aneurysm was successfully

treated by coiling. On day 10, the patient had spontaneous eye opening and weak motor responses to nociceptive stimuli. Verbal response could not be evaluated as the patient was still on mechanical ventilation. The brain MRI (day 7) showed a complete haemorrhagic necrosis of the corpus callosum with a hematoma transfixing the posterior part of the body of the corpus and a bilateral oedema of the cingulate gyri (Figures 4(a)-4(b)). The ventricular system was completely filled with blood in spite of ventricular drainage. No vasospasm or secondary ischaemic lesions could be demonstrated. After the complete weaning from the mechanical ventilation and removal of the tracheostomy (day 22), the patient seemed to understand verbal commands. She was totally mutic and tetraparetic but initiated some movements of the head and neck for "yes" or "no."

Levodopa therapy (125 mg orally t.i.d) was started on day 29 and interrupted on day 48.

The follow-up brain CT scanner after 4 months also demonstrated the integrity of cingulate gyri (Figures 4(c)-4(d)).

Event-related evoked potentials had been performed at the acute phase (day 9) using an oddball auditory paradigm. Only exogenous activities were obtained but were delayed (N100: 170 ms; P200: 250 ms). There were no endogenous activities. The patient was transferred to the rehabilitation ward after one month with persisting akinetic mutism. At 6-month follow-up, the patient had fully recovered speech fluency. She suffered, however, from anxiety and apraxia which was likely related to callosal injury. She was unable to return to work and was transferred to a nursing home. She had regained autonomy for daily life activities but still required some help for postural changes.

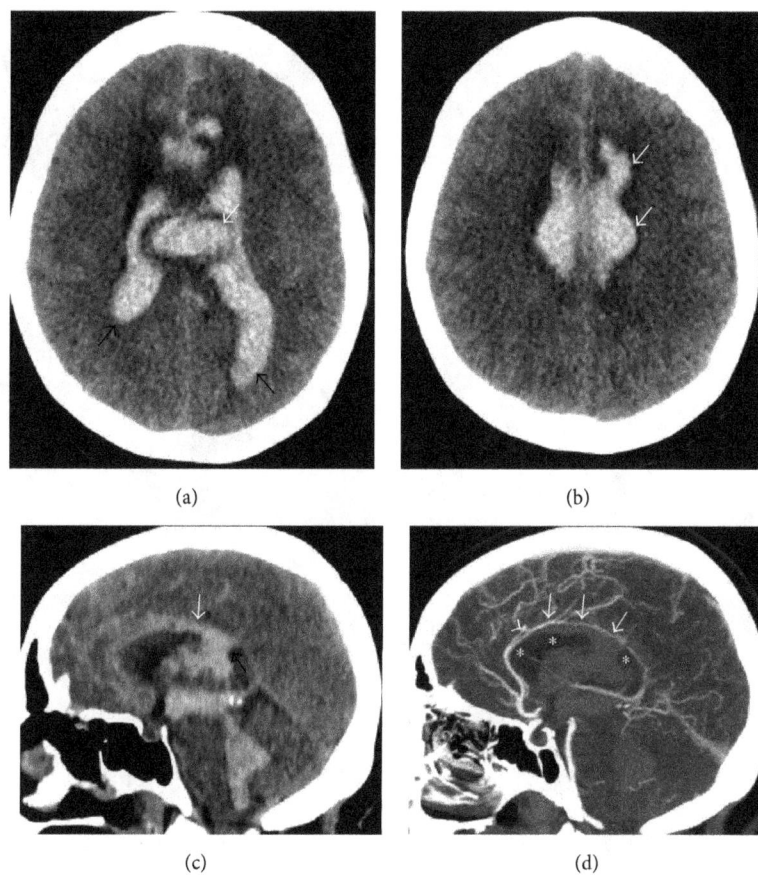

(a)

(b)

(c)

(d)

FIGURE 3: Admission CT scanner work-up of patient 2. (a) Unenhanced axial transverse view through the corpus callosum showing ovoid-shaped hematoma within the mid-posterior area of the body of the corpus (white arrow), anterior interfrontal SAH, and massive haemorrhagic contamination of the whole ventricular system (black arrows). (b) Unenhanced axial transverse view tangent through the cranial aspect of the corpus callosum showing subpial fresh hematoma (arrows). (c) Unenhanced mid-sagittal reformatted view showing filling of the ventricular system by acute hyperintense blood, transgression of the posterior part of the body of the corpus callosum by fresh blood (black arrow), and subpial fresh hematoma at the upper border of the corpus callosum (white arrow). (d) Contrast-enhanced mid-sagittal reformatted view showing the causative RIA of the left ACA (arrowhead) and the subpial hematoma (arrows) on the cranial aspect of the corpus callosum (asterisks). Again, artifactual lowering of the apparent density of the hematoma because of changes in image scaling (window/level) after contrast agent injection (similarly as seen on Figure 1(d)).

A control of brain MRI was planned at 6 months, but the examination had to be interrupted due to uncontrollable anxiety and claustrophobia. We failed to repeat evoked potentials recording for the same reasons. At 12-month follow-up, her condition is relatively unchanged and a new neurocognitive testing is planned.

4. Discussion

The term of "akinetic mutism" (AM) was first introduced by Cairns and coworkers in 1941 to describe a syndrome featured by a lack of responsiveness in spite of apparently preserved vigilance [4]. Clinical examination usually reveals a complete or almost complete immobility and a lack of verbal contact [2]. Anatomically, different brain structures may be involved, with a possible distinction between a telencephalic form (affecting medial frontal lobes, cingulate gyri), a diencephalic form (thalamic/basal ganglia), and a mesencephalic form (upper brainstem reticular activating system). AM is usually observed in the frame of head trauma, brain neoplasia, or ischaemic stroke, but rarely after aneurysmal subarachnoid haemorrhage, and particularly as a presenting feature [1]. A comprehensive literature review performed by Choudhari in 2004 retrieved only a total of 21 published cases of this rare condition [1, 2, 5–15]. Most of the patients usually presented with secondary bilateral infarction in the ACA territory and had poor prognosis. Bilateral damage to anterior cingulate gyri and supplementary motor area, which results in most cases from ischaemic injury in the territories of both ACAs, is often associated with the syndrome. As for hydrocephalus, it has also been implicated in a delayed form of AM following SAH [16]. Only a single previous case of AM without structural lesions, but with bilateral frontal lobe dysfunction demonstrated by single-photon emission computed tomography (SPECT), has been described [5].

Among the neurophysiological tools that can be performed at the bedside, auditory cognitive event-related potentials (ERPs) were rarely explored in patients presenting

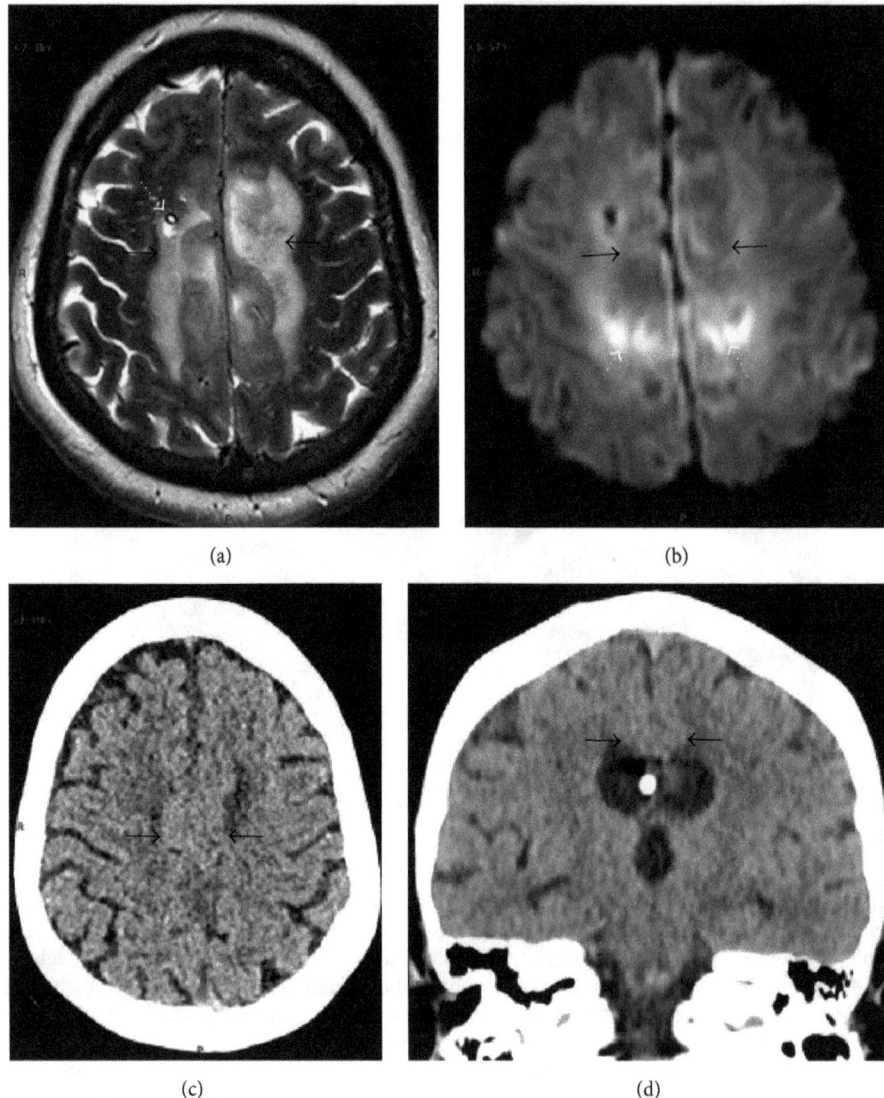

(a)   (b)

(c)   (d)

FIGURE 4: MRI work-up (a-b) at acute phase and delayed (4 months) CT scanner follow-up imaging (c-d) of patient 2. (a) T2-weighted fast-spin echo (FSE) axial transverse view through cingulate gyri demonstrating oedema-related strong hypersignal intensity within them on both sides. Ventricular draining catheter is seen on right frontal area (dotted white arrow). (b) Axial transverse diffusion-weighted (b factor $= 1000\,\text{s/mm}^2$) view in similar slice location failed to reveal hypersignal intensity within the same cingular areas (black arrows), thereby excluding ischaemic cytotoxic oedema. Only false positive artifacts due to adjacent hematoma were seen (arrows). (c-d) CT scanner axial transverse (c) and coronal reformatted (d) images from helical acquisition demonstrating integrity of the cingulate gyri (arrows).

with AM. In a 38-year-old woman with severe AM due to large bilateral ACA infarction due to RIA-related vasospasm, Naccache et al. recorded a "Mismatch Negativity" (MMN) and a larger P300 wave in rare trials than in frequent ones using the passive auditory oddball paradigm [6]. These findings may reflect the persistence of a high level of cognitive integration of current environmental stimuli in case of severe AM and confirmed a similar previous observation [7]. The MMN reflects an automatic preattentive processing stage that seems to be generated in the temporal lobe [8]; the P300 wave is a more complex integrative processing that involves both cortical and subcortical networks [9]. The neural networks involved in the generation of the P300a component are located not only within the frontal cortex

and anterior cingulate gyri but also in parietal, temporal, and occipital regions. The generators of the P300b component originate from the posterior part of the cingulate gyri and also from parietal and temporal lobes [10, 11].

The relevance of MMN and P300 recordings in AM has still not been assessed. One may suggest it could reflect the preservation of a high level of cognitive integration at the acute stage of AM despite poor common neurological testing.

In both cases reported here, no auditory ERPs could be elicited, in contrast to previous reports and despite absence of ischaemic damage of the anterior cingulate gyri and the supplementary motor areas. This is not totally explained by callosal injury or dysfunction, as some authors have documented the preservation of ERPs in patients with callosal disconnection [12, 13]. It could be due to the early timing of the ERP recording but an alternative hypothesis could be that the cortico-subcortical dysfunction involved areas larger than the frontal lobes, thus preventing generation of the P300 components [12, 13]. The discrepancy between the documentation of some orienting reactions to noise or verbal stimuli in both cases and the absence of P300 can be explained by the fact that the ERP stimulus is a pure beep tone in contrast to a richer and more complex auditory stimulus coming from the environment.

The prognosis of AM following SAH is usually poor, expectedly in case of permanent damage to cingulate gyri. In turn, the prognosis appears better when AM is due to hydrocephalus or reversible compression of cingulate gyri similarly to both our patients. There is no existing data that surgical removal of the hematoma could impact on the clinical course. Data regarding the systematic use of dopamine agonists for patients with akinetic mutism are inconclusive. There have been reports that treatment with dopaminergic drugs is useful in akinetic mutism due to lesions at the diencephalon [14]. Dopaminergic agents should be less effective if the lesion is involving the anterior cingulate cortex because dopaminergic receptors would have been destroyed [15]. In our two patients, levodopa withdrawal did not result in clinical deterioration.

Competing Interests

The authors declare that there are no competing interests regarding the publication of this paper.

References

[1] K. A. Choudhari, "Subarachnoid haemorrhage and akinetic mutism," *British Journal of Neurosurgery*, vol. 18, no. 3, pp. 253–258, 2004.

[2] G. Németh, K. Hegedüs, and L. Molnâr, "Akinetic mutism associated with bicingular lesions: clinicopathological and functional anatomical correlates," *European Archives of Psychiatry and Neurological Sciences*, vol. 237, no. 4, pp. 218–222, 1988.

[3] A. O. Ogunyemi, "Akinetic mutism caused by subarachnoid haemorrhage. A case report.," *Central African Journal of Medicine*, vol. 30, no. 2, pp. 273–277, 1984.

[4] H. Cairns, R. C. Oldfield, J. B. Pennybacker, and D. Whitteridge, "Akinetic mutism with an epidermoid cyst of the 3rd ventricle," *Brain*, vol. 64, no. 4, pp. 273–290, 1941.

[5] A. Demirtas-Tatlidede, S. Z. Bahar, and H. Gurvit, "Akinetic mutism without a structural prefrontal lesion," *Cognitive and Behavioral Neurology*, vol. 26, no. 2, pp. 59–62, 2013.

[6] L. Naccache, M. Obadia, S. Crozier et al., "Preserved auditory cognitive ERPs in severe akinetic mutism: a case report," *Cognitive Brain Research*, vol. 19, no. 2, pp. 202–205, 2004.

[7] B. Kotchoubey, M. Schneck, S. Lang, and N. Birbaumer, "Event-related brain potentials in a patient with akinetic mutism," *Neurophysiologie Clinique*, vol. 33, no. 1, pp. 23–30, 2003.

[8] D. von Cramon and M. Albus, "Bilateral anterior infarction and hydrocephalus; complications of a ruptured aneurysm of the anterior communicating artery," *Fortschritte der Medizin*, vol. 98, no. 41, pp. 1602–1606, 1980.

[9] M. Molnár, "On the origin of the P3 event-related potential component," *International Journal of Psychophysiology*, vol. 17, no. 2, pp. 129–144, 1994.

[10] U. Volpe, A. Mucci, P. Bucci, E. Merlotti, S. Galderisi, and M. Maj, "The cortical generators of P3a and P3b: a LORETA study," *Brain Research Bulletin*, vol. 73, no. 4–6, pp. 220–230, 2007.

[11] E. Wronka, J. Kaiser, and A. M. L. Coenen, "Neural generators of the auditory evoked potential components P3a and P3b," *Acta Neurobiologiae Experimentalis*, vol. 72, no. 1, pp. 51–64, 2012.

[12] M. Kutas, S. A. Hillyard, B. T. Volpe, and M. S. Gazzaniga, "Late positive event-related potentials after commissural section in humans," *Journal of Cognitive Neuroscience*, vol. 2, no. 3, pp. 258–271, 1990.

[13] K. Satomi, T. Horai, Y. Kinoshita, and A. Wakazono, "Hemispheric asymmetry of event-related potentials in a patient with callosal disconnection syndrome: a comparison of auditory, visual and somatosensory modalities," *Electroencephalography and Clinical Neurophysiology*, vol. 94, no. 6, pp. 440–449, 1995.

[14] E. D. Ross and R. M. Stewart, "Akinetic mutism from hypothalamic damage: successful treatment with dopamine agonists," *Neurology*, vol. 31, no. 11, pp. 1435–1439, 1981.

[15] O. Combarros, J. Infante, and J. Berciano, "Akinetic mutism from frontal lobe damage responding to levodopa," *Journal of Neurology*, vol. 247, no. 7, pp. 568–569, 2000.

[16] B. Danilewicz, R. Czepko, M. Pyrich, M. Betlej, K. Stachura, and J. Zawiliński, "Immediate and late results of surgical treatment of hydrocephalus after subarachnoid hemorrhage," *Przeglad Lekarski*, vol. 47, no. 10, pp. 678–681, 1990.

20

Corticobasal Syndrome Associated with Antiphospholipid Syndrome Secondary to Systemic Lupus Erythematosus

Ritsuo Hashimoto ⓘ, Tomoko Ogawa, Asako Tagawa, and Hiroyuki Kato

Department of Neurology, International University of Health and Welfare Hospital, Tochigi, Japan

Correspondence should be addressed to Ritsuo Hashimoto; ritsuo@iuhw.ac.jp

Academic Editor: Tapas Kumar Banerjee

We report the case of a 53-year-old woman diagnosed with corticobasal syndrome (CBS) due to antiphospholipid syndrome (APS) secondary to systemic lupus erythematosus. Brain MRI showed marked cortical atrophy, several small infarctions in the deep white matter, and mild white matter changes, all of which were probably due to thrombosis manifestations of APS and could also be related to the CBS. To the best of our knowledge, this is the fourth reported case of CBS due to APS. It is noteworthy that although the common underlying pathologies of the CBS are neurodegenerative diseases, either primary or secondary APS can manifest itself as the CBS.

1. Introduction

Corticobasal syndrome (CBS) is characterized by asymmetric involuntary movements including rigidity, dystonia, tremor, and myoclonus combined with cortical symptoms such as apraxia, cortical sensory loss, and alien limb phenomena [1]. Its underlying pathologies reported so far are diverse and heterogeneous; they include corticobasal degeneration, progressive supranuclear palsy, Alzheimer's disease, Pick's disease, Lew body dementia, motor neuron inclusion body dementia, dementia lacking distinctive histopathology, and Creutzfeldt-Jakob disease [2–4]. In this report, we present a rare case in which a patient developed CBS due to antiphospholipid syndrome (APS) [5–7].

2. Case Report

A 53-year-old right handed woman was referred to our hospital to treat progressive parkinsonism. The patient had experienced convulsions 3 years before her first visit to our hospital and was on medication (diphenylhydantoin 200 mg/day). She developed akinetic-rigid syndrome (dominant on the left side) and a shuffling gait several months after experiencing convulsions. The previous doctor prescribed L-dopa, which proved to have little effect on her condition.

The patient had also demonstrated livedo reticularis of both forearms around the time she presented the akinetic-rigid syndrome. There was no personal history of venous or arterial thrombosis or miscarriage.

On admission, the patient was alert and cooperative, yet she appeared to be slightly depressed. Her speech was easily understandable, albeit slightly hypophonic. Upon examination, she had mild supranuclear gaze palsy showing slight difficulty in looking down. Her horizontal pursuit eye movements were slightly saccadic while the range of motion was normal. Motor power was intact, while exaggerated tendon reflexes were noted on the left side with positive jaw reflex. Babinski sign was negative on either side. Snout reflex was present, yet grasp and palmomental reflexes were negative. There was asymmetric upper limb akinesia and rigidity which was more severe on the left side than on the right. Also, dystonia of the left arm and leg was observed. The gait was slow and stiff with absent arm swing, yet her postural reflexes were relatively well preserved. The patient showed bilateral limb-kinetic apraxia which was prominent on the left side. She could barely use fingers in her right hand to show patterns such as victory sign; however, it was impossible to do so with her left hand. Miming the use of tools and habitual movements such as using a toothbrush, beckoning, and indication of getting away were also difficult for her especially

TABLE 1: Laboratory data of the patient.

WBC	7530/μL	(3500–9700)	Glucose	105 mg/dL	(70–109)
RBC	427×10^4/μL	($376–516 \times 10^4$)	HbA1c (JDS)	5.5%	(4.3–5.8)
Plt	11.5×10^4/μL	($14.0–37.9 \times 10^4$)	CRP	0.25	(0.00–0.30)
PT-INR	1.05	(0.84–1.14)	CH$_{50}$	44	(30–45)
APTT	46.1 sec	Control: 31.6 sec	C3	113	(80–140)
TP	7.7	(6.7–8.3)	C4	25.9	(11–34)
Alb	4.3	(3.9–4.9)	ANA	1280	(<79)
T-Bil	0.3	(0.2–1.2)	DNA/RIA	11.7 IU/mL	(0.0–6.0)
AST	18 IU/L	(8–38)	SS-A	-	
ALT	7 IU/L	(4–44)	SS-B	-	
BUN	20.2 mg/dL	(8.0–20.0)	aCL-IgG	35 U/mL	(0–9)
Cr	0.85 mg/dL	(0.47–0.79)	Urinalysis		
T-CHO	240 mg/dL	(150–219)	Protein	-	
HDL-C	62 mg/dL	(40–90)	OB	-	
Na	142 mEq/L	(135–145)			
K	4.3 mEq/L	(3.5–5.0)			
Cl	105 mEq/L	(98–108)			

( ), normal range; ANA, antinuclear antibody; DNA/RIA, anti-DNA antibody/radioimmunoassay; aCL-IgG, anticardiolipin antibody-IgG; OB, occult blood.

with the left hand which was probably due to the limb-kinetic apraxia. Primary sensations were intact except for loss of joint position sense at her left elbow. There were no cortical sensory deficits such as agraphesthesia and astereognosis. The alien limb phenomenon, neglect syndrome, or myoclonus was not observed. Her mini mental status examination (MMSE) score was 20/30 demonstrating disorientation in time, dyscalculia, mild anterograde amnesia, and decreased digit span.

Laboratory investigations revealed there were thrombocytopenia, slight increased serum creatinine with no proteinuria, elevated activated partial thromboplastin time (APTT), and positive anticardiolipin antibody with IgG titer 35 (positive > 9). Antinuclear antibody was present at a titer of 1:1280 (positive > 79), and anti-DNA antibody was also positive at a titer of 11.7 (positive > 6.0). Test result for SS-A and SS-B antibodies was negative. Complement levels were normal (Table 1). The serological abnormalities including positive anticardiolipin, antinuclear, and anti-DNA antibodies remained, as observed in subsequent tests performed after 3 months. Anticardiolipin antibody was detected in two different times; APS diagnosis was therefore performed. In addition, the present case fulfilled the American College of Rheumatology (ACR) criteria for diagnosing systemic lupus erythematosus (SLE) [8]; she manifested neurological symptoms (convulsions and dementia), and her laboratory data showed hematological involvement (thrombocytopenia), immunological disorder (positive anticardiolipin antibody) and positive antinuclear and anti-DNA antibodies. Brain MRI showed subcortical white matter ischemic changes, marked cortical atrophy that was prominent in the bilateral central areas, and several small infarcts in deep white matter of both hemispheres (Figure 1). Single photon emission tomography using technetium-99m-L, L-ethyl cysteinate dimer (^{99m}Tc-ECD SPECT) showed

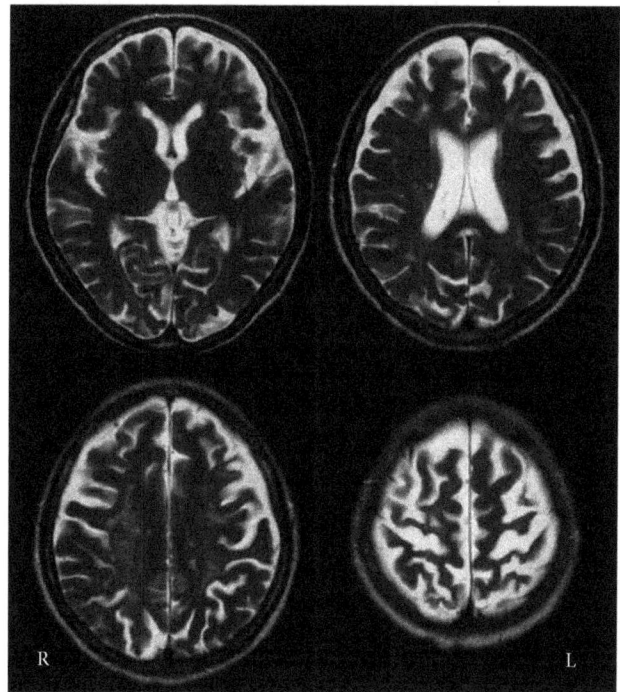

FIGURE 1: Axial T2-weighted magnetic resonance imaging 2 days after admission showing small infarctions in the deep white matter and subcortical high-signal intensities in both hemispheres. Diffuse cortical atrophy that is more prominent in the central areas is also demonstrated. Note that neither ischemic nor atrophic changes are present in the basal ganglia.

decreased cerebral blood flow in the bilateral central areas, which extended to the frontal and parietal areas (Figure 2).

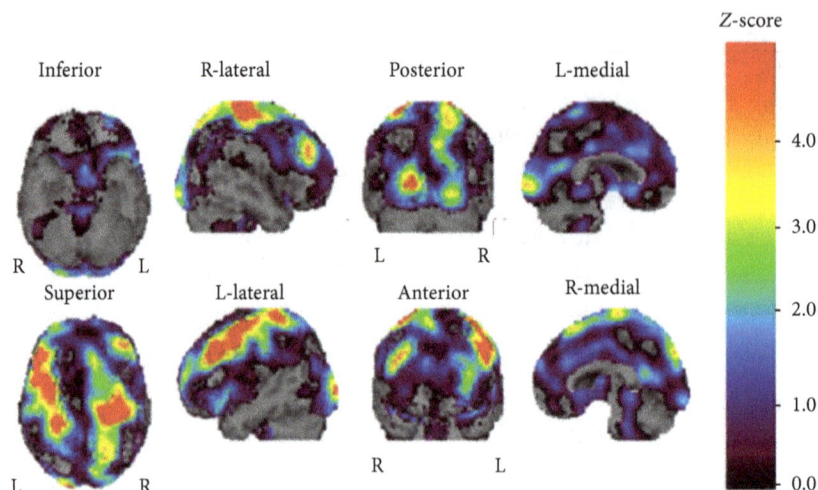

FIGURE 2: ^{99m}Tc-ECD SPECT with easy Z-score Imaging System 10 days after admission showing decreased cerebral blood flow in the bilateral central areas that extends to the frontal and parietal areas.

A diagnosis of CBS due to APS secondary to SLE was made, and aspirin treatment was initiated. Because the patient showed no active systemic disorder other than the neurological manifestations, no therapy was introduced due to SLE. During follow-up, diphenylhydantoin was replaced by zonisamide; however, anticardiolipin, antinuclear, and anti-DNA antibodies tested positive consistently suggesting that the SLE was not induced by diphenylhydantoin. Dabigatran etexilate (75 mg/day) was administered in addition to aspirin at a time; however, APTT prolonged over 3 times that of the contorls' and was discontinued. The patient presented left side dominant akinetic-rigid syndrome and limb-kinetic apraxia over the 8-year follow-up period, both of which changed little in terms of severity. She was ambulant until 61 years of age when she suffered from compression fracture of the 9th thoracic vertebra, which bound her to wheelchair. Repeated MRI scans performed during the follow-up period demonstrated slight progression of diffuse cortical atrophy and subcortical ischemic changes; however, no new infarction was noted. At the age of 62, she died from pneumonia at a local hospital. A postmortem study was not obtained.

3. Discussion

A diagnosis of CBS was made in the present case based on clinical manifestations including left side dominant akinetic-rigid syndrome and limb-kinetic apraxia, both of which were insidious at onset [1]. This case represents the fourth reported description of CBS due to APS. All the previously reported cases had primary APS (APS exists as an independent condition) [5–7]; however, the APS described in the present case was secondary to SLE (Table 2). Thus, this was the first case of CBS due to APS secondary to SLE.

The types of brain MRI lesions observed in the three cases reported previously are as follows: case 1 [5] had multiple infarcts in the cerebral hemispheres and basal ganglia with prominent lesions in the right parietal lobe and head of the left caudate nucleus; case 2 [6] showed extensive white matter changes, marked diffuse cerebral corticosubcortical atrophy, and several infarcts in both hemispheres, involving multiple vascular territories, including the striatum bilaterally; and case 3 [7] demonstrated only diffuse brain atrophy without evidence of cerebral infarction; dopamine transporter imaging studies were normal. Our case had marked cortical atrophy, several small infarctions in the deep white matter, and mild white matter changes; however, neither infarction nor atrophy was noted on either side of the striatum (Table 2). Our case implies that the akinetic-rigid syndrome associated with APS may not necessarily indicate ischemic pathology of the basal ganglia and it may be due to cortical pathology. Overall, it is suggested that in most of the cases APS is related to thrombosis manifestations and could also be related to the CBS. An exception is case 3 [7] who demonstrated only diffuse brain atrophy without evidence of cerebral infarction. The presence of an undetermined antibasal ganglia antibody cannot be ruled out [7, 9].

With regard to the treatment, all patients received anticoagulation and/or antiplatelet treatment. In case reported previously, stabilization of the symptoms was observed in two patients (cases 1, 3) following treatment [5, 7], but one patient (case 2) showed no significant improvement and developed a new infarct at the follow-up performed after 2 years [6]. The patient described in this report exhibited no obvious progression in the symptoms of CBS when using aspirin during the 8-year follow-up. These observations imply that anticoagulation and/or antiplatelet treatment might be effective in preventing progression of symptoms at least in some patients, even if not efficient enough to alleviate them.

In summary, we have reported the fourth case of CBS associated with APS. It must be noted that although the common underlying pathologies of the CBS are neurodegenerative diseases, either primary or secondary APS can manifest itself as the CBS.

TABLE 2: Reported cases of corticobasal syndrome associated with antiphospholipid syndrome.

Case	Authors	APS	Age/sex	Imaging studies	Treatment	Follow-up (period)
1	Lees and Morris [5]	primary	44/F	MRI: multiple infarcts in the cerebral hemispheres and basal ganglia with prominent lesions in the right parietal lobe and head of the left caudate nucleus	Warfarin and aspirin	Moderate improvement in apraxia (3 years)
2	Martino et al. [6]	primary	56/F	MRI: extensive white matter changes, marked diffuse cerebral corticosubcortical atrophy, and several infarcts in both hemispheres involving multiple vascular territories, including the striatum bilaterally	Aspirin and warfarin were separately tried	Progressive deterioration (2 years)
3	Lee et al. [7]	primary	47/M	MRI: only diffuse brain atrophy without evidence of cerebral infarction, and dopamine transporter imaging studies using [^{18}F] FP-CIT PET: normal	Warfarin	No change (6 months)
4	Our case	secondary	53/F	MRI: marked cortical atrophy, several small infarctions in the deep white matter, and mild white matter changes, no infarction nor atrophy in the striatum ^{99m}Tc-ECD SPECT: decreased cerebral blood flow in the bilateral central area extending into the frontal and parietal areas	Aspirin	No significant change (8 years)

APS, antiphospholipid syndrome; [^{18}F] FP-CIT PET, positron emission tomography using ^{18}F-fluorinated N-3-fluoropropyl-2-β-carboxymetholxy-3-β-(4-iodophenyl) nortropane; ^{99m}Tc-ECD SPECT, single photon emission tomography using technetium-99m-L, L-ethyl cysteinate dimer.

Conflicts of Interest

The authors report no conflicts of interest.

References

[1] R. Mathew, T. H. Bak, and J. R. Hodges, "Diagnostic criteria for corticobasal syndrome: A comparative study," *Journal of Neurology, Neurosurgery & Psychiatry*, vol. 83, no. 4, pp. 405–410, 2012.

[2] B. F. Boeve, D. M. Maraganore, J. E. Parisi et al., "Pathologic heterogeneity in clinically diagnosed corticobasal degeneration," *Neurology*, vol. 53, no. 4, pp. 795–800, 1999.

[3] K. A. Josephs, R. C. Petersen, D. S. Knopman et al., "Clinicopathologic analysis of frontotemporal and corticobasal degenerations and PSP," *Neurology*, vol. 66, no. 1, pp. 41–48, 2006.

[4] J. R. Hodges, R. R. Davies, J. H. Xuereb et al., "Clinicopathological correlates in frontotemporal dementia," *Annals of Neurology*, vol. 56, no. 3, pp. 399–406, 2004.

[5] A. J. Lees and H. R. Morris, "Primary antiphospholipid syndrome presenting as a corticobasal degeneration syndrome," *Movement Disorders*, vol. 14, no. 3, pp. 530–532, 1999.

[6] D. Martino, N.-K. Chew, P. Mir, M. J. Edwards, N. P. Quinn, and K. P. Bhatia, "Atypical movement disorders in antiphospholipid syndrome," *Movement Disorders*, vol. 21, no. 7, pp. 944–949, 2006.

[7] D. Lee, S. Eum, C. O. Moon, H. Ma, and Y. J. Kim, "Corticobasal syndrome associated with antiphospholipid syndrome without cerebral infarction," *Neurology*, vol. 82, no. 8, pp. 730-731, 2014.

[8] M. C. Hochberg, "Updating the American College of Rheumatology revised criteria for the classification of systemic lupus erythematosus," *Arthritis & Rheumatology*, vol. 40, no. 9, article 1725, 1997.

[9] M. Carecchio, R. Cantello, and C. Comi, "Revisiting the molecular mechanism of neurological manifestations in antiphospholipid syndrome: Beyond vascular damage," *Journal of Immunology Research*, vol. 2014, Article ID 239398, 2014.

21

Spinal Cord Infarction in a Patient with Hereditary Spherocytosis

Waqar Waheed,[1] Anjali L. Varigonda,[2] Chris E. Holmes,[3] Christopher Trevino,[1] Neil M. Borden,[4] and W. Pendlebury[1]

[1]Department of Neurological Sciences, University of Vermont College of Medicine, Burlington, VT 05401, USA
[2]Department of Psychiatry, University of Vermont College of Medicine, Burlington, VT 05401, USA
[3]Hematology/Oncology Division, Department of Medicine, University of Vermont College of Medicine, Burlington, VT 05401, USA
[4]Department of Radiology, University of Vermont College of Medicine, Burlington, VT 05401, USA

Correspondence should be addressed to Waqar Waheed; waqar.waheed@uvmhealth.org

Academic Editor: Peter Berlit

The etiology of spinal cord infarcts (SCIs), besides being related to aortic perioperative events, in large subset of SCIs, remains cryptogenic. We present a first case of SCI in a patient with hereditary spherocytosis and discuss the potential pathophysiologic considerations for vascular compromise. A 43-year-old woman with a history of hereditary spherocytosis, post splenectomy status, presented with chest, back, and shoulder pain with subsequent myelopathic picture; SCI extending from C4-T2 was confirmed by MRI. Despite aggressive treatment her stroke progressed leading to her demise. Her autopsy confirmed the SCI and revealed some incidental findings, but the cause of SCI remained unidentified. Exclusion of the known etiologies of SCI by extensive negative workup including autopsy evaluation suggested that SCI in our case was related to her history of hereditary spherocytosis. Both venous and arterial adverse vascular events, at a higher rate, have been associated in patients with hereditary spherocytosis who had their spleens removed compared to nonsplenectomized patients. Postsplenectomy increases in the platelet, red blood cell count, leukocyte count, and cholesterol concentrations are postulated to contribute to increased thrombotic risk. Additional prothrombotic factors include continuous platelet activation and adhesion as well as abnormalities of the red blood cell membrane.

1. Introduction

Spinal cord infarcts (SCIs) are very uncommon events that carry immense morbidity and mortality. SCIs encompass less than 1% of all strokes and 5–8% of acute myelopathies [1]. Although the majority of SCIs are associated with perioperative procedures (mostly aortic surgeries) [2], there remains a large subset of SCIs of uncharacterized etiology. This case report serves to shed light on a case of spinal cord infarction in a patient who had hereditary spherocytosis, for which she had undergone splenectomy during childhood. To our knowledge, the example of a spinal cord infarction as a deleterious vascular event in the setting of hereditary spherocytosis has not been previously reported. We will discuss the potential pathophysiologic and clinical considerations of this case.

2. Case Presentation

A 43-year-old woman presented to the emergency department with acute onset of chest, back, and bilateral shoulder and upper arm pain, which started upon rising from a seated position. Subsequent cardiac workup was negative and the pain resolved with ibuprofen, and she was admitted for observation. Over the course of the following day the patient developed bilateral numbness and weakness in her lower extremities, which started sequentially with the right leg progressing to the left leg, and, by the following day, had involvement of the bilateral arms. There was no associated trauma; review of systems was negative for constitutional, cardiopulmonary, or abdominal symptoms.

Past medical and surgical histories were significant for hereditary spherocytosis, morbid obesity, hypertension,

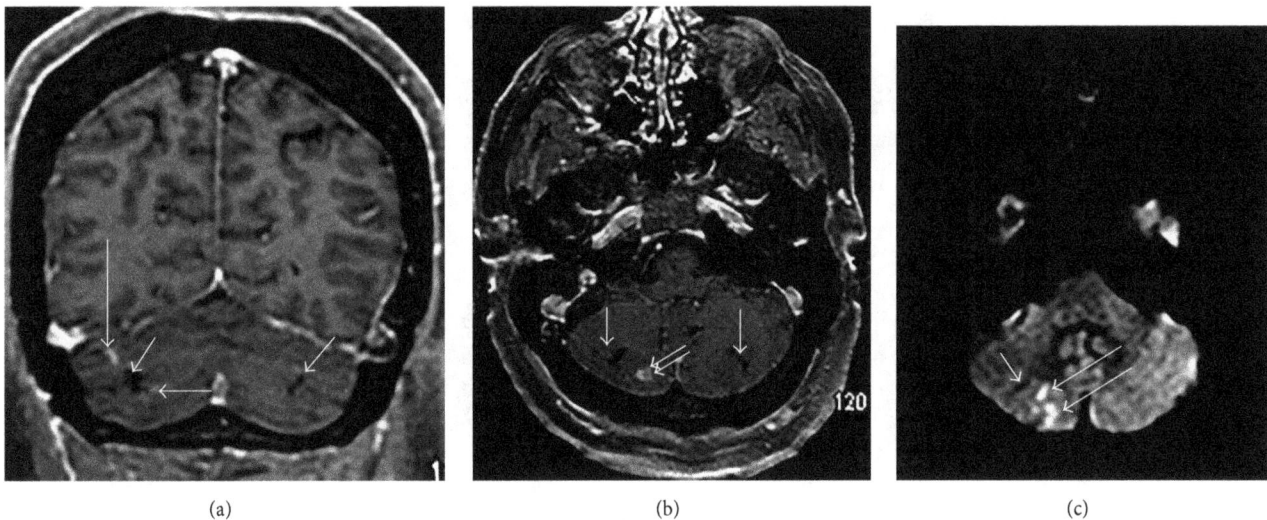

FIGURE 1: (a) Coronal postcontrast T1 weighted magnetic resonance (MR) image shows areas of old (chronic) infarction in the equators of both cerebellar hemispheres (short white arrows) and small, enhancing subacute infarcts in right cerebellum (long white arrows). (b) Axial postcontrast T1 weighted MR image shows areas of old (chronic) infarction in both cerebellar hemispheres (single white arrows) and an enhancing subacute infarct in the right cerebellum (double white arrow). (c) Axial diffusion weighted MR image (DWI) through the posterior fossa shows a small, old right cerebellar infarct (short white arrow) and areas of subacute infarction with diffusion restriction (long white arrows).

primary hyperparathyroidism with associated hypercalcemia and nephrolithiasis, postparathyroidectomy status, borderline diabetes mellitus, mild intellectual disability, and depression. She underwent splenectomy at the age of 14 years for hereditary spherocytosis. She had hematologic follow-up a decade after her splenectomy for persistent leukocytosis and thrombocytosis, attributed to lack of splenic sequestration, further suggested by negative JAK2 and BCR-ABL mutation. About 2 years prior to presentation, she had an unprovoked superficial venous thrombosis of her right lower extremity, for which no hypercoagulability workup was completed.

Home medications included cholecalciferol (Vitamin D3) 2000 IU/day, citalopram 20 mg/day, and lisinopril 10 mg/day. She was a nonsmoker and nonalcoholic with no history of illicit drug use. There was no family history of bleeding or thrombosis disorders.

Her admitting vitals showed pulse of 67/minute, blood pressure of 117/67, and temperature of 36.5°C. Her initial examination in ER showed variable fluctuating weakness and inconsistent sensory findings, confounded by her baseline history of developmental delay; however, subsequent neurologic examination was notable for a myelopathic pattern of weakness, suggested by quadriparesis, legs > arms, hyperreflexia in arms, absent reflexes in legs, loss of pain and temperature in lower extremities with sensory level at T5-6 level, spared proprioception, and vibration as well as loss of sphincter control. Bilateral Babinski signs were negative.

3. Laboratory Data

Magnetic resonance imaging (MRI) of the brain obtained at the time of initial presentation demonstrated areas of old, chronic infarction at the equators of both cerebellar

hemispheres (short white arrows in Figures 1(a) and 1(b)), in the watershed regions between the superior cerebellar and posterior inferior cerebellar artery vascular territories. There were also enhancing areas of subacute infarction in the right cerebellum (long white arrows in Figures 1(a), 1(b), and 1(c)). MRI of the cervical and thoracic spine obtained at this time revealed expansion of the cervical and upper thoracic spinal cord with abnormal increased T2 signal (between the white arrows in Figure 2(a)) with prominent diffusion restriction (between arrows in Figures 2(b) and 2(c)) extending from the inferior C4 level to the mid T2 level. The cord signal abnormality was primarily confined to the central gray matter (asterisks in Figure 2(d)). The clinical presentation and imaging findings were most compatible with anterior spinal artery distribution acute SCI; however, considering the possible patchy enhancement, transverse myelitis remained initially on the differential diagnosis. Lumbar puncture revealed normal results (normal cell count, protein, gram stain, cultures, oligoclonal banding IgG index, and cytology). CT angiogram of her neck and cervical spine was normal with no evidence of dissections or stenosis. A cardioembolic source was excluded with a sinus rhythm EKG and transthoracic echocardiogram demonstrating only mild left ventricular hypertrophy.

Abnormal labs included a complete blood count which showed baseline leukocytosis (34.3, normal 4–12 K/cmm) and thrombocytosis (486, normal 141–320 K/cmm), Hemoglobin A1c (6.3, normal 5.7–6.4%), and C reactive protein (13.9, normal < 1.0 mg/dL). Complete metabolic profile, TSH, Vitamin B12, folic acid, PT, PTT, and urine toxicology screen were normal. Vasculitis markers (ESR, ANA, anti-ds DNA, anti-SSA/SSB and ANCA), anti-NMO, and paraneoplastic panel (Mayo Clinic, Rochester,

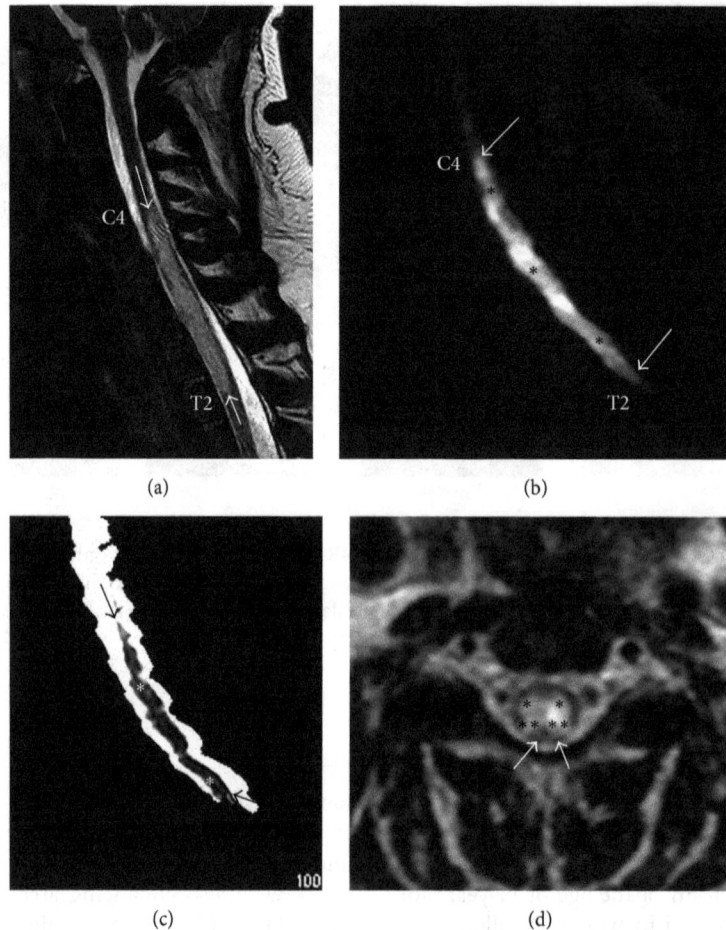

FIGURE 2: (a) Sagittal T2 weighted Fast Spin echo (FSE) MR image shows spinal cord expansion (swelling) with abnormal increased T2 signal extending from the C4 level to the T2 level (between the white arrows). (b) Sagittal DWI trace image shows abnormal increased signal intensity between C4 and T2, corresponding to the abnormal T2 signal noted on Sagittal T2 FSE imaging. (c) Sagittal apparent diffusion coefficient (ADC) map shows abnormal restriction of diffusion (dark signal in spinal cord indicated by arrows and asterisks) indicating that the increased signal on the DWI trace image represents diffusion restriction (not T2 shine through). (d) Axial T2 weighted FSE image at the C4 level shows cord expansion (swelling) and abnormal increased T2 signal within the swollen, edematous central gray matter (single asterisks indicate anterior horns and double asterisks indicate posterior horns of central gray matter). White arrows indicate uninvolved dorsal columns of the spinal cord.

Minnesota, USA) were normal. Her lipid profile revealed cholesterol of 176 mg/dL, LDL of 108 mg/dL, HDL of 43 mg/dL, and triglycerides of 125 mg/dL.

4. Treatment

The patient was started on Aspirin 325 mg/day, atorvastatin 80 mg/day, and subcutaneous enoxaparin deep venous thrombosis prophylaxis dose. Methylprednisolone 1 g intravenous once daily was given for 3 days while the patient was evaluated for a demyelinating disorder.

5. Hospital Course

On second hospitalization day, she was found to be hypotensive (86/54) with low urine output, attributed to low PO input and dehydration; discontinuation of lisinopril and

intravenous fluid administration normalized her blood pressure throughout the remainder of her hospital stay.

On the sixth day of hospitalization, the patient was transferred to ICU for difficulty with clearing secretions and respiratory distress, prompting Chest CT which showed multiple bilateral pulmonary emboli, while venous Doppler ultrasound of the lower extremities was negative for deep venous thrombosis. The patient was started on full dose of anticoagulation with a heparin drip and, after obtaining hematology consultation, folic acid 1 mg for spherocytosis and hypercoagulable workup initiated. Subsequently IgG and IgM anticardiolipin antibodies, anti-beta2-glycoprotein 1 antibodies, dilute Russell's viper venom time, factor V Leiden R506Q mutation by PCR, prothrombin G20210A gene mutation by PCR, PI linked antigen, antithrombin III activity, and protein C activity and protein S activity were within normal limits.

(a)

(b)

(c)

(d)

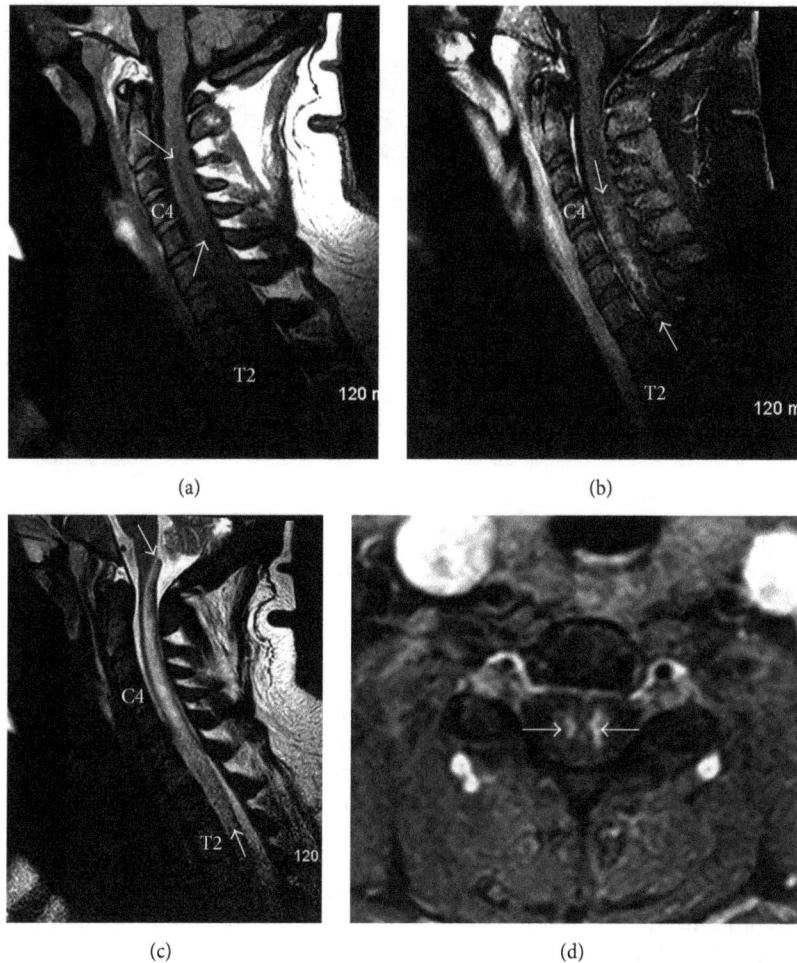

FIGURE 3: (a) Sagittal T1 weighted FSE image shows superior extension of the spinal cord swelling and abnormal decreased signal intensity centrally (between the white arrows). Note normal signal intensity of the osseous vertebral segments. (b) Sagittal T2 weighted FSE image shows superior extension of the spinal cord swelling and abnormal increased signal intensity centrally (between the white arrows) which now extends to the level of the obex. Note normal signal intensity of the osseous vertebral segments. (c) Sagittal postcontrast T1 weighted FSE image shows patchy enhancement within the central portions of the spinal cord (between the white arrows). (d) Axial postcontrast T1 weighted FSE image at the C4 level shows patchy enhancement confined to the central gray matter of the spinal cord, indicated by the white arrows (more prominent on the viewers right).

Despite maximal supportive treatment, the patient continued to progress with repeat imaging obtained 6 days after initial presentation revealed extension of the spinal cord expansion and cord signal abnormality (decreased T1 in Figure 3(a) and increased T2 in Figure 3(b)) which now extended superiorly to the level of the obex, compatible with progressive, superior extension of the spinal cord infarction. Postcontrast imaging revealed patchy areas of enhancement confined to the central gray matter (Figures 3(c) and 3(d)).

A family meeting was held to discuss the likelihood that she would require intubation and would likely require a tracheostomy and ventilator. She ultimately decided to pursue comfort measures instead of intubation and passed away within 24 hours. On autopsy, besides infarction of the anterior two-thirds of the cervical and upper thoracic spinal cord (Figures 4(a) and 4(b)) and left cerebellum, additional findings included two small neuroendocrine carcinoid tumors involving right lung, dilated and hypertrophic cardiomyopathy, two cystic masses of the right kidney, and a ductal plate abnormality involving the liver.

6. Discussion

Our case highlights some known facts of a spinal cord stroke [1–5]. (a) Unlike cerebral infarction, which is usually not painful, most (>80%) spinal infarcts are painful and, like our patient, due to involvement of afferent visceral pathways from the cardiac plexus can be mistaken for cardiac ischemia. (b) The most common clinical presentation (in approximately 95%) of SCI is an anterior spinal artery syndrome with neurologic dysfunction arising from a lesion located in the anterior two-thirds of the spinal cord. Typically, there is involvement of the central gray matter and adjacent white matter tracts, including the corticospinal,

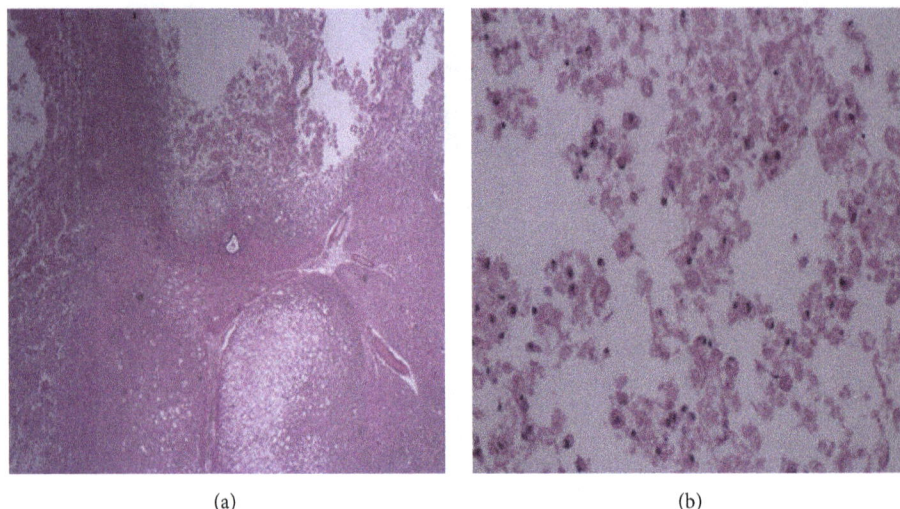

(a)   (b)

FIGURE 4: Low power of the central cervical cord (note central canal) showing cystic areas of acute infarct; 2xb is a low power of the lateral cervical cord with similar changes; high power showing a cystic area with debris and macrophages.

lateral spinothalamic, and autonomic tracts. Infarction with increased T2 signal of the anterior horn of the central gray matter can result in the "owl's eyes" sign described on MRI in anterior spinal artery infarction, though this imaging finding is nonspecific and has been described with other etiologies including infection (poliomyelitis), inflammation (acute idiopathic transverse myelitis), chronic compression myelopathy, and traumatic cord contusion. (c) Depending on the level and territory of spinal cord infarct, patients may develop respiratory distress; in our case C3 to C5 involvement through impairment of diaphragm and the accessory muscles of ventilation, coupled with atelectasis, pulmonary embolism, and caudal brainstem involvement, contributed to respiratory failure. (d) Hemodynamic instability owing to a greater splanchnic nerve palsy (T4–T9 lesion), requiring supportive therapy, can be seen. (e) Imaging of acute SCI related to the anterior spinal artery vascular distribution most often consists of spinal cord swelling (expansion) with abnormal decreased T1 and increased T2 signal involving the central gray matter and adjacent white matter tracts with diffusion restriction. The presence of vertebral body infarction (seen in 4–35% of patients) can provide confirmatory evidence of spinal cord infarction. In the subacute setting patchy contrast enhancement is often present. The main differential consideration for acute spinal cord infarction is transverse myelitis which typically does not demonstrate diffusion restriction and is not associated with vertebral body infarction.

SCI is much less common than cerebral infarction. The possible etiologies include atheromatosis, embolization (cardiogenic, fibrocartilaginous), severe hypotension, pathologic lesions in the aorta (aortic dissection, atherosclerosis, and aortic surgery), venous occlusion, vascular malformation, vasculitis, decompression sickness, vascular neoplasms of the spine (hemangioblastomas and cavernous angiomas), iatrogenicity, and trauma [1, 4, 5]. These etiologies were excluded by appropriate investigations and further verified by autopsy.

Fibrocartilaginous embolism, related to herniation of intervertebral disc material into the spinal vasculature, was suspected clinically based upon severe pain at the onset, a symptom-free interval between the onset of pain and deficits, and evolution of deficits over 15 minutes to 48 hours, which suggests a "spinal stroke in evolution." However, this was excluded by lack of radiological features [6] (prolapsed disk space at the appropriate level or intersomatic disk collapse, Schmorl's nodules) and by lack of pathological evidence of emboli in the spinal vessels on autopsy. Similarly cardioembolic, aortic, and paradoxical embolizations were excluded by normal cardiac echo, telemetry, and CTA head and neck and were further ruled out by autopsy.

The presence of ductal plate abnormalities in the liver and vascular anomalies in the kidney on autopsy suggested that a vascular malformation might have been the cause of our patient's SCI, which through mechanisms of venous hypertension can lead to cord edema and eventually infarction. However, the typical clinical presentation for venous infarction is a gradually progressive myelopathy and MRI features of perimedullary flow voids were absent in our case [7]. The two small bronchial neuroendocrine tumors (NET) identified on autopsy most probably represented an incidental finding due to the lack of associated systemic features and absence of prolonged severe hypotension, which makes NET associated carcinoid crisis an untenable diagnosis [8].

The extensive negative evaluation including autopsy for SCI including hypercoagulable, vasculitis, autoimmune, neoplastic, paraneoplastic, and cardioembolic/aortospinal vasculature workup suggested that a major consideration in the etiology of spinal cord as well as subacute and chronic watershed cerebellar infarcts and pulmonary embolism in our patient was her history of hereditary spherocytosis. Splenectomy, a standard procedure for many hematological conditions including myeloproliferative disorders, hereditary stomatocytosis, thalassemia, sickle cell disease, and sideroblastic anemia, has been associated with postsplenectomy thrombocytosis and increased risk of delayed vascular complications [8–16]. Even though thromboembolic complications have most frequently been reported in thalassemia [17], there have been an increasing body of evidence linking delayed thromboembolic events involving both venous and arterial circulation with hereditary spherocytosis [4, 15–17]. The cumulative incidence of adverse arterial and venous events by the age of 70 was significantly higher in patients with hereditary spherocytosis who had their spleens removed compared to nonsplenectomized patients [18]. In another study, the reported rate of arterial events after age of 40 years was approximately five times higher in hereditary spherocytosis patients without a spleen than in hereditary spherocytosis patients with a spleen. Most of the deaths associated with these events occurred more than fifteen years after splenectomy [19].

Delayed adverse vascular events previously reported in association with postsplenectomy hereditary spherocytosis patients include myocardial infarction, cerebral infarction, pulmonary hypertension, portal vein thrombosis, pulmonary embolism, peripheral venous thrombosis, thrombotic thrombocytopenic purpura, and priapism [9–12, 14–17, 20–24]. Progressive myelopathy due to extramedullary hematopoiesis has also been described in hereditary spherocytosis; it was not confirmed on the neuroimaging studies in our case [13].

The pathophysiology that underpins the increased thrombosis risk in patients with hereditary spherocytosis is not fully elucidated [25]. Postsplenectomy increases in the platelet, hemoglobin, red blood cell count, leukocyte count, C-reactive protein levels, and cholesterol concentrations are postulated to contribute to increased thrombotic risk after splenectomy [25–27]. Continuous platelet activation and adhesion, combined with abnormalities of the red blood cell membrane through increased viscosity and sludging of abnormal red blood cells, may also play a role in increased thrombotic risk [28]. Additional hypercoagulable mechanisms such as increased thrombin generation, a decrease in natural anticoagulants, and an increase in phospholipids such as phosphatidylserine on the abnormal red blood cells have been documented in other congenital anemias but have not been clearly elucidated in patients with hereditary spherocytosis [29, 30].

In conclusion, our case expands the spectrum of adverse vascular events after splenectomy in hereditary spherocytosis and supports an association between splenectomy and increased risk of thrombotic events. Delayed ischemic events in splenectomized patients with hereditary spherocytosis, although not commonly reported, are likely underappreciated. SCI could be a hitherto unreported complication seen after splenectomy in hereditary spherocytosis. Further research is needed to elucidate the pathophysiological mechanisms behind delayed thromboembolic complications in patients with hereditary spherocytosis requiring splenectomy.

Competing Interests

There are no competing interests to report.

References

[1] M. N. Rubin and A. A. Rabinstein, "Vascular diseases of the spinal cord," *Neurologic Clinics*, vol. 31, no. 1, pp. 153–181, 2013.

[2] C. E. Robertson, R. D. Brown Jr., E. F. M. Wijdicks, and A. A. Rabinstein, "Recovery after spinal cord infarcts: long-term outcome in 115 patients," *Neurology*, vol. 78, no. 2, pp. 114–121, 2012.

[3] J. Faig, O. Busse, and R. Salbeck, "Vertebral body infarction as a confirmatory sign of spinal cord ischemic stroke: report of three cases and review of the literature," *Stroke*, vol. 29, no. 1, pp. 239–243, 1998.

[4] C. Masson, J. P. Pruvo, J. F. Meder et al., "Spinal cord infarction: clinical and magnetic resonance imaging findings and short term outcome," *Journal of Neurology, Neurosurgery and Psychiatry*, vol. 75, no. 10, pp. 1431–1435, 2004.

[5] A. A. Rabinstein, "Vascular myelopathies," *CONTINUUM Lifelong Learning in Neurology*, vol. 21, pp. 67–83, 2015.

[6] T. P. Duprez, L. Danvoye, D. Hernalsteen, G. Cosnard, C. J. Sindic, and C. Godfraind, "Fibrocartilaginous embolization to the spinal cord: serial MR imaging monitoring and pathologic study," *American Journal of Neuroradiology*, vol. 26, no. 3, pp. 496–501, 2005.

[7] K. Jellema, L. R. Canta, C. C. Tijssen, W. J. van Rooij, P. J. Koudstaal, and J. van Gijn, "Spinal dural arteriovenous fistulas: clinical features in 80 patients," *Journal of Neurology, Neurosurgery and Psychiatry*, vol. 74, no. 10, pp. 1438–1440, 2003.

[8] S. Fischer, M. Kruger, K. McRae, N. Merchant, M. S. Tsao, and S. Keshavjee, "Giant bronchial carcinoid tumors: a multidisciplinary approach," *The Annals of Thoracic Surgery*, vol. 71, no. 1, pp. 386–393, 2001.

[9] J. J. Van Hilten, J. Haan, A. R. Wintzen et al., "Cerebral infarction in hereditary spherocytosis," *Stroke*, vol. 20, no. 12, pp. 1755–1756, 1989.

[10] D. L. Becton, M. Kletzel, W. C. Arnold, and D. H. Berry, "Thrombotic thrombocytopenic purpura in an asplenic patient with hereditary spherocytosis: failure of plasmapheresis, antiplatelet therapy, and corticosteroids," *American Journal of Pediatric Hematology/Oncology*, vol. 10, no. 1, pp. 5–8, 1988.

[11] W. McGrew and G. R. Avant, "Hereditary spherocytosis and portal vein thrombosis," *Journal of Clinical Gastroenterology*, vol. 6, no. 4, pp. 381–382, 1984.

[12] C. Sparwasser, B. Danz, and W. F. Thon, "Segmental unilateral priapism—a case report," *Der Urologe*, vol. 27, no. 5, pp. 266–268, 1988.

[13] A. I. De Backer, P. Zachee, I. J. Vanschoubroeck, K. J. Mortele, P. R. Ros, and M. M. Kockx, "Extramedullary paraspinal hematopoiesis in hereditary spherocytosis," *JBR-BTR*, vol. 85, pp. 206–208, 2002.

[14] J. E. Hayag-Barin, R. E. Smith, and F. C. Tucker Jr., "Hereditary spherocytosis, thrombocytosis, and chronic pulmonary emboli: a case report and review of the literature," *American Journal of Hematology*, vol. 57, no. 1, pp. 82–84, 1998.

[15] G. W. Stewart, J. A. L. Amess, S. W. Eber et al., "Thromboembolic disease after splenectomy for hereditary stomatocytosis," *British Journal of Haematology*, vol. 93, no. 2, pp. 303–310, 1996.

[16] K. H. Scholz, C. Herrmann, U. Tebbe, J. M. Chemnitius, U. Helmchen, and H. Kreuzer, "Myocardial infarction in young patients with Hodgkin's disease—potential pathogenic role of radiotherapy, chemotherapy, and splenectomy," *The Clinical Investigator*, vol. 71, no. 1, pp. 57–64, 1993.

[17] Y. T. Tai, Y. L. Yu, C. P. Lau, and P. C. Fong, "Myocardial infarction complicating postsplenectomy thrombocytosis, with early left ventricular mural thrombus formation and cerebral embolism—a case report," *Angiology*, vol. 44, no. 1, pp. 73–77, 1993.

[18] R. F. Schilling, R. E. Gangnon, and M. I. Traver, "Delayed adverse vascular events after splenectomy in hereditary spherocytosis," *Journal of Thrombosis and Haemostasis*, vol. 6, no. 8, pp. 1289–1295, 2008.

[19] C. D. Robinette and J. F. Fraumeni Jr., "Splenectomy and subsequent mortality in veterans of the 1939–45 war," *The Lancet*, vol. 2, no. 8029, pp. 127–129, 1977.

[20] S. C. Tso, T. K. Chan, and D. Todd, "Venous thrombosis in haemoglobin H disease after splenectomy," *Australian and New Zealand Journal of Medicine*, vol. 12, no. 6, pp. 635–638, 1982.

[21] P. J. Broe, C. L. Conley, and J. L. Cameron, "Thrombosis of the portal vein following splenectomy for myeloid metaplasia," *Surgery Gynecology & Obstetrics*, vol. 152, no. 4, pp. 488–492, 1981.

[22] P. Macchia, F. Massei, M. Nardi, C. Favre, E. Brunori, and V. Barba, "Thalassemia intermedia and recurrent priapism following splenectomy," *Haematologica*, vol. 75, no. 5, pp. 486–487, 1990.

[23] J. Hirsh and J. V. Dacie, "Persistent post-splenectomy thrombocytosis and thrombo-embolism: a consequence of continuing anaemia," *British Journal of Haematology*, vol. 12, no. 1, pp. 44–53, 1966.

[24] D. H. Gordon, D. Schaffner, J. M. Bennett, and S. I. Schwartz, "Postsplenectomy thrombocytosis: its association with mesenteric, portal, and/or renal vein thrombosis in patients with myeloproliferative disorders," *Archives of Surgery*, vol. 113, no. 6, pp. 713–715, 1978.

[25] F. Rodeghiero and M. Ruggeri, "Short- and long-term risks of splenectomy for benign haematological disorders: should we revisit the indications?" *British Journal of Haematology*, vol. 158, no. 1, pp. 16–29, 2012.

[26] S. E. Crary and G. R. Buchanan, "Vascular complications after splenectomy for hematologic disorders," *Blood*, vol. 114, no. 14, pp. 2861–2868, 2009.

[27] M. P. Westerman, "Hypocholesterolaemia and anaemia," *British Journal of Haematology*, vol. 31, no. 1, pp. 87–94, 1975.

[28] R. F. Schilling, "Spherocytosis, splenectomy, strokes, and heart attacks," *The Lancet*, vol. 350, no. 9092, pp. 1677–1678, 1997.

[29] N. Goldschmidt, G. Spectre, A. Brill et al., "Increased platelet adhesion under flow conditions is induced by both thalassemic platelets and red blood cells," *Thrombosis and Haemostasis*, vol. 100, no. 5, pp. 864–870, 2008.

[30] K. de Jong, S. K. Larkin, S. Eber, P. F. H. Franck, B. Roelofsen, and F. A. Kuypers, "Hereditary spherocytosis and elliptocytosis erythrocytes show a normal transbilayer phospholipid distribution," *Blood*, vol. 94, no. 1, pp. 319–325, 1999.

22

Atypical Features in a Large Turkish Family Affected with Friedreich Ataxia

Semiha Kurt,[1] Betul Cevik,[1] Durdane Aksoy,[1] E. Irmak Sahbaz,[2]
Aslı Gundogdu Eken,[2] and A. Nazli Basak[2]

[1]Department of Neurology, Gaziosmanpasa University Faculty of Medicine, 60100 Tokat, Turkey
[2]Suna and Inan Kıraç Foundation Neurodegeneration Research Laboratory, Molecular Biology and Genetics Department,
 Bogazici University, 34342 Istanbul, Turkey

Correspondence should be addressed to Semiha Kurt; gsemihakurt@hotmail.com

Academic Editor: Dominic B. Fee

Here, we describe the clinical features of several members of the same family diagnosed with Friedreich ataxia (FRDA) and cerebral lesions, demyelinating neuropathy, and late-age onset without a significant cardiac involvement and presenting with similar symptoms, although genetic testing was negative for the GAA repeat expansion in one patient of the family. The GAA repeat expansion in the frataxin gene was shown in all of the family members except in a young female patient. MRI revealed arachnoid cysts in two patients; MRI was consistent with both cavum septum pellucidum-cavum vergae and nodular signal intensity increase in one patient. EMG showed demyelinating sensorimotor polyneuropathy in another patient. The GAA expansion-negative 11-year-old female patient had mental-motor retardation, epilepsy, and ataxia. None of the patients had significant cardiac symptoms. Description of FRDA families with different ethnic backgrounds may assist in identifying possible phenotypic and genetic features of the disease. Furthermore, the genetic heterogeneity observed in this family draws attention to the difficulty of genetic counseling in an inbred population and to the need for genotyping all affected members before delivering comprehensive genetic counseling.

1. Introduction

Friedreich ataxia (FRDA) is an autosomal recessive neurodegenerative disorder and the most common hereditary ataxia. The FRDA locus was detected on chromosome 9 in 1988 [1]. The frataxin gene, which encodes a protein that probably acts as a mitochondrial iron transporter, was detected in 1996 [1]. Most mutations appear to be unstable expansions of a GAA repeat in the first intron of the gene [1].

Harding described the essential clinical features as (1) autosomal recessive inheritance, (2) onset before 25 years of age, (3) progressive limb and gait ataxia, (4) absent tendon reflexes in the lower extremities, (5) electrophysiological signs of axonal sensory neuropathy (within 5 years of onset), (6) dysarthria, (7) areflexia at all four extremities, (8) distal loss of position and vibration sense, (9) extensor plantar reflex, and (10) muscle weakness in the lower extremities [2].

The "typical" or "classic" form of the disease is defined as a disease form exhibiting all the clinical features listed by Harding [2, 3]. Disease forms which do not meet these criteria are referred to as atypical Friedreich ataxia. Skeletal deformities, cardiomyopathy, and diabetes are the most common systemic conditions associated with FRDA [4]. The disease is characterized by clinical variability regarding the age at onset, the rate of progression, and presence/absence of areflexia, muscle weakness, or cardiomyopathy. However, the clinical manifestations tend to be similar in affected siblings in the same family [4], indicating the crucial role of genetic factors for phenotypic expression of the disease.

In FRDA patients, magnetic resonance imaging scans reveal spinal cord atrophy along with normal brainstem, cerebellum, and cerebrum [2]. Demyelinating neuropathy and late disease onset after the age of 25 years are the manifestations excluding the classical form of FRDA [1, 3]. Cardiac involvement occurs in most of the patients with FRDA [2]. Similar symptoms related to multiple diseases are also rare in the same family [5].

Here, we describe the atypical clinical features of several members of the same family diagnosed with Friedreich ataxia (FRDA) and cerebral lesions, demyelinating neuropathy, and late-age onset without a significant cardiac involvement and presenting with similar symptoms, although genetic testing was negative for the GAA repeat expansion in one patient of the family.

2. Patients and Methods

Our index case was a 37-year-old man admitted to our outpatient clinic following a history of ataxia. Family members with similar symptoms were identified in Tokat, a city in the Middle Black Sea region of Turkey. This study was performed in accordance with the Helsinki Declaration. All adult participants provided written informed consent. Parents of participating minors provided written informed consent; literate minors who could write also provided signed assent. All subjects received a detailed explanation of the study and genetic counseling as appropriate. A pedigree was prepared in the field. A detailed history was obtained from each subject, and each subject received a detailed neurological examination. All available previous tests and imaging studies of the patients were recorded in detail.

Five stages of disease disability were distinguished: stage 0: patients at risk with normal examination results; stage 1: clinical signs of FRDA found at clinical exam; stage 2: functional signs but able to walk unaided; stage 3: clinical and functional signs, unable to walk without help; stage 4: confined to wheelchair, able to stand but not to walk; stage 5: bedridden: unable to stand [1].

Electrophysiological Examination. Electrophysiological studies were performed using standard nerve conduction techniques with Medelec-Oxford EMG equipment. Sensory nerve conduction studies were performed orthodromically on median and ulnar nerves and antidromically on the sural and superficial peroneal nerves. Motor nerve conduction studies were conducted on the median, ulnar, tibial, and peroneal nerves. Electromyography was performed on at least two proximal and distal muscles from the upper and lower extremities.

DNA Sample Collection and Genetic Analysis. Blood samples were taken from the cubital vein into EDTA-containing tubes during field work. DNA was isolated using the Magna Pure Compact System from Roche, followed by PCR analysis.

3. Results

Figure 1 shows the pedigree structure of the family. Blood samples were obtained from five symptomatic and 15 asymptomatic family members during family screening. Neurological examination of 15 asymptomatic family members did not reveal any abnormal finding. Ten out of these fifteen family members were carriers of GAA repeat expansion.

Clinical, electrophysiological, and neuroradiological data were obtained from two male and two female family members suffering from ataxia (Table 1). One male patient was evaluated clinically and genetically. Patients I.1 (the index patient) and II.5 were brothers, and Patient III.5 was their niece. Patients II.10 and II.11 were siblings and first cousins of Patients II.1 and II.5.

4. Clinical Presentation of the Family

4.1. Patient II.5 (Index Case). The 37-year-old male patient presented with a history of imbalance and numbness in hands and feet starting from the age of 18 without any other previous complaints. Although numbness in the hands and feet has improved in time, the imbalance had worsened. Following the increasing deterioration of the writing hand, muscle weakness in the hands and feet increased. Speech disturbance started about 6-7 years ago. 2-3 years ago, he started to require unilateral aid to walk due to the increased risk of fall. The patient defined similar complaints in his brother, in a female and male cousins, and in his niece. His neurological examination revealed dysarthric speech and a mild effacement of the left nasolabial fold, diffuse weakness and atrophy in the legs, and a mild distal atrophy in the hands. Deep tendon reflexes were absent in the upper and lower extremities. He had a moderate dysmetria and dysdiadochokinesia. His gait was ataxic in spite of unilateral walking aid. Joint-position sense was impaired in the toes. Plantar reflexes were absent on both sides. A mild thoracic scoliosis, pes cavus, and hammer toes were detected in his examination. The results of routine hematological and biochemical investigations were normal. He had no clinical symptoms of a cardiac disease and ECG was normal. In the electrophysiological studies, sensory action potentials were absent in the sural, superficial peroneal, median, and ulnar nerves. Median nerve conduction velocity (NCV) was 38.7 m/s, terminal latency (TL) was 4.3 ms, and F latency was 36.5 ms. Ulnar NCV was 33.45 m/s, TL was 4 ms, and F latency was 37.3 ms. Peroneal NCV was 27.3 m/s, TL was 6.2 ms, and F latency was 68.5 ms. Tibial NCV was 25.4 m/s, TL was 6.55 ms, and F latency was 64.4 ms. Conduction abnormalities matched demyelinating neuropathy criteria [6]. Brain MRI scans revealed an image of arachnoid cyst approximately 25 mm in diameter in posterior vermian area (Figure 2(a)).

4.2. Patient II.1. The 47-year-old male patient stated imbalance that started at the age of 27. Later on, speech disturbance was added to his complaints. Both imbalance and speech disturbance have gradually worsened and he was barely able to take a few steps with bilateral walking aid for the last 5-6 years, usually using a wheelchair. His neurological examination revealed dysarthric speech and bilateral horizontal nystagmus, a mild loss of muscle strength in the lower extremities in spite of normal muscle strength in the upper extremities, a normal superficial sensation and loss of vibration sense in the distal foot, absent deep tendon reflexes, and extensor plantar responses on both sides. Dysmetria

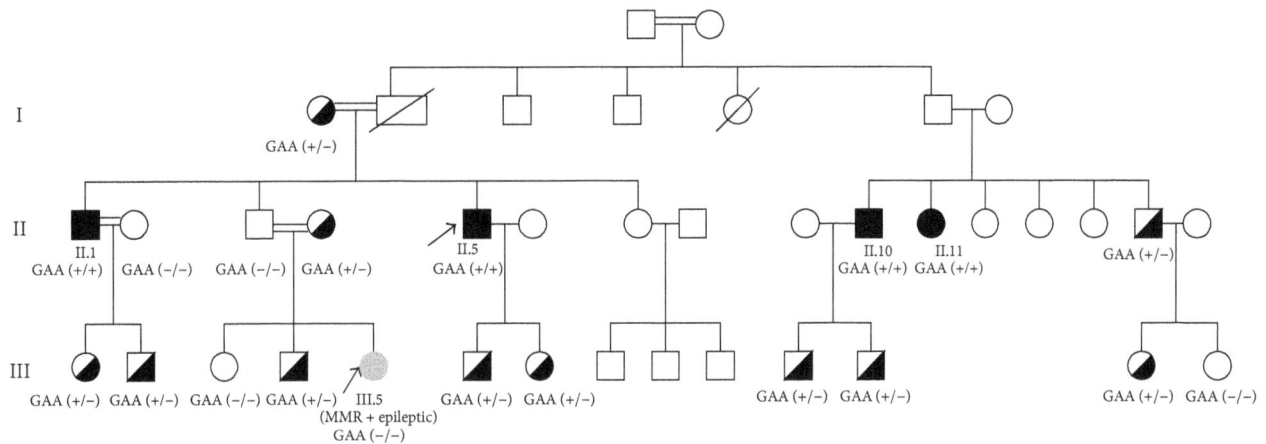

FIGURE 1: Pedigree of a family with FRDA. Black boxes indicate affected FRDA patients. The index case is indicated by an arrow. Semiblack boxes indicate FRDA carriers. The FRDA(−) case is indicated by grey box and the number III.5.

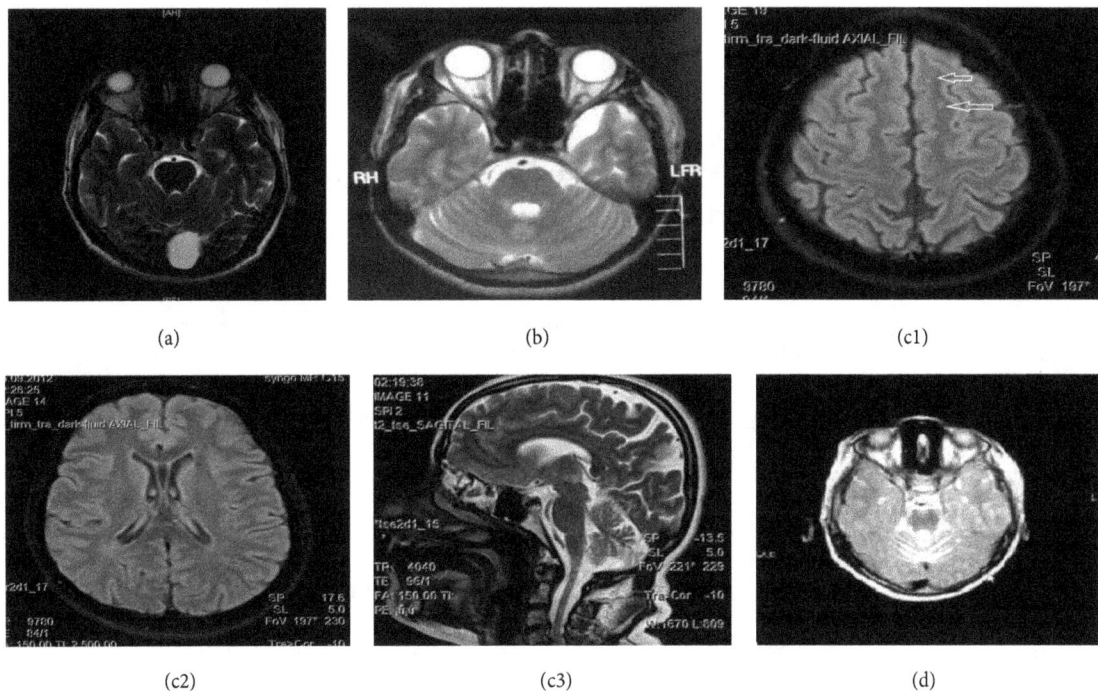

(a) (b) (c1)

(c2) (c3) (d)

FIGURE 2: Arachnoid cyst in posterior vermian area in Patient II.5 (a); left temporal arachnoid cyst in Patient II.1 (b); multiple nodular (white arrows) lesions (c1), cavum septum pellucidum-cavum vergae variation (c2), and cerebellar atrophy in Patient II.11 (c3); cerebellar atrophy in Patient III.5 (d).

and dysdiadochokinesia were detected in the upper limbs. He was barely able to stand and take a few steps. The results of routine hematological and biochemical investigations were normal. He had no clinical symptoms of cardiac disease and ECG was normal. Echocardiography revealed a mild diastolic dysfunction. On electrophysiological examination, sensory action potentials were absent in the sural nerve and moderately reduced in amplitude and velocity in the median and ulnar nerves. The median, ulnar, peroneal, and tibial motor conduction studies were normal.

Patient's previous MRI scans of the brain revealed a left temporal CSF-isointense lesion consistent with arachnoid cyst (Figure 2(b)) and previous MRI and X-ray of the thoracolumbar spine showed S-shaped scoliosis.

4.3. Patient II.10. The 52-year-old male patient stated gait imbalance and speech disturbance first started when he was sixteen. He became wheelchair-bound in 1997 due to gradually increased ataxia. His neurological examination revealed severe dysarthria, bilateral horizontal nystagmus, a normal superficial sensation, and reduced sense of vibration and position in the distal foot. There was no significant loss of muscle strength. Triceps and biceps reflexes were

TABLE 1: Clinical and laboratory characteristics of the patients.

Feature	Patient II.5	Patient II.1	Patient II.10	Patient II.11	Patient III.5
Age at evaluation	37	47	52	40	11
Age at onset	18	27	16	16	Infant
Duration of the disease	19	20	36	24	11
Sex	M	M	M	F	F
First symptom	Ataxia, paresthesia	Ataxia	Ataxia	Ataxia	MMR
Ataxia	++	+++	+++	+++	+++
Dysarthria	+	++	++	++	++
Muscle weakness					
Upper limbs	+	−	−	+	++
Lower limbs	+	+	−	+++	+++
Deep tendon reflexes					
Upper limbs	Absent	Absent	Diminished	Absent	Absent
Lower limbs	Absent	Absent	Absent	Absent	Absent
Joint position/vibration sense abnormalities					
Upper limbs	−	−	−	+	NP
Lower limbs	+	+	+	+	NP
Babinski sign	Absent	Extensor	Flexor	Extensor	Extensor
Extraneurological findings	Scoliosis, hammer toes	Scoliosis	Scoliosis	Scoliosis	Scoliosis
Cardiomyopathy	−	−	−	−	−
Cranial MRI	Arachnoid cyst	Arachnoid cyst	NP	CV, CSP, NL, and C-Ce atrophy	Ce-atrophy
NCS	Demyelinating neuropathy	Sensorial neuropathy	NP	Sensorial neuropathy	Sensorial neuropathy
Functional score	Unable to walk without help	Confined to wheelchair	Confined to wheelchair	Confined to wheelchair	Confined to wheelchair

M: male, F: female, MMR: mental motor retardation, NP: not performed, NL: nodular lesions, CV: cavum vergae, CSP: cavum septum pellucidum, C: cerebral, and Ce: cerebellar. +++: severe; ++: moderate; +: mild; −: no.

diminished while other deep tendon reflexes were absent too. Flexor plantar responses were obtained on both sides and severe bilateral dysmetria and dysdiadochokinesia were detected predominantly on the left side and he was unable to stand. Scoliosis was noted by visual inspection. The patient had no cardiac complaints and did not accept to undergo investigations other than genetic analysis.

4.4. Patient II.11. The 40-year-old female patient first started to have difficulty in walking when she was sixteen. The gait disorder was followed by a speech disturbance and loss of muscle strength particularly in the lower limbs, and she became wheelchair-bound at the age of 25. Her neurological examination revealed dysarthria, bilateral horizontal nystagmus, and muscle strength of 4/5 in the upper extremities and 0/5 in the lower limbs apart from muscle strength of 2/5 in the dorsiflexion and plantar flexion of the toes, on both sides. Muscle tone was reduced in the lower extremities. Vibration sense was reduced in the distal parts of the hands and foot, in addition to the glove-stocking hypoesthesia. Deep tendon reflexes were absent and an extensor plantar response

was obtained on both sides. Severe bilateral dysmetria and dysdiadochokinesia were detected predominantly on the left side and she was unable to stand even with bilateral assistance. Moderate thoracic scoliosis was evident. The results of routine hematological and biochemical investigations were normal. She had no clinical symptoms of a heart disease and ECG was normal. On electrophysiological examination, sensory action potentials were absent in the sural, superficial peroneal, median, and ulnar nerves. The median, ulnar, peroneal, and tibial motor conduction studies were normal. MRI scan of the brain of the patient revealed signal changes of the white matter indicating multiple nodular lesions in the cerebral parenchyma at the level of corona radiata, centrum semiovale, a congenital cavum septum pellucidum, cavum vergae variation in the interventricular space, and cerebral and cerebellar atrophy (Figures 2(c1), 2(c2), and 2(c3)).

4.5. Patient III.5. The 11-year-old female patient with motor and mental retardation was born by Cesarean section for breech presentation at term. She kept her head steady at 8 months of age and sat without support at the age of three, crawled at the age of four and started to walk at the age of five. Subsequently, she has gradually developed a gait ataxia and required the assistance of a walker and then she became unable to walk. She had her first seizure when she was 6 months old. First valproic acid was started and then it was switched to lamotrigine. The seizures were taken under control by lamotrigine and the treatment was discontinued following two years of seizure-free period of time. It was reported that she was unable to talk in sentences but she could speak a few words and she was partly able to understand. In the neurological examination, she was capable of forming words in a dysarthric pattern. She was not oriented and poorly cooperative. Gross examination of the cranial nerves revealed no abnormality. Muscle strength was determined as 4/5 in the proximal parts of upper extremities and 3/5 in the distal parts and as 3/5 in the proximal parts of lower extremities and 0/5 in the distal parts. Muscle tone was reduced. Sensory and cerebellar tests could not be performed. Deep tendon reflexes were absent and plantar responses were extensor. Previous routine blood biochemistry and hematological tests were within normal limits. Amino acid levels were found to be within normal limits in an AA analysis using tandem MS (LC-MS-MS) method. C8/C12 ratio was found to be mildly elevated in the acylcarnitine/carnitine analysis; however, the result of the repeat test was normal. Serum levels of vitamin E, AFP, lactate, IgA, IgE, IgG, and IgM were found to be within normal levels. Urine organic acid assessment revealed an excretion of 50 mmol/mol of succinic acid. The excretion of oxalic acid was equal to the internal standard and the excretion of homovanillic acid and vanillylmandelic acid was equal to half of the internal standard along with elevated excretion of pyruvic acid, 3-OH isobutyric acid, ethylmalonic acid, adipic acid, 3-indol acetic acid, and 3-OH propionic acid and trace amount of erythrov 4,5 diOH hexanoate lactone, tiglylglycine, and methyl citrate. The excretion of other organic acids was within normal limits. Increased SCA-specific CAG repeat was not found in any of the SCA 1, 2, 3, 6, and 7 loci. Personal-social development was determined at the level of 18.5 months of age, fine motor skills were found at the level of 14–19 months, language skills were found at the level of 22–30 months of age, and gross motor development was found to be at the level of 12 months in the Denver II developmental screening test. ECG and echocardiography tests were normal. Previous EEGs reported a slow background activity and sharp waves in the right temporooccipital regions and some of them were reported as normal. Motor nerve conduction studies were normal in the lower extremities and no response could be obtained from the sural nerve in the EMG which was interpreted as a technical issue. Cerebellar atrophy was reported in the MRI scan of the brain (Figure 2(d)). The repeat EEG was normal. Sensory nerve action potentials could not be obtained from the sural and superficial peroneal nerves and sensory nerve action potential amplitudes of the median and ulnar nerves were reduced in the repeat EMG study. Motor conduction studies were normal. The patient had scoliosis concave to the left.

5. DNA Analysis

PCR analysis for the GAA repeat in the frataxin gene revealed the homozygous presence of the GAA repeat in all four affected members of generation II. The young Patient III.5 did not have GAA repeat in this locus. The analysis of her parents validated the result, since her mother was a carrier, whereas the father was normal for the GAA repeat.

6. Discussion

In patients with Friedreich ataxia, MRI scans of the spine show thinning of the cervical spinal cord and signal abnormalities in the posterior and lateral columns [7]. Cerebellar atrophy is not a common finding in CT or MRI images; however, the presence of cerebellar atrophy indicates a severe, advanced disease [7, 8]. Brain MRI may be a useful diagnostic procedure, since the absence of cerebellar atrophy may point out other forms of hereditary recessive ataxia rather than Friedreich ataxia [2, 7]. However, as far as we know, no intracranial lesions have been reported in FRDA. Arachnoid cyst was reported in two of our patients and cavum septum pellucidum and cavum vergae variation and nodular signal changes were detected in Patient II.11. Arachnoid cysts and congenital intra-axial midline cysts (cavum septum pellucidum, cavum vergae, and cavum velum interpositum) are nonneoplastic neurological cysts [9]. Arachnoid cysts are fluid-filled duplications or splittings of the arachnoid layer with a content mildly different from the cerebrospinal fluid [10]. They may occur sporadically as isolated variations or may be associated with other malformations or diseases [10]. Usually arachnoid cysts are incidentally detected on imaging studies of the brain [11]. Although most cases are sporadic, intracranial arachnoid cysts in several members of the same family have been reported in a few publications [11]. In one of these reports, arachnoid cysts were accompanied by a deletion in chromosome 16 in the same family [11]. Jadeja and Grewal presented an unusual association of genetic myopathy, oculopharyngeal muscular dystrophy, and arachnoid cysts in the same family [12]. Değerliyurt et al. described two siblings with porencephaly, hemiparesis, epilepsy, and atrophic kidney associated with an arachnoid cyst in one of the siblings and in the asymptomatic mothers. Col4A1 gene mutation screening revealed a novel mutation in mother and both children [13]. Bayrakli et al. presented an intracranial arachnoid cyst family from southern Turkey with six out of seven offspring with intracranial arachnoid cysts in different localizations [14]. Arachnoid cyst was found to be present in two male siblings with FRDA in our study.

When a septum pellucidum has a separation between its two leaflets, it is referred to as cavum septum pellucidum (CSP). This condition takes place when there is separation between the leaflets of the septum pellucidum and posterior extension to the splenium of the corpus callosum. The anterior columns of the fornix separate the anterior cavum septum pellucidum and the posterior cavum vergae (CV). CSP may persist in up to 20% of adults. CV is present in up to 30% of newborns, although it may persist in less than 1% of the adult individuals. CV cysts are usually associated with

CSP [9]. The CSP and CV cyst association was detected also in our patient.

Preadolescent onset is commonly regarded as crucial for the diagnosis of FRDA. Harding revised the diagnostic criteria in order to include patients with late onset up to the age of 25 years [3]. The complaints of Patient II.1 started after the age of 25. Late onset Friedreich ataxia, defined by symptom onset after the age of 25, accounts for 14% of the cases, while very late onset Friedreich ataxia, characterized by disease onset after the age of 40, is very rare [15].

Nerve conduction studies reveal axonal sensory neuropathy along with small or absent sensory action potentials in FRDA patients [2]. Motor conduction velocities are normal or mildly reduced in comparison to the sensory nerve potentials [2]. Nerve conduction studies of Patients II.1 and II.11 shared these characteristics; however, the motor nerve studies of our index case revealed demyelinating characteristics. According to Harding's criteria, a marked reduction of motor nerve conduction velocities is a finding that may exclude the diagnosis of FRDA [3]. However, Panas et al. reported three unrelated families with four affected children who suggested a hereditary motor and sensory neuropathy according to the clinical findings; however, the molecular genetic analysis was consistent with FRDA [16]. They claimed that the mutation identified in all four patients supports that these cases are representatives of a "variant" form of FRDA [16]. Similarly, Benomar et al. also reported that, in four out of seven FRDA patients, electromyography revealed a severe demyelinating neuropathy and severe demyelination and axonal neuropathy in the other three patients [1].

Cardiomyopathy is present in two-thirds of the patients with FRDA which is primarily symmetric concentric hypertrophic cardiomyopathy; in addition, some patients exhibit asymmetric septal hypertrophy [2]. Electrocardiogram reveals widespread T wave inversions and signs of ventricular hypertrophy [2]. The Acadian Type (Louisiana Form), which is observed in a specific population of French origin living in North America, was distinguished from typical FRDA by its milder course and lower incidence of cardiomyopathy [2]. Similarly to the Acadian Type, no significant cardiomyopathy was detected in our cases.

The EMG patterns and ages of onset were heterogeneous in our cases. The interfamilial clinical variability in FRDA patients was explained by mutation heterogeneity before the elucidation of the molecular basis of FRDA. The knowledge that almost all cases of FRDA are caused by the same dynamic mutation provided another way to interpret phenotypic heterogeneity [16]. According to Illarioshkin et al., the cooccurrence of distinct clinical variants of the disorder is associated with different combinations of the mutated alleles inherited from parents [4].

The genetic study of Patient III.5 was negative for FRDA. Bouhlal et al. have described three distinct gene defects leading to an autosomal recessive ataxia in a consanguineous Tunisian family [5]. A study conducted by Zlotogora asserted that a chance phenomenon, the migration of families with affected patients or a digenic inheritance, might be responsible for the genetic heterogeneity observed in some autosomal recessive disease. However, these explanations are not persuasive in most cases. Although the selection mechanism was demonstrated to explain most of the observations, it is difficult to prove [17]. The hypothesis of a coincidental association seemed to be the most logical explanation; however, it is also difficult to explain it on a statistical basis [5].

Description of FRDA families with different ethnic backgrounds may assist in identifying possible phenotypic and genetic features of the disease. Furthermore, the genetic heterogeneity observed in this family draws attention to the difficulty of genetic counseling in an inbred population and to the need for genotyping all affected members before delivering a comprehensive genetic counseling.

Competing Interests

All authors declare that they have no conflicts of interest in the present study.

References

[1] A. Benomar, M. Yahyaoui, F. Meggouh et al., "Clinical comparison between AVED patients with 744 del a mutation and Friedreich ataxia with GAA expansion in 15 Moroccan families," *Journal of the Neurological Sciences*, vol. 198, no. 1-2, pp. 25–29, 2002.

[2] G. Alper and V. Narayanan, "Friedreich's ataxia," *Pediatric Neurology*, vol. 28, no. 5, pp. 335–341, 2003.

[3] A. E. Harding, "Friedreich's ataxia: a clinical and genetic study of 90 families with an analysis of early diagnostic criteria and intrafamilial clustering of clinical features," *Brain*, vol. 104, no. 3, pp. 589–620, 1981.

[4] S. N. Illarioshkin, G. K. Bagieva, S. A. Klyushnikov, I. V. Ovchinnikov, E. D. Markova, and I. A. Ivanova-Smolenskaya, "Different phenotypes of Friedreich's ataxia within one 'pseudo-dominant' genealogy: relationships between trinucleotide (GAA) repeat lengths and clinical features," *European Journal of Neurology*, vol. 7, no. 5, pp. 535–540, 2000.

[5] Y. Bouhlal, M. Zouari, M. Kefi, C. Ben Hamida, F. Hentati, and R. Amouri, "Autosomal recessive ataxia caused by three distinct gene defects in a single consanguineous family," *Journal of Neurogenetics*, vol. 22, no. 2, pp. 139–148, 2008.

[6] S. J. Oh, *Clinical Electromyograhy Nerve Conduction Studies*, Lippincott Williams & Wilkins, Philadelphia, Pa, USA, 3rd edition, 2003.

[7] J. B. Schulz, S. Boesch, K. Bürk et al., "Diagnosis and treatment of Friedreich ataxia: a European perspective," *Nature Reviews Neurology*, vol. 5, no. 4, pp. 222–234, 2009.

[8] M. Anheim, C. Tranchant, and M. Koenig, "The autosomal recessive cerebellar ataxias," *The New England Journal of Medicine*, vol. 366, no. 7, pp. 636–646, 2012.

[9] R. S. Tubbs, S. Krishnamurthy, K. Verma et al., "Cavum velum interpositum, cavum septum pellucidum, and cavum vergae: a review," *Child's Nervous System*, vol. 27, no. 11, pp. 1927–1930, 2011.

[10] T. Westermaier, T. Schweitzer, and R.-I. Ernestus, "Arachnoid cysts," *Advances in Experimental Medicine and Biology*, vol. 724, pp. 37–50, 2012.

[11] G. Arriola, P. De Castro, and A. Verdú, "Familial arachnoid cysts," *Pediatric Neurology*, vol. 33, no. 2, pp. 146–148, 2005.

[12] K. J. Jadeja and R. P. Grewal, "Familial arachnoid cysts associated with oculopharyngeal muscular dystrophy," *Journal of Clinical Neuroscience*, vol. 10, no. 1, pp. 125–127, 2003.

[13] A. Değerliyurt, G. Ceylaner, H. Koçak et al., "A new family with autosomal dominant porencephaly with a novel COL4A1 mutation. Are arachnoid cysts related to COL4A1 mutations?" *Genetic Counseling*, vol. 23, no. 2, pp. 185–193, 2012.

[14] F. Bayrakli, A. I. Okten, U. Kartal et al., "Intracranial arachnoid cyst family with autosomal recessive trait mapped to chromosome 6q22.31-23.2," *Acta Neurochirurgica*, vol. 154, no. 7, pp. 1287–1291, 2012.

[15] M. B. Delatycki and L. A. Corben, "Clinical features of Friedreich ataxia," *Journal of Child Neurology*, vol. 27, no. 9, pp. 1133–1137, 2012.

[16] M. Panas, N. Kalfakis, G. Karadima, P. Davaki, and D. Vassilopoulos, "Friedreich's ataxia mimicking hereditary motor and sensory neuropathy," *Journal of Neurology*, vol. 249, no. 11, pp. 1583–1586, 2002.

[17] J. Zlotogora, "Multiple mutations responsible for frequent genetic diseases in isolated populations," *European Journal of Human Genetics*, vol. 15, no. 3, pp. 272–278, 2007.

23

Another Case of Multilevel Cervical Disconnection Syndrome Presenting as Neonatal Encephalopathy

Kaylan M. Brady,[1] **Jonathan A. Blau,**[2] **Spencer J. Serras,**[3]
Jeremy T. Neuman,[4] **and Richard Sidlow** ⓘ[5]

[1]*Department of Pediatrics, Staten Island University Hospital-Northwell Health, Staten Island, NY, USA*
[2]*Division of Neonatology, Department of Pediatrics, Staten Island University Hospital-Northwell Health, Staten Island, NY, USA*
[3]*Division of Neuroradiology, Department of Radiology, Staten Island University Hospital-Northwell Health, Staten Island, NY, USA*
[4]*Division of Pediatric Radiology, Department of Radiology, Staten Island University Hospital-Northwell Health,*
Staten Island, NY, USA
[5]*Division of Pediatric Hospitalist Medicine, Department of Pediatrics, Staten Island University Hospital-Northwell Health,*
Staten Island, NY, USA

Correspondence should be addressed to Richard Sidlow; rich.sidlow@gmail.com

Academic Editor: Andreas K. Demetriades

Multilevel cervical disconnection syndrome (MCDS) is a rare malformation of the cervical spine previously documented in two toddlers. We present a case of a newborn first thought to have hypoxic-ischemic encephalopathy who was subsequently diagnosed with MCDS. The possibility of in utero presentation of the syndrome in this patient and the categorization of this syndrome in the spectrum of basilar skull/upper cervical malformation syndromes is discussed.

1. Introduction

Most congenital cervical spine anomalies are asymptomatic and, if ever, present well after birth or are found incidentally on radiographic imaging. These known anomalies, including basilar impression, occipitocervical synostosis, odontoid anomalies, and Klippel-Feil syndrome, can present with neck pain, weakness, and upper extremity numbness. These anomalies, however, are not known to cause symptoms at birth, in the neonatal period, or even in infancy.

Two childhood cases of symptomatic cervical spine anomalies have been reported, both distinct from other known anomalies, in which the authors coined the term "multilevel cervical disconnection syndrome (MCDS)" [1]. Both cases presented due to clinical symptoms of spinal cord compression as toddlers. Neither of these cases, however, presented with symptoms at birth.

We present below a case of a baby boy born with MCDS causing spinal cord compression and encephalopathy at birth.

2. Case Description

A baby boy was born at 38 weeks and six days gestation to a primigravid woman. The mother was followed by a high-risk obstetrician due to SSRI use during the initial months of pregnancy. Otherwise, the maternal history was unremarkable, and the prenatal history was significant only for breech presentation. The mother presented to labor and delivery due to a four-week history of decreased fetal movements. A nonstress test was performed which was reactive with good fetal heart rate; however, a biophysical profile performed immediately afterwards was 6/10 due to lack of fetal movement/fetal tone. The mother was admitted for an emergent cesarean section delivery.

Once delivered, the baby was floppy, apneic, pallid, and bradycardic. Neonatal Resuscitation Protocol was initiated and after no response to tactile stimulation and positive pressure ventilation (PPV), a Code 100 was called. Chest compressions were begun and the baby was intubated. Apgar scores were two at one minute and five at five minutes, respectively. Two doses of epinephrine were given via the endotracheal tube (ET) and an umbilical venous catheter was placed emergently. A normal saline bolus was given due to poor perfusion, pallor and bradycardia. The Apgar score at ten minutes was seven. The baby was then given PPV through the ET tube during transportation to the neonatal intensive care unit (NICU).

Upon arrival to the NICU, the baby was flaccid, hypothermic, bradycardic, apneic, and hypoxic. The baby had no spontaneous respirations. The neurological examination revealed absent cry, Moro, gag, suck, swallow and grasp reflexes, and decreased tone throughout with intermittent twitching of the left upper and lower extremities. The spine was grossly normal. Arterial blood gases on admission revealed a mixed respiratory and metabolic acidosis (pH 6.92 (nl 7.38-7.42)/pCO2 78 mmHg (nl 38-42 mmHg)/pO2 92 mmHg (nl 94-98 mmHg)/HCO3 16.2 mEq/L (nl 23-27 meq/L)/BE-16.4 (nl -2-2)). Since the physical examination findings and presentation were consistent with hypoxic-ischemic encephalopathy (HIE), a 72-hour neonatal whole body cooling protocol was begun at hour 6 of life [2]. The baby was also started on ampicillin and gentamicin for presumed sepsis, which were discontinued after 48 hours once the blood culture result was negative.

While being cooled, the baby began to have inconsistent symmetric spontaneous movements of his extremities, withdrawal of all extremities, and symmetric facial movements in response to painful stimuli. There was no spontaneous eye opening, but he resisted eye opening. Patellar and bicep reflexes were I/IV and toes were down going. Video electroencephalogram revealed mild slowing initially, but normalized by day three of life with no slowing or epileptiform activity. The baby remained ventilator dependent and failed multiple apnea tests.

On day of four of life, the baby was rewarmed with improvement in overall tone, a now inconsistent gag reflex, strong withdrawal to painful stimuli, and II/IV reflexes throughout. Despite the baby's slightly improved neurological exam, he remained ventilator dependent with no spontaneous respirations.

Magnetic resonance imaging (MRI) of the brain performed on day five of life revealed no definitive evidence of acute infarct or hypoxic/anoxic injury, but revealed an abnormality of the cervical spine. MRI of the cervical spine revealed spinal cord compression at the level of the foramen magnum secondary to a craniocervical junction anomaly with severe kyphosis of the upper cervical spine at the level of C3-C4 (Figure 1). Computerized tomography of the cervical spine confirmed the diagnosis along with occipitalization and assimilation of the atlas and absent ossifications centers of the upper cervical spine (Figures 2 and 3).

Upon the diagnosis of spinal cord compression, the baby was transferred for urgent neurosurgical evaluation and treatment. Despite surgical intervention with suboccipital craniotomy and posterior cervical laminectomy with rib graft spinal fusion, no improvement was noted and the baby had no purposeful movements postoperatively. He later underwent tracheostomy for persistent respiratory failure. The patient was discharged to a specialty rehabilitation center where he

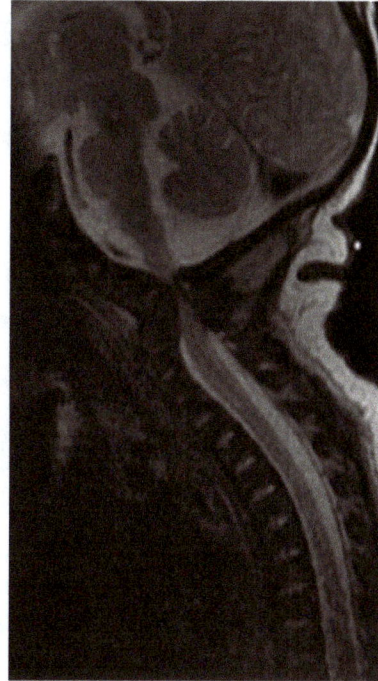

FIGURE 1: MRI of cervical spine: spinal cord compression at level of the foramen magnum secondary to craniocervical junction anomaly with focal severe kyphosis of the upper cervical spine (C3-C4).

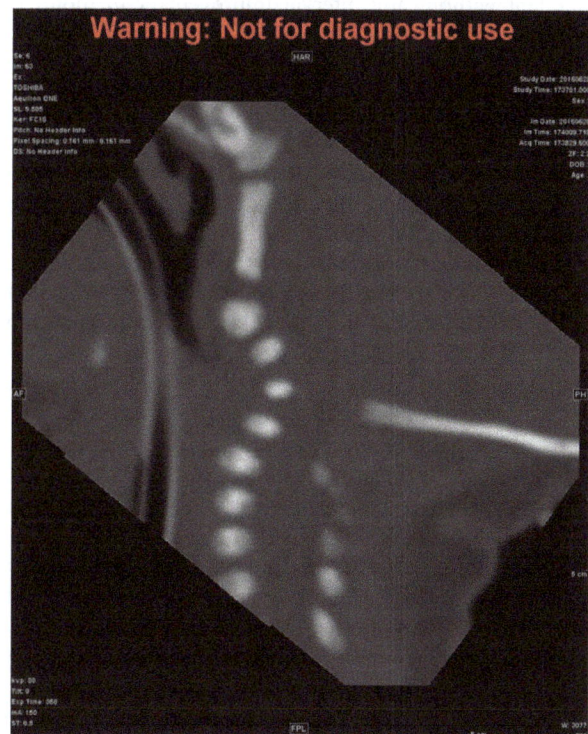

FIGURE 2: CT of cervical spine: occipitalization/assimilation of the atlas with severe kyphoscoliosis of the upper cervical spine, resulting in severe spinal canal stenosis with spinal cord compression. Incomplete/absent ossification centers of the upper cervical spine.

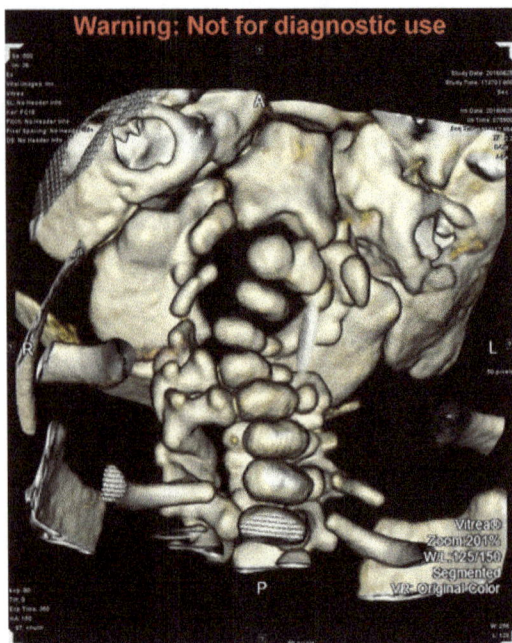

FIGURE 3: 3D image of MRI of cervical spine: absent pedicle in the midcervical spine.

remained for nine months and was subsequently discharged home. The patient has remained quadriplegic and ventilator dependent without any interval improvement in motor or respiratory function.

3. Discussion

The incidence of congenital anomalies of the cervical spine is much less common than HIE, the former occurring in approximately 1 in 40,000 to 42,000 births versus 1.5 per 1,000 live births in the United States [3, 4]. Basilar impression, occipitocervical synostosis, odontoid anomalies, and Klippel-Feil syndrome do not present symptomatically at birth and are not known to cause severe spinal cord compression requiring mechanical ventilation [5]. Therefore, cervical spine anomalies and spinal cord compression were not in the differential diagnosis of this baby at the time of presentation or during his initial clinical course. Retrospectively, the encephalopathic presentation of this baby can be explained by the combination of phrenic nerve palsy and the neurological sequelae resulting from high cervical spinal cord compression. Additionally, given the absence on physical examination of other facial, orthopedic, and cardiac findings, no syndromic explanation (e.g., Larsen Syndrome) was considered.

Two childhood cases with similar radiographic findings have been reported by Klimo et al., one in a 22-month-old female with myelopathy and a neck deformity and another in a three-year-old male with upper and lower extremity weakness. Both patients were previously healthy and had no significant birth history. Radiographic imaging of the cervical spine in both cases showed multilevel abnormalities of the cervical pedicles, cervical kyphosis, and spinal cord compression. The authors termed this condition "multilevel cervical disconnection syndrome (MCDS)", due to the apparent disconnect between the anterior and posterior column. Both cases were repaired surgically in a similar fashion with improvement of symptoms postoperatively. These two cases, however, presented as toddlers, were normal at birth and had a much less severe component of cervical kyphosis and spinal cord compression [1].

The above authors believed that the embryological cause of the abnormalities in the cervical spine was due to a defect in ossification and chondrification at the level of the cervical pedicles [1]. Others have theorized that Chiari-1 malformation, cervical spina bifida occulta, cervical scoliosis, Klippel-Feil deformity, atlantoaxial assimilation, atlantooccipital fusion, and basilar invagination may be developmental variants along a spectrum of severity common to the base of the skull and upper cervical spine [6]. In patients without collagenopathies, mutations in the genes GDF3 and GDF6 which code for osseous growth differentiation factors, defects of postotic neural crest (PONC) cells, or subclavian artery supply disruption sequence (SASDS) have been proposed as explanations for the anomalies previously listed [7–9]. We would add (MCDS) to this list and invoke these same explanations as possible etiologies of this syndrome.

Our case had similar radiographic findings with at least one missing pedicle at the level of the midcervical spine along with obvious cervical kyphosis and incomplete/absent ossification centers (Figure 3). The profound in utero presentation of this baby was likely caused by the apex of cervical kyphosis being at the level of C4 compressing the spinal cord down to approximately one millimeter in diameter early on in development.

This is the first case of MCDS documented in a neonate and with symptoms documented in utero. Spinal cord compression due to cervical spine anomalies, although rare, should therefore be kept in the differential diagnosis of a newborn suspected of having neonatal encephalopathy, as it can present with respiratory failure due to phrenic nerve palsy with neurological sequelae. Additional imaging of the cervical spine is needed for diagnosis and can be performed concomitantly with the brain imaging necessary to confirm HIE. This also expands the differential diagnosis to include additional structural abnormalities other than vertebral bony anomalies at the level of the cervical spine that could cause spinal cord compression and phrenic nerve palsy, such as an arteriovenous malformation (AVM). One case has been documented in a full-term baby born with flaccid quadriparesis that remained ventilator dependent, found on MRI to have an epidural hematoma compressing the cervical cord, later attributed to an AVM on postpartum examination [10].

4. Conclusion

Although extremely rare, spinal cord compression due to cervical spine anomalies should be kept in the differential diagnosis of a baby presenting with encephalopathy, as it can cause phrenic nerve palsy resulting in respiratory failure and neurological sequelae. Radiologic imaging can be performed early in the clinical course in conjunction with the ongoing workup for neonatal encephalopathy. This can allow for a more rapid diagnosis and treatment plan and ultimately confirm or eliminate a potential cause for the neonate's symptoms.

Conflicts of Interest

The authors report no conflicts of interest concerning the materials or methods used in this study or the findings specified in this paper.

References

[1] P. Klimo Jr., R. C. E. Anderson, and D. L. Brockmeyer, "Multilevel cervical disconnection syndrome: Initial description, embryogenesis, and management: Report of two cases," *Journal of Neurosurgery*, vol. 104, no. 3, pp. 181–187, 2006.

[2] S. Shankaran, A. R. Laptook, R. A. Ehrenkranz et al., "Whole-body hypothermia for neonates with hypoxic-ischemic encephalopathy," *The New England Journal of Medicine*, vol. 353, no. 15, pp. 1574–1584, 2005.

[3] P. Klimo Jr., G. Rao, and D. Brockmeyer, "Congenital Anomalies of the Cervical Spine," *Neurosurgery Clinics of North America*, vol. 18, no. 3, pp. 463–478, 2007.

[4] J. J. Kurinczuk, M. White-Koning, and N. Badawi, "Epidemiology of neonatal encephalopathy and hypoxic-ischaemic encephalopathy," *Early Human Development*, vol. 86, no. 6, pp. 329–338, 2010.

[5] Medscape, "Medscape: Congenital spinal deformity. New York, USA, 2017," https://emedicine.medscape.com/article/1260442 -overview#a6.

[6] S.-L. Wong, D. C. Paviour, and R. E. Clifford-Jones, "Chiari-1 malformation and the neck-tongue syndrome: Cause or coincidence?" *Cephalalgia*, vol. 28, no. 9, pp. 994-995, 2008.

[7] J. N. B. Bavinck and D. D. Weaver, "Subclavian artery supply disruption sequence: hypothesis of a vascular etiology for Poland, Klippel-Feil, and Möbius anomalies," *American Journal of Medical Genetics*, vol. 23, no. 4, pp. 903–918, 1986.

[8] C. A. Markunas, K. Soldano, K. Dunlap et al., "Stratified whole genome linkage analysis of chiari type i malformation implicates known klippel-feil syndrome genes as putative disease candidates," *PLoS ONE*, vol. 8, no. 4, Article ID e61521, 2013.

[9] T. Matsuoka, P. E. Ahlberg, N. Kessaris et al., "Neural crest origins of the neck and shoulder," *Nature*, vol. 436, no. 7049, pp. 347–355, 2005.

[10] D. M. Coulter, H. Zhou, and L. B. Rorke-Adams, "Catastrophic intrauterine spinal cord injury caused by an arteriovenous malformation," *Journal of Perinatology*, vol. 27, no. 3, pp. 186–189, 2007.

24

Differential Diagnosis and Management of Incomplete Locked-In Syndrome after Traumatic Brain Injury

Lauren Surdyke, Jennifer Fernandez, Hannah Foster, and Pamela Spigel

Brooks Rehabilitation Hospital, 3599 University Blvd S, Jacksonville, FL 32216, USA

Correspondence should be addressed to Lauren Surdyke; lauren.surdyke@brooksrehab.org

Academic Editor: Samuel T. Gontkovsky

Locked-in syndrome (LIS) is a rare diagnosis in which patients present with quadriplegia, lower cranial nerve paralysis, and mutism. It is clinically difficult to differentiate from other similarly presenting diagnoses with no standard approach for assessing such poorly responsive patients. The purpose of this case is to highlight the clinical differential diagnosis process and outcomes of a patient with LIS during acute inpatient rehabilitation. A 32-year-old female was admitted following traumatic brain injury. She presented with quadriplegia and mutism but was awake and aroused based on eye gaze communication. The rehabilitation team was able to diagnose incomplete LIS based on knowledge of neuroanatomy and clinical reasoning. Establishing this diagnosis allowed for an individualized treatment plan that focused on communication, coping, family training, and discharge planning. The patient was ultimately able to discharge home with a single caregiver, improving her quality of life. Continued evidence highlights the benefits of intensive comprehensive therapy for those with acquired brain injury such as LIS, but access is still limited for those with a seemingly poor prognosis. Access to a multidisciplinary, specialized team provides opportunity for continued assessment and individualized treatment as the patient attains more medical stability, improving long-term management.

1. Introduction

It has been estimated that approximately 10 million people across the world are affected by traumatic brain injury (TBI) annually with nearly half of those individuals remaining moderately to severely disabled one year out from injury [1]. Due to the extensive care for these patients, their total burden of care costs across the lifespan has been estimated at $200 million per year when considering acute management through long-term placement [1]. Rates of misdiagnosis in patients with a disorder of consciousness (DOC) from TBI have been reported to be as high as 43% [2–5]. This rate of misdiagnosis is highest when performed by nonspecialized physicians and rehabilitation teams [5, 6]. Persons with locked-in syndrome (LIS), akinetic mutism (AM), and spinal cord injury (SCI) can also have very similar presentation making differential diagnosis complex. One of these differentials, LIS, is a rare outcome of cerebral damage that is both debilitating and complex to diagnose. Traumatic LIS only accounts for 10% of etiologies, with the most frequent

cause being interruption of the motor pathways in the ventral pons by basilar artery occlusion [7]. Other reported causes include but are not limited to ALS, tumors or abscesses, and postoperative complications [7].

LIS was originally introduced by Plum and Posner in 1966 as a condition associated with lesion of the ventral pons, disrupting the corticospinal and corticobulbar pathways without involvement of the cortex [8]. In 1979, Bauer et al. introduced the notion that instead of one typical presentation of the syndrome, three varieties exist including the classical variety, incomplete variety, and total variety [9]. The classical variety manifests as quadriplegia, lower cranial nerve paralysis, and mutism with preservation of vertical gaze and, most notably, intact consciousness indicated by abilities to communicate via eye movements. The incomplete variety is similar in presentation to the classical variety; however, the patient presents with additional voluntary movements that vary on a case-by-case basis. The total variety describes a patient with no voluntary movement and closed eyes [9]. Despite the lack of apparent awareness in these patients, indications of conscious mental activity have been shown through use of technology such as EEG, which can correlate brain activity in relation to stimuli [10].

Much of the recent literature supports a need for standardized diagnostic procedures to confirm LIS; however, this is often reliant on imaging which may not show pathological changes even when a clinical picture of LIS is present [11, 12]. Several obstacles exist in correlating clinical presentations to anatomical pathology, including but not limited to the varied underlying patient characteristics (age, baseline cognitive status and orientation, previous neurological disorders, and comorbidities), as well as the diversity in size and nature of the lesion itself [13]. Oftentimes in acute care, patients are too sedated and are seen for such brief periods of time that does not allow for thorough clinical assessment.

Over the past 10 years, a growing body of literature has investigated highly dependent patients such as those with a DOC or LIS and how they may benefit from inpatient rehabilitation. Increased reports suggest that highly dependent individuals after TBI can benefit from comprehensive inpatient rehabilitation despite an initial seemingly poor prognosis and that specialized care units improve outcomes [1, 13, 14].

However, due to limited funding and the strength of research to support the need for this comprehensive level of care, many patients are not given such an opportunity. As a result, days or months often go by before an accurate diagnosis of LIS is made. León-Carrión et al. reported that the diagnosis of LIS is not usually made until approximately two months after onset [7]. This complexity increases in trauma patients where there may be multiple injures leading to greater increases in time until an accurate diagnosis [15, 16].

Clinicians can use their knowledge of neuroanatomy and expected clinical presentations to isolate a suspected lesion location and thus aid in early diagnostics when imaging is not readily available. The purpose of this paper is to describe the clinical differential diagnosis process that occurred in the inpatient rehabilitation setting for a patient presenting with quadriplegia and mutism following traumatic etiology. A secondary purpose of this paper is to highlight how access to this level of care and an accurate diagnosis impacted outcomes for this patient.

2. Case Description

A 32-year-old female was admitted to a specialized inpatient rehabilitation program utilizing a comprehensive rehab team focused on assessing patients with severe traumatic brain injury with the goal of providing accurate diagnosis, family training, and intensive therapy to promote best outcomes. The team included a physician, neuropsychologist, physical therapist, cognitive therapist, speech therapist, occupational therapist, and nurse. This multidisciplinary team collaborated towards the final diagnosis described here and together established a personalized plan of care and discharge recommendations.

Acute care records showed patient had undergone CT of the brain revealing right frontal parenchymal contusion and a diffuse area of subarachnoid blood. No midline

TABLE 1: Examination findings.

Expressive communication	No verbalizations or facial gestures, able to establish communication via blinking, 75% accuracy regarding orientation
Visual tracking	All directions, nystagmus and ocular bobbing noted
Arousal/attention	Awake, alert, focused on examiner throughout
Auditory response	No motor response to commands except ocular
Object manipulation	No motor response or grasp reflex noted
Motor response	No head control, righting reactions, or protective extension. No withdrawal to pain.
Reflexes	VOR and pupillary light intact

TABLE 2: FIM scoring.

FIM scores	Evaluation	Discharge
Self-care	8/56	8/56
Mobility	5/35	5/35
Communication and cognition	5/35	17/35
Total	18/126	30/126

shift, herniation, or mass effect was identified. Other acute comorbidities included right subcondylar mandible fracture requiring her jaw to be wired shut, further complicating assessment during her inpatient stay. No reports regarding MRI or angiography were received from the acute care setting which may have expedited diagnostics prior to admission to inpatient rehabilitation.

Initial team evaluation in the specialized program focuses on identifying and differentiating purposeful and generalized responses to stimuli using a combination of testing components derived from the Western, CRS-R, and Glasgow [16]. Observations of purposeful activity during initial evaluation were not observed due to lack of any spontaneous movement of the patient; however, the patient appeared generally awake based on observation of open eyes and spontaneous visual tracking. Ocular bobbing, which is characterized by a fast down beat of the eyes and slow return to baseline, was observed in addition to a distinct sustained and direction-changing nystagmus [17]. The functional independence measure (FIM) was used to capture the patient's disability and how much assistance the patient required to perform activities of daily living. Refer to Table 1 for further examination findings and Table 2 for FIM scoring.

Based on the patient's wakefulness and consistent meaningful and purposeful interactions with the environment through eye gaze communication, a disorder of consciousness was ruled out. Further, understanding of the anatomy of the described reflexes and presentation guided the team towards isolation of a ventral pons lesion location and the suspected diagnosis of LIS, with need for further work-up to confirm.

TABLE 3: Differential diagnosis: acute onset of quadriplegia and mutism.

Diagnoses considered		Key finding to rule out	
Disorder of consciousness	↓	Assessment revealing patient wakefulness and ability to communicate via eye gaze	×
Upper cervical spinal cord injury	↓	Observation of normal, quiet respiration and impairment of supraspinal muscles	×
Akinetic mutism	↓	Lack of automatic protective extension/equilibrium reactions and no withdrawal to pain	×
Locked-in syndrome		Primary suspected diagnosis by exclusion of other likely diagnoses	√

TABLE 4: Primary classifications for disorders of consciousness.

Specific disorder of consciousness	Defining features
Coma	Unconscious and unaware with disruption of the reticular activating system of the brainstem.
Unresponsive wakefulness	Partially conscious and no awareness, with preservation of brainstem structures.
Minimally conscious state	Limited but clear evidence for awareness of self/environment with inconsistent but reproducible goal-directed behaviors. Brainstem structures intact.

3. Differential Considerations

Based on the team evaluation, differential diagnosis aimed to include diagnoses that may match the patient presentation of acute onset of quadriplegia and mutism following trauma. The working list of diagnoses included LIS, DOC, AM, and an upper cervical SCI. Since LIS was the primary suspected diagnosis, the goal of further assessment was to rule out all other suspected diagnoses in order to confirm by exclusion. See Table 3 for a schematic of the overall differential diagnosis process.

3.1. Disorders of Consciousness. There are three primary classifications for DOC including coma, unresponsive wakefulness, and minimally conscious state. Consciousness is defined by being both alert and aware. Alertness depends on normal functioning of the reticular formation, thalamus, and cortex while awareness requires higher ordering processing that integrates both sensory and motor information [17]. In a DOC, some degree of impairment exists within these structures; see Table 4 for the classifications of DOC.

In the presented case of traumatic etiology, the diagnostic process was complicated by frontal lobe brain injury confirmed by CT from acute care stay. Inappropriate or absent responses could be due to language impairments, initiation impairments, or other associated impairments more likely related to the brain injury as opposed to locked-in syndrome. Based on the patient's demonstration of arousal and consistent means of communicating a level of orientation, the diagnosis of a DOC was ruled out.

3.2. Upper Cervical Spinal Cord Injury. An upper cervical SCI was included due to the presentation of quadriplegia. All key muscles defined by the International Standards for Neurologic Classifications of Spinal Cord Injury Association (ISNCSI) in the standard motor exam were scored zero out of five bilaterally, leading to the notion that the injury must be above the level C5 at which the motor exam begins [18]. Sensory testing was completed, using a modified method due to communication impairments. The patient was instructed to open her eyes when light touch was detected, and this was used to test all key sensory points. Light touch was detected at all key points using this method, but examination was unable to determine if the sensation was altered to any degree with this method. Additionally, sharp dull differentiation was deferred due to communication impairments and time limitations.

With an upper cervical SCI, there is also reasonable expectation for demonstration of labored breathing or need for mechanical ventilation support with injuries above C5 [19]. Our patient demonstrated quiet respiration with no abnormal patterns of inhalation. Additionally, both facial expression (controlled by cranial nerve VII in the brainstem) and head/neck control were impaired in this individual, indicating a supraspinal lesion and reducing the likelihood that the patient presentation was due to SCI.

3.3. Akinetic Mutism. AM is a condition characterized by diminished neurologic drive with a decrease in nearly all motor functions including facial expression, gestures, and speech output but with some degree of alertness and intact spontaneous visual tracking [20]. In this condition, individuals typically maintain normal muscle tone and reflexes; however, due to the decreased spontaneous movement a perceived paralysis could allow it to be mistaken as LIS. A study of AM following stroke revealed that eight patients with AM identified the frontal lobe as the most frequent location of lesion [20]. The frontal lobe plays an important role in the initiation of behavior and speech, and its dysfunction produces lack of spontaneity and reduced motor output. Based on the role of the frontal lobe in initiation, protective extension and equilibrium reactions would remain intact, even if delayed due to the nature of these reactions being initiated automatically and involuntarily in the brainstem [21].

In this case, these reactions were persistently impaired throughout the course of the patient's stay in addition to a lack of any withdrawal to pain. In AM, the patient should demonstrate some evidence for motoric abilities through self-initiated tasks. For example, patients with AM may be observed performing automatic motor tasks such as swatting a fly. The telephone effect has also been described in patients with AM in which the patient spontaneously answers a ringing phone with a verbal "hello" [22]. This patient did not reveal any of these characteristics of AM. In addition, the patient demonstrated initiation and the ability to follow some motor commands through specific visual activation and eye opening/closing without any delay. Over the course of care, the patient also began to demonstrate some recovery of more distal voluntary movements (trace toe and finger movements, bilateral head turning, and head lifting to midline) with the ability to initiate movement on command once movement potentials were established. Based on the presented rationale, the diagnosis of AM was ruled out.

3.4. Locked-In Syndrome. Clinical reasoning allowed for exclusion of above working diagnoses, supporting the likelihood that the patient presentation was due to LIS. She presented with the classical symptoms of quadriplegia, mutism, intact consciousness, and ability to communicate via eye gaze movements. Reading comprehension was determined to be intact later in her stay, further supporting the diagnosis of LIS where patients typically remain cognitively intact [23]. She also demonstrated the ability to sequence three step commands via eye gaze movements and was oriented to situational and personal questions with 100% accuracy by week five of her inpatient stay.

Knowledge of anatomy and correlation to presentation further strengthened the diagnosis of LIS by helping isolate where the suspected lesion was. The presentation of motor versus sensory impairments indicated a more likely ventral lesion [21]. The vestibular ocular reflex, which was intact, uses dorsally located connections with cranial nerves III and VI, again indicating a more ventral lesion. To further isolate a ventral lesion, a positive Babinski sign supported corticospinal tract damage [21]. Based on ISNCSI testing, the lesion was likely above C5. Absence of facial expression, which is controlled by cranial nerve VII in the brainstem, further indicates a more cephalic lesion. The pupillary light reflex was intact. This reflex descends to the pretectal area in the midbrain before reaching the oculomotor nucleus and achieving its motor output [10]. An intact pupillary light reflex indicated the lesion was likely below the midbrain. By using the above rational based on patient presentation, the lesion location was isolated to the ventral pons further confirming the diagnosis of LIS. The patient was classified under the incomplete variety due to her recovery of additional voluntary movements, which included active movement of toes, head turning and maintaining midline, and facial expression [9].

4. Outcomes

The highly skilled rehabilitation team was able to confirm diagnosis through clinical assessment at week five after injury, with imaging affirming a small pontine injury at week six. The patient was cared for initially in an acute care hospital with limited therapy for four weeks and no confirmed diagnosis, prior to her five-week inpatient rehabilitation admission. With a five-week stay in inpatient rehabilitation came the time that allowed for accurate and timely assessment, recognizing that the diagnosis of LIS is not usually made until two months after onset [7]. Imaging was performed early on in the patient's course of care; however, the initial CT showed no lesion associated with the ventral pons. This CT was performed without contrast and arguably too early to show the corresponding lesion associated with LIS [10]. MRI, which may have been more sensitive in detecting the lesion, was not performed until week six after injury with no reports as to why this was not performed in the acute care hospital.

Establishing the diagnosis of LIS allowed for treatment approaches and goals to shift in order to maximize functional patient participation and family training. Aggressive mobilization demonstrated limited motor recovery and decreased expectation of such with the diagnosis of LIS warranted treatment focused on improving communication to more efficiently identify and address the patient's needs. Augmentative and alternative communication was trialed via the Tobii; however, the patient was not able to functionally use this device due to difficulties associated with calibration from her resting nystagmus. Mobility training became compensatory with focus on use of a head switch power wheelchair and family training to safely assist in transfers.

Upon discharge, the patient was able to use a head controlled device to alert caregivers when she required assistance, reducing her required level of supervision. She was able to direct her care with the ability sequence multistep commands, reducing the required level of education and experience of future caregivers. She was more efficient with her altered means of communication, allowing her to interact and participate in life more. With improved communication, cognition, and postural control, the patient was also able to engage in initial phases of learning how to operate a head control power chair. Though the patient did not achieve independence with wheelchair mobility, she continued to show potential for improved functional use of a power chair with continued reinforcement of steering skills and safe obstacle negotiation. Upon discharge, she was able to navigate straight paths and wide turns; however, due to inconsistent performance and distance modifiers, she required total assistance based on the FIM.

Despite these meaningful functional changes, the patient's FIM scores did not adequately highlight what was achieved through rehabilitation (Table 2). She required total assistance for all self-care and mobility items with minimal but meaningful communication and cognitive progressions. Refer to Figure 1 for a review of this patient's stay, highlighting timing and outcomes.

5. Discussion

Access to inpatient rehabilitation in this case facilitated an early and accurate diagnosis, which streamlined the patient's individualized plan of care. Extensive family training, increased patient mobility through wheelchair propulsion,

| Week 1 | Week 2 | Week 3 | Week 4 | Week 5 | Week 6 | Week 7 | Week 8 | Week 9 | Week 10 |

Week 1
(i) MVA resulting in initial injury
(ii) Admission to acute care
(iii) CT of brain

Week 3
(i) Acute care PT & ST initiated

Week 5
(i) BWSTT
(ii) 100% oriented
(iii) LIS confirmed

Week 7
(i) Reading comprehension
(ii) Practice head control WC

Week 9
(i) Jaw wire bands removed
(ii) Smiling on command
(iii) Single word vocalizations

Week 2
(i) R mandibular condyle fracture
(ii) CT nondisplaced L4 TP fracture and internal injuries

Week 4
(i) Admit inpatient
(ii) Total assist ×3 for all mobility
(iii) Communication via blinking system

Week 6
(i) Trace toe activation = LIS incomplete variety
(ii) MRI = no SCI, small pontine injury
(iii) Attempted AAC Tobii; calibration limited by nystagmus

Week 8
(i) Lift head on command
(ii) Maintain head in midline
(iii) Trace finger activation

Week 10
(i) DC home
(ii) Total assist ×1
(iii) WC mobility

MVA: motor vehicle accident
R: right
TP: transverse process
PT: physical therapy
ST: speech therapy

BWSTT: body weight support treadmill training
LIS: locked-in syndrome
WC: wheelchair
DC: discharge

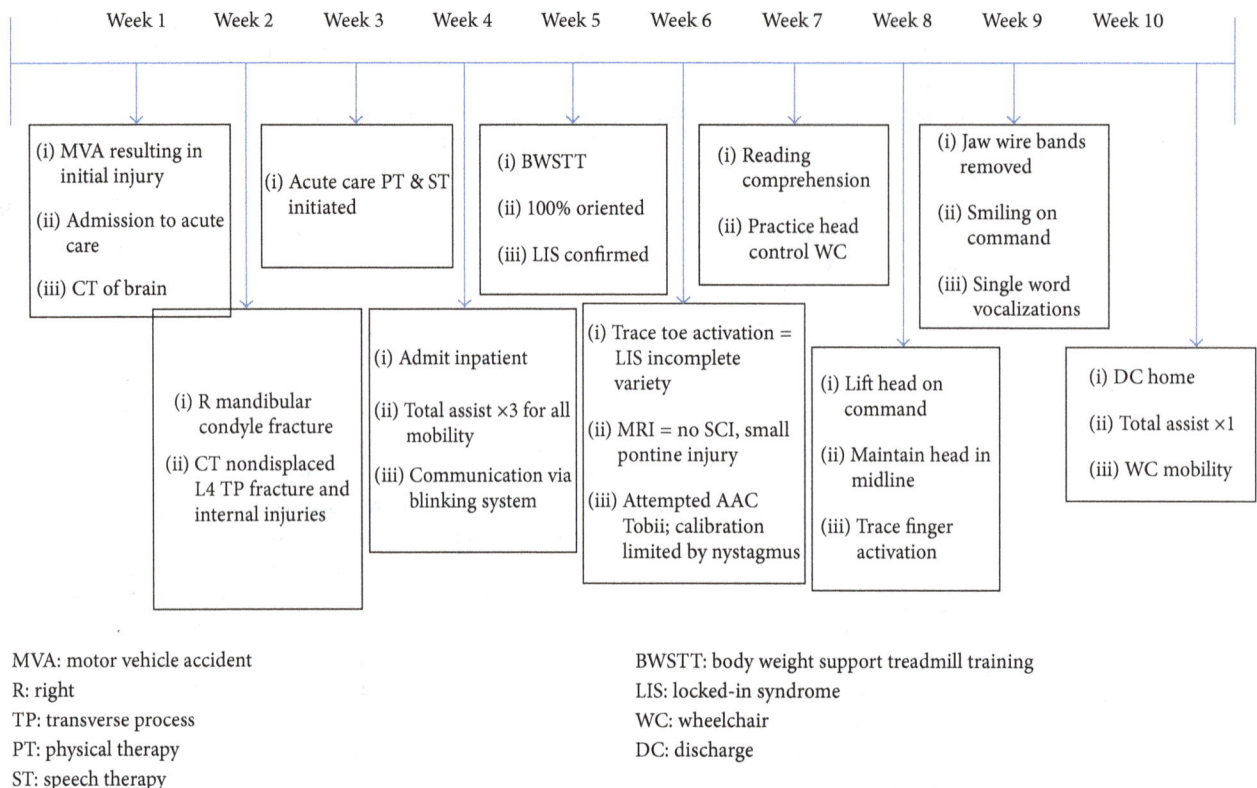

FIGURE 1: Patient course of care timeline.

and improved communication allowed this patient to return home with family ten weeks after injury instead of requiring institutional care. The patient was further able to make decisions and direct her care, increasing her current and future autonomy. This is of great significance as these patients are often placed in long-term care facilities and at the same time are living longer [24]. Considering lifelong costs has become more important due to the reported longer life expectancy in those with LIS, understanding that up to 83% will live ten years after onset [11, 25]. Current research has demonstrated that by simplifying care needs and providing family training, inpatient rehabilitation can reduce long-term costs and in this case it did [26, 27]. Longer life expectancy additionally brings to consideration quality of life (QOL), with research to support that physical disability alone does not predict a lesser QOL [11, 25]. This patient achieved improved autonomy as stated above and was able to return home, both of which are positively associated with greater quality of life in those with LIS.

As displayed above, outcomes in this case were positively impacted by access to a comprehensive rehab program. Clinicians with expertise in treating patients with disorders of consciousness allowed for accurate assessment and diagnosis which guided individualized treatment of this particular patient. It took a multidisciplinary team effort to ensure carryover of therapeutic interventions and to reduce the likelihood of secondary complications. Imaging was performed early on in the patient's course of care; however, the initial CT showed no lesion associated with the ventral

pons. This CT was performed without contrast and arguably too early to show the corresponding lesion associated with LIS. Kotchoubey and Lotze reported 22 patients with severe occlusive defect of the basilar artery in which CT did not show any pathological changes during the acute stage, reporting that hypodensity typically cannot be seen until 2 weeks after the infarct [10]. MRI, which is reported to be the most sensitive method in diagnosis of structural disorders in LIS, was not performed until week six, shortly after the patient's admission to inpatient rehabilitation. It has been reported that MRI can reveal a distinct lesion that was not visualized on CT and is particularly important for cases of nonvascular etiology, as in this case of traumatic etiology [10]. The MRI cleared the patient for SCI damage and showed a small pontine injury. Even still, in some cases in which the patient presents with clinical signs of LIS, MRI and CT scans may show no pathological changes, warranting the need for the adjunct clinical based assessment to guide treatment [28, 29].

Since reimbursement is directly tied to FIM gains, those with such a severe brain injury are not often given the opportunity to participate in inpatient rehabilitation and undergo this level of assessment. The FIM has floor effects in highly dependent individuals, which was particularly evident in this case warranting the need for more sensitive measures [13]. Research supports that an early and intensive multidisciplinary treatment plan for patients with LIS, begun within one month of onset, improved health status and decreased the chances for mortality [24] Even still, access to an inpatient rehabilitation team is limited and when provided the opportunity, pressure exists for early discharge leading to higher chances of institutionalization [13, 26]. Literature continues to support that lifelong costs are lowest following TBI with supervised home placement after rehabilitation [1]. It is then our responsibility as health care professionals to advocate for these individuals to maximize access and ultimate outcomes following diagnosis of LIS.

6. Conclusion

Continued research is needed to better define what low level patients can gain from inpatient rehabilitation and health care providers must recognize the importance of accurate diagnosis for plan of care development, noting that an individualized and team approach are critical in the management of poorly responsive patients. Limitations in health care coverage and funding for high level studies will make this challenging, with high rates of misdiagnosis further confounding research. New models of assessment and care for these patients must be established to maximize their opportunity for making functional and meaningful progress to lessen their burden of care and public cost impacts. There is an identified need for a more standardized approach and more sensitive means of tracking functional progress in these patients to obtain reimbursement. Though case reports alone will not be strong enough to facilitate development of standards of care, well researched case reports can continue to build the body of literature upon which future research can grow.

Conflicts of Interest

The authors declare that there are no conflicts of interest regarding the publication of this paper.

References

[1] I. Humphreys, R. L. Wood, C. J. Phillips, and S. Macey, "The costs of traumatic brain injury: a literature review," *ClinicoEconomics and Outcomes Research*, vol. 5, no. 1, pp. 281–287, 2013.

[2] K. Andrews, L. Murphy, R. Munday, and C. Littlewood, "Misdiagnosis of the vegetative state: retrospective study in a rehabilitation unit," *British Medical Journal*, vol. 313, no. 7048, pp. 13–16, 1996.

[3] C. Schnakers and et al., "Accuracy of diagnosis of persistent vegetative state," *Neurology*, vol. 43, no. 8, pp. 1465–1467, 2006.

[4] C. Schnakers, J. Giacino, K. Kalmar et al., "Does the FOUR score correctly diagnose the vegetative and minimally conscious states? [1]," *Annals of Neurology*, vol. 60, no. 6, pp. 744–745, 2006.

[5] C. Schnakers, A. Vanhaudenhuyse, J. Giacino et al., "Diagnostic accuracy of the vegetative and minimally conscious state: clinical consensus versus standardized neurobehavioral assessment," *BMC Neurology*, vol. 9, article 35, 2009.

[6] N. L. Childs, W. N. Mercer, and H. W. Childs, "Accuracy of diagnosis of persistent vegetative state," *Neurology*, vol. 43, no. 8, pp. 1465–1467, 1993.

[7] J. León-Carrión, P. Van Eeckhout, M. D. R. Domínguez-Morales, and F. J. Pérez-Santamaría, "The locked-in syndrome: A syndrome looking for a therapy," *Brain Injury*, vol. 16, no. 7, pp. 571–582, 2002.

[8] F. Plum and J. B. Posner, *The Diagnosis of Stupor and Coma*, Davis Co, Philadelphia, Pa, USA, 1966.

[9] G. Bauer, F. Gerstenbrand, and E. Rumpl, "Varieties of the locked-in syndrome," *Journal of Neurology*, vol. 221, no. 2, pp. 77–91, 1979.

[10] B. Kotchoubey and M. Lotze, "Instrumental methods in the diagnostics of locked-in syndrome," *Restorative Neurology and Neuroscience*, vol. 31, no. 1, pp. 25–40, 2013.

[11] M.-C. Rousseau, S. Pietra, M. Nadji, and T. Billette De Villemeur, "Evaluation of quality of life in complete locked-in syndrome patients," *Journal of Palliative Medicine*, vol. 16, no. 11, pp. 1455–1458, 2013.

[12] L. Snoeys, G. Vanhoof, and E. Manders, "Living with locked-in syndrome: an explorative study on health care situation, communication and quality of life," *Disability and Rehabilitation*, vol. 35, no. 9, pp. 713–718, 2013.

[13] L. Turner-Stokes, S. Paul, and H. Williams, "Efficiency of specialist rehabilitation in reducing dependency and costs of continuing care for adults with complex acquired brain injuries," *Journal of Neurology, Neurosurgery and Psychiatry*, vol. 77, no. 5, pp. 634–639, 2006.

[14] R. J. Jox, J. L. Bernat, S. Laureys, and E. Racine, "Disorders of consciousness: Responding to requests for novel diagnostic and therapeutic interventions," *The Lancet Neurology*, vol. 11, no. 8, pp. 732–738, 2012.

[15] R. Carrai, A. Grippo, S. Fossi et al., "Transient post-traumatic locked-in syndrome: A case report and a literature review," *Neurophysiologie Clinique*, vol. 39, no. 2, pp. 95–100, 2009.

[16] C. Beaulieu, *The Response Evaluation Program*, Brooks Rehabilitation Hospital, Jacksonville, Fla, USA, 2014.

[17] H. Blumenfeld, *Neuroanatomy through Clinical Cases*, Sinauer Associates, Inc, Sunderland, Mass, USA, 2002.

[18] American Spinal Cord Injury Association, 2015, http://www.asia-spinalinjury.org/elearning/ISNCSCI.php.

[19] W. Urmey, S. Loring, J. Mead et al., "Upper and lower rib cage deformation during breathing in quadriplegics," *Journal of Applied Physiology*, vol. 60, no. 2, pp. 618–622, 1985.

[20] N. Nagaratnam, K. Nagaratnam, K. Ng, and P. Diu, "Akinetic mutism following stroke," *Journal of Clinical Neuroscience*, vol. 11, no. 1, pp. 25–30, 2004.

[21] L. Lundy-Ekman, *Neuroscience Fundamentals for Rehabilitation*, Saunders, St. Louis, Mich, USA, 3rd edition, 2007.

[22] B. C. Yarns and D. K. Quinn, "Telephone effect in akinetic mutism from traumatic brain injury," *Psychosomatics*, vol. 54, no. 6, pp. 609–610, 2013.

[23] N. Neumann and B. Kotchoubey, "Assessment of cognitive functions in severely paralysed and severely brain-damaged patients: neuropsychological and electrophysiological methods," *Brain Research Protocols*, vol. 14, no. 1, pp. 25–36, 2004.

[24] E. Casanova, R. E. Lazzari, S. Lotta, and A. Mazzucchi, "Locked-in syndrome: Improvement in the prognosis after an early intensive multidisciplinary rehabilitation," *Archives of Physical Medicine and Rehabilitation*, vol. 84, no. 6, pp. 862–867, 2003.

[25] M.-C. Rousseau, K. Baumstarck, M. Alessandrini, V. Blandin, T. Billette De Villemeur, and P. Auquier, "Quality of life in patients with locked-in syndrome: evolution over a 6-year period," *Orphanet Journal of Rare Diseases*, vol. 10, no. 1, article 88, 2015.

[26] L. Turner-Stokes, "Cost-efficiency of longer-stay rehabilitation programmes: can they provide value for money?" *Brain Injury*, vol. 21, no. 10, pp. 1015–1021, 2007.

[27] J. Whyte and R. Nakase-Richardson, "Disorders of conscious-
      ness: outcomes, comorbidities, and care needs," *Archives of
      Physical Medicine and Rehabilitation*, vol. 94, no. 10, pp. 1851–
      1854, 2013.

[28] P. Dollfus, P. L. Milos, A. Chapuis, P. Real, M. Orenstein, and J.
      W. Soutter, "The locked-in syndrome: a review and presentation
      of two chronic cases," *Paraplegia*, vol. 28, no. 1, pp. 5–16, 1990.

[29] E. L. Luxenberg, F. D. Goldenberg, J. I. Frank, R. Loch Mac-
      donald, and A. J. Rosengart, "Locked-in syndrome from rostro-
      caudal herniation," *Journal of Clinical Neuroscience*, vol. 16, no.
      2, pp. 333-334, 2009.

25

Bilateral Hypoglossal Nerve Palsy due to Brainstem Infarction: A Rare Presentation of Presumed Pyogenic Meningitis

A. G. T. A. Kariyawasam ⓘ,[1] **C. L. Fonseka** ⓘ,[2,3] **S. D. A. L. Singhapura,**[3] **J. S. Hewavithana,**[3] **H. M. M. Herath** ⓘ,[2,3] **and K. D. Pathirana**[4]

[1]*Registrar in Medicine, University Medical Unit, Teaching Hospital Karapitiya, Sri Lanka*
[2]*Consultant Physician, Department of Internal Medicine, Faculty of Medicine, University of Ruhuna, Sri Lanka*
[3]*Consultant Physician, University Medical Unit, Teaching Hospital, Karapitiya, Galle, Sri Lanka*
[4]*Professor in Neurology, Department of Internal Medicine, Faculty of Medicine, University of Ruhuna, Sri Lanka*

Correspondence should be addressed to A. G. T. A. Kariyawasam; thiliniaro88@gmail.com

Academic Editor: Norman S. Litofsky

Background. Cranial nerve palsies are well-known complications of basal meningitis, especially in patients with tuberculous meningitis. However, a minority of bacterial meningitis gets complicated with cranial nerve palsies. Although cerebral infarctions are known to occur with acute bacterial meningitis, infarctions occurring in the brainstem are infrequently described. *Case Presentation.* We report a 46-year-old healthy female who presented with dysarthria with fever, headache, and vomiting and was diagnosed to have acute pyogenic meningitis complicated with a brainstem infarction resulting in bilateral hypoglossal palsy. Her MRI revealed an infarction in the lower part of the medulla oblongata, probably involving the bilateral hypoglossal nuclei. *Conclusion.* Isolated bilateral hypoglossal nerve palsy is an extremely rare cranial nerve palsy, secondary to pyogenic meningitis. To our knowledge, this should be the first reported case of isolated bilateral hypoglossal nerve palsy due to a brainstem infarct in the background of pyogenic meningitis.

1. Introduction

Despite the current advanced treatment, meningitis still carries a substantial morbidity and mortality [1]. Fever, headache, and neck stiffness are considered as the hallmarks of meningitis. Presence of focal signs in meningitis points towards an unfavourable outcome [2]. Cranial nerve palsies are one of such focal signs associated with meningitis. In general, the cranial nerve involvement in meningitis is associated with a higher risk of mortality and disability and 5-10% of patients with acute bacterial meningitis can get complicated with cranial nerve involvement in the early course of the illness [3]. Multiple cranial nerve involvement is usually considered as an indicator of basilar meningitis and is thought to be a result of compression caused by oedematous brain or meningeal inflammation resulting in perineuritis. Third, fourth, sixth, and seventh nerves are the commonest nerves to get affected [3] and the involvement of the hypoglossal nerve is very rarely described in literature.

We herewith report a rare case of bilateral hypoglossal nerve palsy due to posteromedial infarction in the medulla oblongata secondary to acute bacterial meningitis. As far as we are aware, this is the first reported case of isolated bilateral hypoglossal nerve palsy, secondary to acute bacterial meningitis.

2. Case Presentation

A 46-year-old previously healthy female developed an insidious onset severe persistent headache, most prominent in the occipital region lasting for 10 days. Six days after the onset, she experienced dysarthria and a difficulty in moving her tongue within the mouth with a difficulty in eating and drinking. She did not complain of nasal regurgitation of food or nasal quality of speech. After admission, she was found to have a high-grade fever. She was otherwise healthy and denied symptoms of cough, decreased appetite, weight loss, or past history of tuberculosis. On admission, she was found

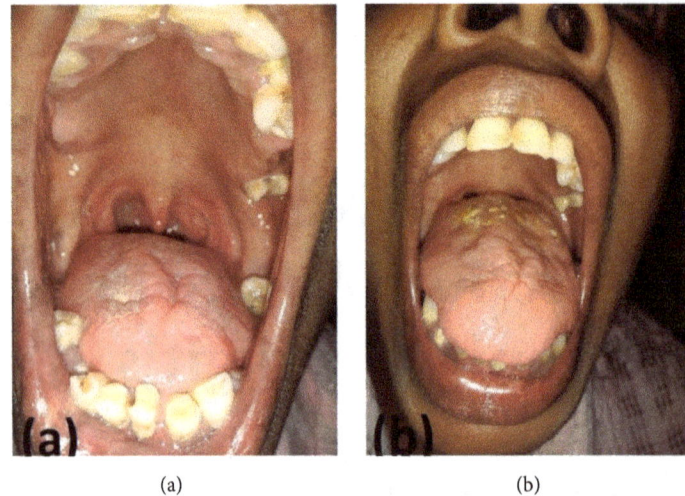

(a)   (b)

FIGURE 1: Bilateral tongue wasting: (a) resting position; (b) on protrusion.

to be ill with elicitable neck stiffness. Neurological examination revealed bilateral hypoglossal nerve palsy with marked tongue atrophy, more prominent in the left side (Figure 1) with tongue fasciculations and without other cranial nerve palsies or pyramidal weakness. Her eye movements were saccadic with a broad-based ataxic gait without other signs of cerebellar involvement.

Her blood tests revealed a haemoglobin of 12.5g/dl with a neutrophil leukocytosis (19,000/μL; 92.2% of neutrophils) with elevated ESR (100 1st Hr) and CRP (195 u/L). Her blood cultures were negative. Noncontrast CT brain did not reveal any abnormality. Cerebrospinal fluid (CSF) biochemistry revealed significant elevation of protein (111 mg/dL) with 59 polymorphs and 8 lymphocytes per cubic millimetre with reduced CSF glucose (29 mg/dL). CSF for GeneXpert for tuberculosis and staining for acid-fast bacillus (AFB) and fungal and atypical cells were negative. Pyogenic, mycobacterial, and fungal CSF cultures were negative and CSF for Meningococcus, Haemophilus, and Pneumococcus antigens were also negative. Her chest radiograph did not reveal any changes suggestive of pulmonary tuberculosis or sarcoidosis. Syphilis (VDRL & THPA), HIV serology, and autoimmune markers for vasculitis (rheumatoid factor, ANA (IF), and p & c-ANCA) were negative.

We initiated her on empirical treatment as for pyogenic meningitis with ceftriaxone and vancomycin for which she had a gradual improvement of general status with improvement of fever, meningism, gaze, and gait abnormalities while tongue weakness and atrophy persisted. Since we considered tuberculous meningitis as a possibility, we deferred treatment with steroids. Her rapid recovery in the absence of steroids or antituberculous drugs further supported our presumed diagnosis of pyogenic meningitis. Subsequently, she underwent MRI of brain and brainstem, which revealed a posteromedial infarction in the lower part of the medulla oblongata without leptomeningeal enhancement and did not show a significant cerebral oedema (Figure 2). At the end of three weeks of antibiotics, inflammatory markers and repeat CSF analysis

reached normal levels. After discharge, we reviewed her at one month and three & six months and she was free of fever with good general condition and had normal inflammatory markers. However, she had persistent tongue atrophy with difficult speech from which she was gradually recovering with the help of physiotherapy.

3. Discussion

Hypoglossal nerve palsy (HNP) is an uncommon cranial nerve palsy comparing to other commoner cranial nerves such as 3rd, 6th, and 7th cranial nerves [4]. Kean et al. in a case series described 100 patients with HNP either isolated or together with other cranial nerve palsies. In nearly 50 percent, HNP was secondary to either primary or secondary intracranial malignancy [5]. Therefore, it was concluded that HNP is a sign of intracranial malignancy indicating poor prognosis. Some years later, Panagariya et al. described a case series containing 12 clinical cases of isolated HNP and found that 33% had intracranial tuberculosis which were treated with antituberculous therapy. Other causes were sarcoidosis (8%), idiopathic (25%), and atlantooccipital dislocation (8%) and the overall recovery rate was nearly 60% [6].

Rocholt et al. described a patient with meningitis due to *Neisseria Meningitidis* complicated with obstructive hydrocephalus who had isolated unilateral HNP which resolved over 5 months [3]. Although unilateral HNP was infrequently reported with pyogenic meningitis, we could not find cases where bilateral HNP was reported.

A recent retrospective study was conducted in patients affected with acute bacterial meningitis (ABM) or tuberculous meningitis (TBM); the predictive value of each neurological sign on the diagnosis of above was analysed. They observed that the presence of cranial nerve palsies was the most important neurological predictor favouring TBM over ABM (OR = 1.980, CI 95%: 1.161-3.376) [2]. Since tuberculosis is commonly encountered in Sri Lanka, we strongly suspected TB meningitis. But, considering her

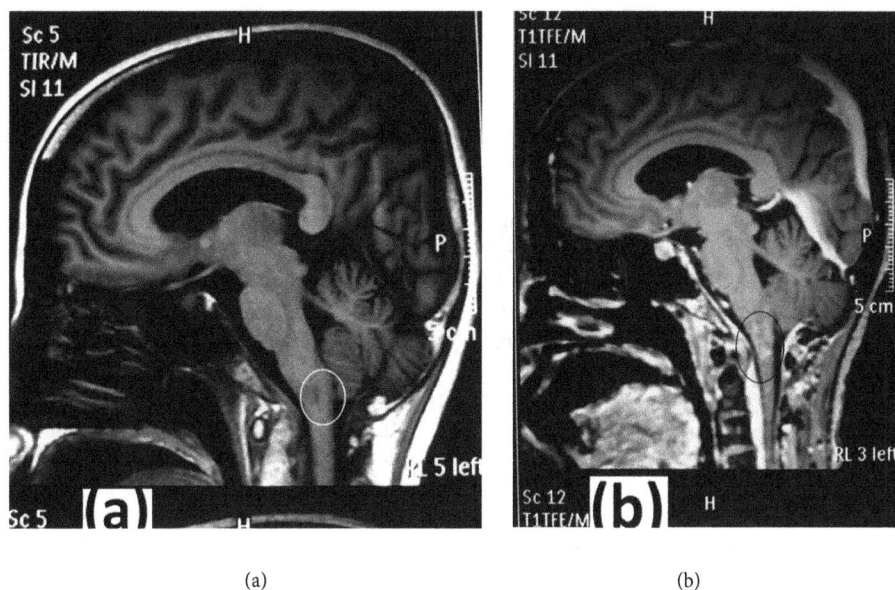

(a)   (b)

Figure 2: T1-weighted MRI of brainstem involving medulla oblongata demonstrating an infection: (a) without contrast; (b) postcontrast.

acute presentation, absence of constitutional symptoms, and CSF finding of polymorphic cell predominance, we initiated treatment as pyogenic meningitis. We continued to investigate further to exclude possible tuberculosis. The GeneXpert test in CSF which is nearly 60% sensitive and CSF AFB (sensitivity 10-20%) and TB cultures (sensitivity 50-60%) [7] were all negative. Our patient did not show meningeal enhancement or basal exudates in MRI brain, which is the most sensitive radiological feature, found in 90% of CNS tuberculosis [8].

With treatment, our patient showed a significant clinical improvement and inflammatory markers became normal. In addition, repeat CSF analysis two weeks later showed complete resolution of CSF abnormalities. All these findings stabilized the diagnosis of acute pyogenic meningitis. We attributed the uncommon presentation of bilateral tongue involvement to a posteromedial medullary infarction which was observed in the MRI scan of the brain (Figure 2).

For several decades, attention has been paid to the neurological complications of meningitis including cerebral infarctions. Diederik van de Beek et al. in a review described that 15-20% of community-acquired bacterial meningitis is complicated with infarctions of the brain matter [9].

According to another Danish population-based cohort study, 14% infarctions were observed in the course of ABM [10]. Many similar studies have proven that cerebral infarctions do occur as a complication in a significant proportion of patients with ABM [11]. Instances where such ischemic strokes occurring in the brainstem though rare are reported in the literature [12–14]. The patient had significant atrophy of the tongue. We assumed that this is due to denervation atrophy secondary to the brainstem infarction, although it is an uncommon finding in acute cases, due to the fact

that the subacute nature of presentation atrophy could be expected. The hypoglossal nerve is the sole motor innervator of the tongue; denervation atrophy of the tongue can result in significant changes of the tongue [15].

Apart from the involvement of bilateral HNP, our patient had other brainstem signs such as saccadic eye movements and cerebellar ataxia which got completely resolved with treatment. According to an animal experimental study carried out to explain the pathophysiology of eye saccades, it was suggested that the saccade palsy could have resulted from an insult to the lower pons [16]. This is supposed to be due to damage to caudal paramedian-pontine reticular formations (PPRF). When PPRF is damaged bilaterally, inputs from caudal PPRF to the rostral interstitial nucleus of the medial longitudinal fasciculus are greatly affected through the direct ascending anatomic pathway between them. This is supposed to result in oculomotor signs [17]. Although MRI did not show a definite pontine lesion in our patient, it could occur due to brain oedema or incomplete ischemia extending to the lower pons [17]. Complete recovery of other brainstem signs suggests the possible transient damage of other brainstem areas due to oedema or incomplete ischemia as a result of inflammatory response induced by the basilar meningitis.

4. Conclusions

Isolated bilateral hypoglossal nerve palsy is extremely rare cranial nerve palsy secondary to pyogenic meningitis. Brainstem infarcts involving the medial medullary region of the medulla oblongata can lead to a presentation of bilateral hypoglossal nerve palsy. To our knowledge, this is the first reported case of bilateral hypoglossal nerve palsy due to a brainstem infarct in the background of pyogenic meningitis.

Conflicts of Interest

The authors declare that there are no conflicts of interest.

Authors' Contributions

A. G. T. A. Kariyawasam, C. L. Fonseka, S. D. A. L. Singhapura, J. S. Hewavithana, and K. D. Pathirana investigated the case. C. L. Fonseka, H. M. M. Herath, and A. G. T. A. Kariyawasam planned radiological investigation and prepared the manuscript. All the authors got involved in editing the content and approved then final version for publication.

References

[1] M. A. Rabbani, A. A. Khan, S. S. Ali, B. Ahmad, S. M. Baig, and M. A. Khan, "Spectrum of complications and mortality of bacterial meningitis: an experience from a developing country," *Journal of Pakistan Medical Association*, vol. 53, no. 12, pp. 580–583, Dec 2003.

[2] A. Moghtaderi, R. Alavi-Naini, and S. Rashki, "Cranial nerve palsy as a factor to differentiate tuberculous meningitis from acute bacterial meningitis," *Acta Medica Iranica*, vol. 51, no. 2, pp. 113–118, 2013.

[3] M. Rockholt and C. Cervera, "Hypoglossal nerve palsy during meningococcal meningitis," *The New England Journal of Medicine*, vol. 371, no. 15, p. e22, 2014.

[4] J. R. Keane, "Multiple cranial nerve palsies: Analysis of 979 cases," *JAMA Neurology*, vol. 62, no. 11, pp. 1714–1717, 2005.

[5] J. R. Keane, "Twelfth-nerve palsy. Analysis of 100 cases," *JAMA Neurology*, vol. 53, no. 6, pp. 561–566, 1996.

[6] B. Sharma, P. Dubey, S. Kumar, A. Panagariya, and A. Dev, "Isolated Unilateral Hypoglossal Nerve Palsy: A Study of 12 cases," *Journal of neurology*, vol. 2, no. 1, 2010.

[7] N. C. Bahr, S. Marais, M. Caws et al., "GeneXpert MTB/Rif to Diagnose Tuberculous Meningitis: Perhaps the First Test but not the Last," *Clinical Infectious Diseases*, vol. 62, no. 9, pp. 1133–1135, 2016.

[8] M. Sanei Taheri, M. A. Karimi, H. Haghighatkhah, R. Pourghorban, M. Samadian, and H. Delavar Kasmaei, "Central Nervous System Tuberculosis: An Imaging-Focused Review of a Reemerging Disease," *Radiology Research and Practice*, vol. 2015, Article ID 202806, 8 pages, 2015.

[9] E. S. Schut, M. J. Lucas, M. C. Brouwer, M. D. I. Vergouwen, A. Van Der Ende, and D. Van De Beek, "Cerebral infarction in adults with bacterial meningitis," *Neurocritical Care*, vol. 16, no. 3, pp. 421–427, 2012.

[10] J. Bodilsen, M. Dalager-Pedersen, H. C. Schønheyder, and H. Nielsen, "Stroke in community-acquired bacterial meningitis: A Danish population-based study," *International Journal of Infectious Diseases*, vol. 20, no. 1, pp. 18–22, 2014.

[11] D. van de Beek, J. de Gans, A. R. Tunkel, and E. F. M. Wijdicks, "Community-acquired bacterial meningitis in adults," *The New England Journal of Medicine*, vol. 354, no. 1, pp. 44–53, 2006.

[12] J. Z. Willey, S. Prabhakaran, and R. DelaPaz, "Retroperitoneal infection complicated by bacterial meningitis and ventriculitis with secondary brainstem infarction," *Neurocritical Care*, vol. 6, no. 3, pp. 192–194, 2007.

[13] R. Garg, H. Malhotra, M. Jain, N. Kumar, G. Lachuryia, and L. Mahajan, "Brainstem infarct as a rare complication of coagulase-negative staphylococcus meningitis," *Neurology India*, vol. 65, no. 3, pp. 621–623, 2017.

[14] S. B. Lee, L. K. Jones, and C. Giannini, "Brainstem infarcts as an early manifestation of Streptococcus anginosus meningitis," *Neurocritical Care*, vol. 3, no. 2, pp. 157–160, 2005.

[15] L. Junquera and L. Gallego, "Denervation atrophy of the tongue after hypoglossal-nerve injury," *The New England Journal of Medicine*, vol. 367, no. 2, p. 156, 2012.

[16] V. Henn, W. Lang, K. Hepp, and H. Reisine, "Experimental gaze palsies in monkeys and their relation to uman pathology," *Brain*, vol. 107, no. 2, pp. 619–636, 1984.

[17] K. Toyoda, Y. Hasegawa, T. Yonehara, J. Oita, and T. Yamaguchi, "Bilateral medial medullary infarction with oculomotor disorders," *Stroke*, vol. 23, no. 11, pp. 1657–1659, 1992.

26

Rapid Ascending Sensorimotor Paralysis, Hearing Loss, and Fatal Arrhythmia in a Multimorbid Patient due to an Accidental Overdose of Fluoxetine

Matthew Herrmann, Prissilla Xu, and Antonio Liu

White Memorial Medical Center Department of Internal Medicine, Los Angeles, CA, USA

Correspondence should be addressed to Matthew Herrmann; herrmann.matthew7@gmail.com

Academic Editor: Peter Berlit

Background. Common side effects of selective serotonin reuptake inhibitors (SSRIs) include tachycardia, drowsiness, tremor, nausea, and vomiting. Although SSRIs have less toxic side effects compared to more traditional antidepressants, serious and life threatening cases of SSRI overdose have been reported. We describe a 24-year-old multimorbid female who presented to the emergency department with rapid onset ascending sensorimotor paralysis, complicated by respiratory and cardiac arrest, found to have fatal levels of fluoxetine by toxicological analysis, not taken in a suicidal act. *Results.* Autopsy was performed at the Los Angeles County Medical Examiner's Office of a female with no evidence of traumatic injury. Toxicological analysis revealed lethal levels of fluoxetine, toxic levels of diphenhydramine, and multiple other coingested substances at nontoxic levels. Neuropathological examination of the brain and spinal cord revealed no evidence of Guillain-Barre paralysis. *Conclusions.* Lethal levels of fluoxetine and multiple potential drug-to-drug interactions in our patient likely contributed to her unique signs and symptoms. This is the first case reporting neurologic signs and symptoms consisting of rapid onset ascending sensorimotor paralysis, hearing loss, respiratory failure, cardiac arrest, and death in a patient with lethal levels of fluoxetine.

1. Introduction

Selective serotonin reuptake inhibitors (SSRIs) are commonly used to treat depression and anxiety disorders and are some of the most widely prescribed antidepressants today [1]. Multiple case studies have reported that SSRIs are associated with a less toxic side effect profile and fewer reported deaths have been attributed to overdose compared to more traditional antidepressants, such as tricyclic antidepressants [2, 3]; however, serious and life threatening sequelae have been reported. Additionally, among SSRIs, fluoxetine has been reported to be the least toxic by hazard index measures [3]. The largest published case series on fluoxetine overdoses found that the most common effects were signs of serotonin syndrome such as tachycardia, drowsiness, tremor, nausea, and vomiting [4]. Other significant sequelae include seizures, cardiac toxicity, and death [2, 5]. We report abnormal symptomatology of a young woman due to an accidental fatal fluoxetine overdose, consisting of rapid onset, ascending sensorimotor paralysis,

bilateral hearing loss, respiratory failure, cardiac arrest, and eventual death.

2. Case Report

A 24-year-old Hispanic female with diabetes mellitus type 1, anemia, hypertension, chronic pancreatitis with partial pancreatectomy, cholecystectomy, and splenectomy presented to the emergency department (ED) with abdominal pain not relieved by oral pain medications. She recalled her home medications to be mirtazapine 30 mg orally nightly, fluoxetine unknown dose orally three times a day, carbamazepine 200 mg orally twice daily, insulin glargine 15–20 units subcutaneously nightly, morphine sulfate 30 mg orally twice daily, tramadol 50 mg orally four times a day, hydromorphone 4 mg orally six times a day as needed for pain, and hydrocodone/acetaminophen 325/10 mg orally six times a day as needed for pain, and she had been taking them to relieve her pain. She was discharged from the ED but returned on the same day with worsening abdominal pain, loss of sensation in lower extremities, lips, and hands, and ascending paralysis. The patient was noted to have a leukocytosis with bandemia, fever, and tachycardia suspicious for sepsis. Computed tomography (CT) of the abdomen was significant for small bowel edema and ascites. The patient continued to deteriorate with worsening ascending paralysis, bilateral hearing loss, hypotension, and respiratory failure with subsequent endotracheal intubation. She underwent two rounds of cardiopulmonary resuscitation (CPR) for a total of approximately 109 minutes but ultimately expired.

An autopsy was performed and documented a well-developed woman with no evidence of traumatic injuries. Postmortem serum analysis revealed fatal levels of heart blood fluoxetine concentration of 2.3 mcg/mL.

The cause of death was thought to be multiple medication intoxication with fatal levels of fluoxetine. A neuropathologist was consulted who agreed with the diagnosis and thought that her symptoms were primarily due to overmedication with fluoxetine. She had no known history of suicidal ideation or attempt but did have chronic pain. Thus, the favored mode of death was accident. Contributory factors to death included acute on chronic, culture negative pancreatitis with abscess formation, and likely sepsis.

3. Experimental

3.1. Specimens. All specimens were analyzed and collected at autopsy at Los Angeles County Medical Examiner's Office. Submitted specimens included heart ventricles and septum, left lung, right lung, liver, right kidney, small bowel and colon, and head of pancreas. The neuropathological specimens consisted of formalin fixed brain, spinal cord with attached dura mater, and complete cranial dura mater.

4. Results

Positive findings on gross and microscopic pathology revealed evidence of chronic pancreatitis with superimposed acute pancreatitis with abscess, culture negative for three days after death, and surgical absent pancreatic tail. The spleen and gall bladder were also surgically absent. The cut surface of the pancreas was pale, fibrotic, and gritty, with loss of normal lobular appearance. Rare small punctate hemorrhages were present, with a single ~0.5 cm possible abscess cavity present centrally in fibrotic area with no communication to the surface. Other microscopic findings revealed acute pneumonia of the left lung, mild emphysematous changes of bilateral lungs, few hypertrophic myocytes of the heart septum and left ventricle, and mild nonspecific chronic hepatitis. There was no evidence of septic emboli.

Gross impression of neuropathological specimens revealed brain swelling, cavum septum pellucidum, external rotation of left hippocampus, beaking of the inferior frontal lobe, cerebral vermis atrophy, and no gross atrophy of the nerves and spinal cord, with no spinal cord lesions noted on cross section. The meninges were clear and there was no gross evidence of meningitis. Neuropathological examination of the brain and spinal cord revealed no evidence of Guillain-Barre paralysis and findings consistent with hypoxic-ischemic encephalopathy. The findings of cerebellar atrophy and hippocampal neuronal dropout suggested a chronic seizure disorder, which was not noted on history.

4.1. Toxicological Analysis. Toxicology tests revealed a lethal level of fluoxetine, 1.8 mcg/mL, in the femoral blood, and 2.3 mcg/mL in the heart blood, as well as 0.81 mcg/mL of norfluoxetine in the femoral blood and 1.1 mcg/mL of norfluoxetine in the heart blood. Diphenhydramine was also found at toxic levels, 0.78 mcg/mL, in the femoral blood. Other medications present at nontoxic levels included metoclopramide, mirtazapine, nortramadol, tramadol, midazolam, lidocaine, carbamazepine, hydrocodone, codeine, morphine, and hydromorphone in her heart and femoral blood. Levels of ethanol, barbiturates, cocaine and metabolites, fentanyl, methamphetamine and methlenedioxymethamphetamine, free phencyclidine, free oxycodone, and free oxymorphine were not detected

5. Discussion

Fluoxetine, one of the SSRI antidepressants, was introduced into clinical practice over 25 years ago and has remained one of the most popular and safe [6–8] antidepressants in the United States [9]. While approximately half of fluoxetine intoxications remain asymptomatic [4, 9], symptoms of fluoxetine overdose are "minimally toxic" and include tachycardia, drowsiness, tremor, nausea, and vomiting [10]. However, more serious sequelae have also been reported, such as seizures [10–16], cardiac conduction abnormalities [16], CNS depression, respiratory arrest, and even death [5]. Our patient whose toxicological analysis revealed lethal levels of fluoxetine presented with tachycardia and, uniquely, loss of sensation in her lower extremities, lips, and hands and developed rapidly ascending paralysis with respiratory arrest, cardiac arrest, and eventual death.

The patient reported taking fluoxetine, unknown dose, three times a day despite the recommended dose of between 20 and 80 mg per day [17]. It was unclear for how long she had been taking this dose. There was no indication from her history or from the pathologist's report that this was a suicidal attempt. Mode of death determined to be accidental from multiple medication intoxication. The toxicologist report revealed multiple drugs present in her femoral and heart blood, with diphenhydramine, fluoxetine, and norfluoxetine at toxic levels. Our review of the literature revealed that our patient presented with neurologic findings that are first to be described in association with fluoxetine ingestion.

The pathomechanism by which toxic levels of fluoxetine could have caused these unique symptoms is described in, in vitro, animal and human studies. Multiple experimental studies have showed that at hypertherapeutic and overdose concentrations of fluoxetine, fluoxetine demonstrates evidence of cytotoxicity, antiproliferative effects, and mitochondrial dysfunction. Specifically, these studies noted inhibition of mitochondrial function and depletion of cellular ATP levels with significantly increased lactate production, activation of

TABLE 1: Drugs found in patient's blood by toxicological analysis, site of metabolism, reference range, and documented drug-drug interactions.

Medication	Blood site	Measured concentration (mcg/mL)	Metabolism	Reference range	Drug-drug interactions	Comment
Diphenhydramine	Femoral/heart	0.78/0.63 (toxic level)	50% liver metabolism to diphenylmethane, which suggests a large first-pass effect	Antihistamine effects at levels >0.025 mcg/mL Drowsiness at levels 0.03–0.04 mcg/mL Mental impairment at levels >0.06 mcg/mL Toxic: >0.1 mcg/mL Therapeutic: not established	Metabolism/transport effects inhibit CYP2D6 (moderate) and CYP1A2, 2C9, and 2C19 (minor)	May increase fluoxetine level via inhibition of CYP2D6
Fluoxetine	Femoral/heart	1.8/2.3 (toxic level)	CYP450 (extensive P450 CYP2D6 inhibitor, demethylation) Active metabolite: norfluoxetine	Therapeutic: fluoxetine: 0.1–0.8 mcg/mL Toxic: fluoxetine plus norfluoxetine: >2 mcg/mL	Metabolism/transport effects substrate of CYP1A2 (minor), 2B6 (minor), 2C9 (major), 2C19 (minor), 2D6 (major), 2E1 (minor), and 3A4 (minor) It inhibits CYP1A2 (moderate), 2B6 (weak), 2C9 (weak), 2C19 (moderate, 2D6 (strong), and 3A4 (weak)	Avoid concomitant use with MAO inhibitors Increased effect/toxicity of serotonin reuptake inhibitor/antagonist, carbamazepine, CNS depressants, CYP1A2 substrates, CYP2C19 substrates, CYP2D6 substrates, serotonin modulators
Norfluoxetine	Femoral/heart	0.81/1.1 (toxic level)	Active metabolite of fluoxetine	Therapeutic: norfluoxetine (active metabolite): 0.1–0.6 mcg/mL Toxic: fluoxetine plus norfluoxetine: >2.0 mcg/mL		Patient had combined fluoxetine + norfluoxetine 3.3 mcg/ml in heart blood, over the toxic limit 2.0 mcg/ml
Metoclopramide	Femoral/heart	0.10/0.10	Hepatic: minimal, via simple conjugation	N/A	Metabolism/Transport effects substrate of (minor) CYP1A2, 2D6; it inhibits CYP2D6 (weak)	May increase fluoxetine level via inhibition of CYP2D6

TABLE 1: Continued.

Medication	Blood site	Measured concentration (mcg/mL)	Metabolism	Reference range	Drug-drug interactions	Comment
Mirtazapine	Femoral/heart	0.19/0.11	CYP450 extensively hepatic via CYP2D6, CYP1A2, CYP2C9, and CYP3A4 Metabolites: 8-hydroxyl metabolite, N-desmethyl, and N-oxide metabolites	N/A	Metabolism/transport effects substrate of CYP1A2 (major), 2C9 (minor), 2D6 (major), and 3A4 (major) It inhibits CYP1A2 (weak), 3A4 (weak)	*May increase levels/effects of CNS depressants Serotonin modulators* The level/effects of mirtazapine may be increased by CYP1A2 inhibitors (strong), 2D6 inhibitors (moderate), CYP3A4 inhibitors (moderate)
Tramadol	Femoral/heart	0.2/0.17	Extensively hepatic via demethylation, glucuronidation, and sulfation Pharmacologically active metabolite formed by CYP2D6 (M1; O-demethyl tramadol)	0.1–0.3 mcg/mL However, serum level monitoring is not required	Metabolism/transport effects substrate of CYP2D6 (major), 3A4 (major)	*May increase levels/effects of CNS depressants; MAOI; SSRIs;* Serotonin modulators The level/effects of tramadol may be increased by CYP2D6 inducers (moderate), 3A4 inhibitors (strong) The levels/effects of tramadol may be decreased by CYP2D6 inhibitors (moderate), 3A4 inducers (strong)
Nortramadol	Femoral/heart	0.82/0.84	Active metabolite of tramadol	0.1–0.3 mcg/mL However, serum level monitoring is not required		
Lidocaine	Heart	<0.5	CYP450 90% hepatic metabolism via CYP1A2 Active metabolites: Monoethylglycinexylidide (MEGX) Glycinexylidide (GX)	Therapeutic: 1.5–5 mcg/mL Potentially toxic levels: >6 mcg/mL Toxic: >9 mcg/mL	Metabolism/transport effects substrate of CYP1A2 (minor), 2A6 (minor), 2B6 (minor), 2C9 (minor), 2D6 (major), and 3A4 (major); it inhibits CYP 1A2 (strong), 2D6 (moderate), and 3A4 (moderate)	Lidocaine may decrease the levels/effects of tramadol *May increase fluoxetine level via inhibition of CYP2D6*

TABLE 1: Continued.

Medication	Blood site	Measured concentration (mcg/mL)	Metabolism	Reference range	Drug-drug interactions	Comment
Midazolam	Heart	0.105	Metabolized in the liver and gut via biotransformation mediated by CYP3A4	N/A	Metabolism/transport effects substrate of CYP2B6 (minor), 3A4 (major) and it inhibits CYP 2C8 (weak), 2C9 (weak), and 3A4 (weak)	*The levels/effects of midazolam may be increased by SSRIs* The levels/effects of midazolam may be decreased by carbamazepine and CYP3A4 inducers (strong)
Carbamazepine	Heart	5.0	CYP450 Primarily via CYP3A4 Active metabolites: Carbamazepine-10,11-epoxide (partly responsible for intoxication)	Therapeutic levels: 4–12 mcg/mL Toxic level: >15 mcg/mL	Metabolism/transport effects substrate of CYP2C8 (minor), 3A4 (major), It induces CYP 1A2 (strong), 2B6 (strong), 2C8 (strong), 2C9 (strong), 2C19 (strong), and 3A4 (strong)	*May increase the levels/effects of CNS depressants* *The levels/effects of carbamazepine may be increased by CYP3A4 inhibitors and SSRIs (i.e., fluoxetine*
Hydrocodone	Heart	Free hydrocodone level 0.06	Liver metabolism by N-demethylation (catalyzed by CYP3A4, 2B6, and 2C19), 0-demethylation (catalyzed by CYP2B6 and 2C19), and 6-keto reduction to the corresponding 6-alpha and 6-beta hydroxyl metabolites Active metabolites: Norhydrocodone (major) Hydromorphone (minor)	N/A	Metabolism/transport effects substrate of CYP3A4 (major)	*May increase the levels/effects of CNS depressants and SSRIs (i.e., fluoxetine)*

TABLE 1: Continued.

Medication	Blood site	Measured concentration (mcg/mL)	Metabolism	Reference range	Drug-drug interactions	Comment
Codeine	Heart	Presumptive+	CYP450 Primarily via CYP2D6, CYP3A4, and UDP-glucuronosyl-transferase 2B7 and 2B4	Therapeutic: not established Toxic: >1.1 mcg/mL	Metabolism/transport effects substrate of CYP2D6 (major) and CYP3A4 (minor) It inhibits CYP2D6 (weak)	*May increase the levels/effects of CNS depressants and SSRIs (i.e., fluoxetine) May increase fluoxetine level via CYP2D6 inhibition*
Morphine	Heart	Presumptive+	Liver metabolism by N-demethylation, N-dealkylation, 0-dealkylation, conjugation, and hydrolysis Active metabolite: Morphine-3-glucuronide (M3G) Morphine-6-glucuronide (M6G)	Therapeutic: surgical anesthesia: 65–80 ng/mL Toxic: 200–5000 ng/mL	Metabolism/ transport effects substrate of CYP2D6 (minor)	*May increase the levels/effects of CNS depressants and SSRIs (i.e., fluoxetine)*
Hydromorphone	Heart	Presumptive+	Extensive liver first-pass metabolism primarily via glucuronidation Inactive metabolite: Hydromorphone-3-glucuronide	N/A	Not a significant substrate of inhibitor of CYP450	*May increase the levels/effects of CNS depressants and SSRIs*

apoptosis, and evidence of redox stress and DNA damage [18–22].

The drug-drug interactions which potentially contributed to our patient's toxic levels of fluoxetine and unique symptomatology include fluoxetine with metoclopramide, carbamazepine, tramadol, mirtazapine, codeine, hydrocodone, and morphine. Fluoxetine, diphenhydramine, and metoclopramide are all inhibitors CYP2D6, one of the cytochrome P450 enzymes necessary for detoxification of foreign chemicals and metabolism of drugs. Inhibitor of this enzyme likely contributed to the toxic levels noted in her blood. Also, it is well documented that the concurrent use of fluoxetine with codeine, hydrocodone, hydromorphone, mirtazapine, morphine, and tramadol, and the use of concurrent carbamazepine with codeine, hydromorphone, and mirtazapine may result in increased risk of serotonin syndrome [23–25]. Overall, our patient's unique symptomatology could be explained by the damaging effects of toxic levels of fluoxetine as well as the multiple drug-drug interactions as outline in Table 1.

Most fatalities due to fluoxetine exposure are reported either with extremely large doses (greater than 150 times the daily dose) or with the presence of coingestants such as ethanol or benzodiazepines [4, 6]. In 2014, the NDPS reported that the range of fluoxetine blood concentrations in listed fatalities ranged from 0.68 mcg/ml to 2.2 mcg/L, which is significantly greater than the typical steady state therapeutic concentration of 0.25 mcg/mL. To put this into perspective, toxicological analysis on our patient revealed fatal levels of heart blood fluoxetine and norfluoxetine concentrations at 2.3 mcg/mL and 1.1 mcg/mL, respectively, well above the therapeutic limit. It is important to note that, in one study of antidepressant overdose, no correlation between fluoxetine level and mental status was found, while another study of fluvoxamine overdose found no correspondence between drug levels and symptom severity [17, 18], suggesting that each patient presenting with an SSRI overdose, despite quantity consumed, can have unique symptomatology.

Although most patients recover from fluoxetine overdose, high dose ingestions can lead to cardiovascular and neurologic complications, including death. In this case, the patient had lethal levels of fluoxetine noted in her blood, as well as levels of multiple other medications with known drug-drug interactions to fluoxetine, possibly contributing to her unique symptomatology. However, this patient's presenting neurologic signs and symptoms are unique and have yet to be described in current reports of fatal levels of fluoxetine ingestions or coingestions involving fluoxetine.

Conflicts of Interest

The authors have no conflicts of interest to report.

References

[1] S. H. Preskorn, H. P. Feighner, C. Y. Stanga, and R. Ross, *Antidepressants: Past, Present and Future*, 2004, Past, Present and Future.

[2] G. K. Isbister, S. J. Bowe, A. Dawson, and I. M. Whyte, "Relative toxicity of selective serotonin reuptake inhibitors (SSRIs) in overdose," *Journal of Toxicology—Clinical Toxicology*, vol. 42, no. 3, pp. 277–285, 2004.

[3] N. White, T. Litovitz, and C. Clancy, "Suicidal antidepressant overdoses: a comparative analysis by antidepressant type.," *Journal of medical toxicology : official journal of the American College of Medical Toxicology*, vol. 4, no. 4, pp. 238–250, 2008.

[4] D. J. Borys, S. C. Setzer, L. J. Ling, J. J. Reisdorf, L. C. Day, and E. P. Krenzelok, "Acute fluoxetine overdose: A report of 234 cases," *American Journal of Emergency Medicine*, vol. 10, no. 2, pp. 115–120, 1992.

[5] M. W. Lai, W. Klein-Schwartz, G. C. Rodgers et al., "2005 Annual report of the American association of poison control centers' national poisoning and exposure database," *Clinical Toxicology*, vol. 44, no. 6-7, pp. 803–932, 2006.

[6] J. T. Barbey and S. P. Roose, "SSRI safety in overdose," *Journal of Clinical Psychiatry*, vol. 59, suppl. 15, pp. 42–48, 1998.

[7] H. A. Spiller, S. Morse, and C. Muir, "Fluoxetine ingestion: a one year retrospective study," *Veterinary and Human Toxicology*, vol. 32, article 153, 1990.

[8] W. Chiang, M. Ford, P. Wax, R. Hoffman, M. Howland, and L. Goldfrank, "Prospective evaluation of fluoxetine ingestions," *Veterinary and Human Toxicology*, vol. 32, article 348, 1991.

[9] Top 200 generic drugs by unit in 2007. Drug Topics, June 2017, http://drugtopics.modernmedicine.com/drug-topics/news/modernmedicine/modern-medicine-feature-articles/top-200-generic-drugs-unit-2007.

[10] J. J. Weber, "Seizure activity associated with fluoxetine therapy," *The Journal of Clinical Pharmacology*, pp. 8:296–8:296, 1989.

[11] R. Hargrave, D. Martinez, and A. J. Bernstein, "Fluoxetine-induced seizures," *Psychosomatics*, vol. 33, no. 2, pp. 236-237, 1992.

[12] V. P. Prasher, "Seizures associated with fluoxetine therapy," *Seizure*, vol. 2, no. 4, pp. 315–317, 1993.

[13] M. R. Ware and R. B. Stewart, "Seizures Associated with Fluoxetine Therapy," *DICP*, vol. 23, no. 5, pp. 428-428, 2016.

[14] G. Braitberg and S. C. Curry, "Seizure after isolated fluoxetine overdose," *Annals of Emergency Medicine*, vol. 26, no. 2, pp. 234–237, 1995.

[15] R. Gross, P. N. Dannon, E. Lepkifker, J. Zohar, and M. Kotler, "Generalized seizures caused by fluoxetine overdose," *American Journal of Emergency Medicine*, vol. 16, no. 3, pp. 328-329, 1998.

[16] A. Graudins, C. Vossler, and R. Wang, "Fluoxetine-induced cardiotoxicity with response to bicarbonate therapy," *American Journal of Emergency Medicine*, vol. 15, no. 5, pp. 501–503, 1997.

[17] G. Gartlehner, R. A. Hansen, L. C. Morgan et al., "Comparative benefits and harms of second-generation antidepressants for treating major depressive disorder: An updated meta-analysis," *Annals of Internal Medicine*, vol. 155, no. 11, pp. 772–785, 2011.

[18] E. Elmorsy, A. Al-Ghafari, F. M. Almutairi, A. M. Aggour, and W. G. Carter, "Antidepressants are cytotoxic to rat primary blood brain barrier endothelial cells at high therapeutic concentrations," *Toxicology in Vitro*, vol. 44, pp. 154–163, 2017.

[19] A. L. Hansson, Z. Xia, M. C. Berglund, A. Bergstrand, J. W. Depierre, and L. Nässberger, "Reduced cell survival and morphological alterations induced by three tricyclic antidepressants in human peripheral monocytes and lymphocytes and in cell lines derived from these cell types," *Toxicology in Vitro*, vol. 11, no. 1-2, pp. 21–31, 1997.

[20] T. S. Davies and W. M. Kluwe, "Erratum: Preclinical toxicological evaluation of sertraline hydrochloride (Drug and Chemical Toxicology)," *Drug and Chemical Toxicology*, vol. 21, no. 4, pp. 521–537, 1998.

[21] A. Carvajal Garcia-Pando, J. Garcia del Pozo, A. Sanchez et al., "Hepatoxicity associated with new antidepressants," *Journal of Clinical Psychiatry*, pp. 135–137, 2002.

[22] Y. Li, L. Couch, M. Higuchi, J.-L. Fang, and L. Guo, "Mitochondrial dysfunction induced by sertraline, an antidepressant agent," *Toxicological Sciences*, vol. 127, no. 2, pp. 582–591, 2012.

[23] C. Lacy, L. Armstrong, M. P. Goldman, and L. L. Lance, *Drug Information Handbook*, 20th edition.

[24] http://www.micromedexsolutions.com.

[25] http://www.globalrph.com.

27

Late-Onset Pompe Disease with Nemaline Bodies

E. Frezza ⓘ, C. Terracciano, M. Giacanelli, E. Rastelli, G. Greco, and R. Massa ⓘ

Neuromuscular Diseases Unit, Department of Systems Medicine, University of Rome Tor Vergata, Rome, Italy

Correspondence should be addressed to R. Massa; massa@uniroma2.it

Academic Editor: Isabella Laura Simone

Pompe disease is an autosomal recessive disorder characterized by deficiency of alpha-glucosidase, a lysosomal enzyme, which can lead to glycogen accumulation in skeletal muscle, heart, and nervous system. Clinical presentation is highly variable, with infantile and late-onset (LOPED) forms. Although muscle biopsy findings are rather stereotyped, atypical features have been described. A 52-year-old man without a family history of muscle disorders presented with slowly progressing upper and lower limb girdle weakness and hyperCKemia. At needle EMG, a diffuse neurogenic pattern was detected. Muscle biopsy showed a selective type 1 fiber atrophy with vacuoles of various sizes, filled with PAS and acid phosphatase positive material, confirmed to be glycogen by electron microscopy (EM). Many atrophic fibers contained foci of myofibrillar material recognized as nemaline bodies (NBs) at EM. Low level of alpha-glucosidase activity in blood and molecular genetic testing confirmed the diagnosis of late-onset Pompe disease (LOPED). Major causes of hereditary and acquired NB myopathy were ruled out. In conclusion, NBs represent a novel histological finding in LOPED and characterize the atypical presentation of our case.

1. Introduction

Pompe disease is an autosomal recessive genetic disorder characterized by deficiency of the enzyme alpha-glucosidase. Onset and phenotypic spectrum of Pompe disease are wide and vary from the early infantile onset (IOPD) (0-1 year) to the late onset form that may present with different phenotypes, ranging from a symptomless to a severe form (LOPED) [1].

LOPED clinical spectrum is heterogeneous and includes fatigue, exercise intolerance, obstructive sleep apnea syndrome (OSAS), axial and proximal muscular weakness, and restrictive respiratory failure.

Muscle biopsy findings of LOPED differ considerably between patients and range from normal to highly abnormal. They usually comprise a vacuolar myopathy with abnormal glycogen accumulation. Vacuolization may affect preferentially either type 1 or type 2 fibers. Other findings are neurogenic-like pattern and the presence of necrotic fibers.

To confirm the suspicion of Pompe disease the quantitation of alpha-glucosidase activity is mandatory and, in case of positivity, molecular genetic testing provides finalization of the diagnosis.

2. Case Report

A 52-year-old man, without a history of neurological or muscle disorders, presented with slowly progressing upper and lower limb girdle weakness lasting for about 7-8 years. In particular, he complained of difficulties in going up- and downstairs and in carrying weights. He also complained of dyspnea, even with mild efforts. No dysphagia or dysphonia was reported. A recent check-up blood test showed mild hyperCKemia (CK= 468 UI/L; n. v. 10-167 UI/L).

At neurological examination he presented lumbar hyperlordosis, abdominal breath, and waddling gait. Manual muscle test (MRC) revealed bilateral and symmetric weakness of *deltoid* (4, R+L), *pectoralis* (3, R+L), *biceps b.* (4, R+L), *triceps b.* (4, R+L), *ileo-psoas* (4, R+L), and *quadriceps* (4, R+L). All remaining muscles had normal strength. Hypotrophy was evident in the axial musculature, with the presence of winged scapulae.

On blood tests, CK was slightly elevated and serum protein electrophoresis was normal.

Functional respiratory test showed a moderate restrictive ventilatory deficit.

Nerve conduction studies were unremarkable. By concentric needle EMG, abundant fibrillation potentials and

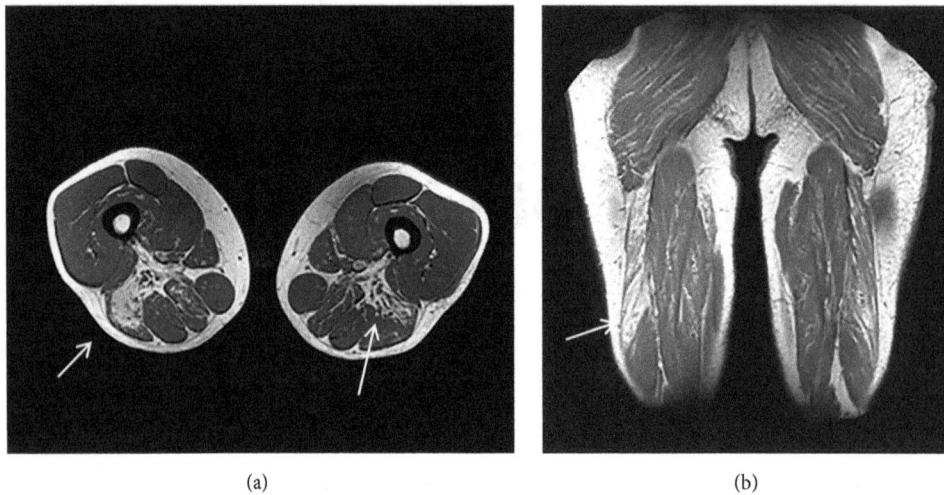

(a)   (b)

FIGURE 1: MRI of the thighs in axial T2 (a) and coronal T2 (b) sections shows bilateral fibroadipose degeneration of the *adductor* and *biceps femoris* muscles.

positive sharp waves, associated with sporadic fasciculation potentials and complex repetitive discharges with MUPs of increased amplitude, duration, and polyphasic aspect, were detected in *tibialis anterior* muscles. Other muscles (L *deltoid* and R *vastus*) showed milder signs of neurogenic MUPs remodeling. Only in R *infraspinatus*, MUPs of reduced amplitude and duration were found, indicating a myopathic pattern.

MRI of the thighs showed a bilateral fibro-adipose degeneration of the *adductor* and *biceps femoris* muscles, together with hypertrophy of the *gracilis* muscles (Figure 1).

The patient underwent a muscle biopsy of the left *vastus lateralis* that showed few necrotic and numerous atrophic fibers, the majority of which containing small, medium, and large vacuoles. At the PAS reaction, performed on cryostat and, for a better resolution, resin sections [2], these vacuoles appeared filled with polysaccharide material that showed glycogen structure at electron microscopy (EM) observation. By the acid phosphatase reaction, all optically visible vacuoles, plus a large number of small, intracytoplasmic foci, stained positively, indicating a lysosomal nature of the vacuoles. ATPase histochemistry revealed that vacuoles were present almost exclusively in type 1 fibers, which were also diffusely atrophic, as opposed to the normal appearance of type 2 fibers. Furthermore, many of these atrophic fibers (7% of all fibers contained in transverse sections) displayed numerous, discrete, deposits of basophilic material, located centrally within the fiber cytoplasm or, in some instances, in a subsarcolemmal position (Figure 2). By EM, this material was distributed in multiple, cigar-shaped, stereotyped formations oriented consistently with the longitudinal axis of the fibers and representing nemaline bodies (NBs). These were composed of myofibrillar material in apparent continuity with Z-bands (Figure 3). No cores, or other typical alterations seen in congenital myopathies, were observed.

In order to substantiate a diagnosis of Pompe disease, we performed alpha-glucosidase (GAA) assay by mass spectrometry on dry blood spots which showed GAA 0.27

μmol/L/h (n.v. 1.86–21.9 μmol/L/h); alpha-galactosidase, as control enzyme, was within normal limits (8.13 μmol/L/h; n.v. 5.71–49.02 μmol/L/h). Consistently, GAA value in blood lymphocytes was also very low (1 nM/mg/h; n.v. 13-32 nM/mg/h). Enzymatic assay on muscle biopsy was not performed due to shortage of tissue.

Diagnosis was finally confirmed by molecular analysis, which showed a compound heterozygosis for the known c.-32-13 T>G splice mutation and the known c.2544delC deletion (p.Lys849fs) in the *GAA* gene.

3. Discussion

The clinical presentation of LOPED spans a wide range of severity, from asymptomatic to seriously impaired patients. In our case, the degree of clinical involvement could be placed in the middle of this range, with a muscle distribution typical of LOPED.

EMG findings are usually suggestive of a myopathy, although neurogenic changes were described in some cases. The almost "pure" neurogenic features of our patient may represent a less frequent EMG pattern, possibly indicating secondary neurogenic modifications induced by a chronic myopathic process.

Classic LOPED histopathology shows a vacuolar myopathy with abnormal glycogen accumulation, which may affect preferentially either type 1 or type 2 fibers, and increased staining for acid phosphatase activity. Atypical features have been reported as the presence of reducing bodies-like globular inclusions, lobulated fibers, COX-negative fibers, and ragged-red fibers [3].

In addition to the common histopathological alterations, in the present case we found abundant NBs grouped in the cytoplasm of a high percentage of muscle fibers, mainly of type 1.

The coexistence of glycogen-filled vacuoles, NB, and fiber atrophy with an overwhelming prevalence among type 1 fibers indicates that, for unknown reasons, this fiber type is

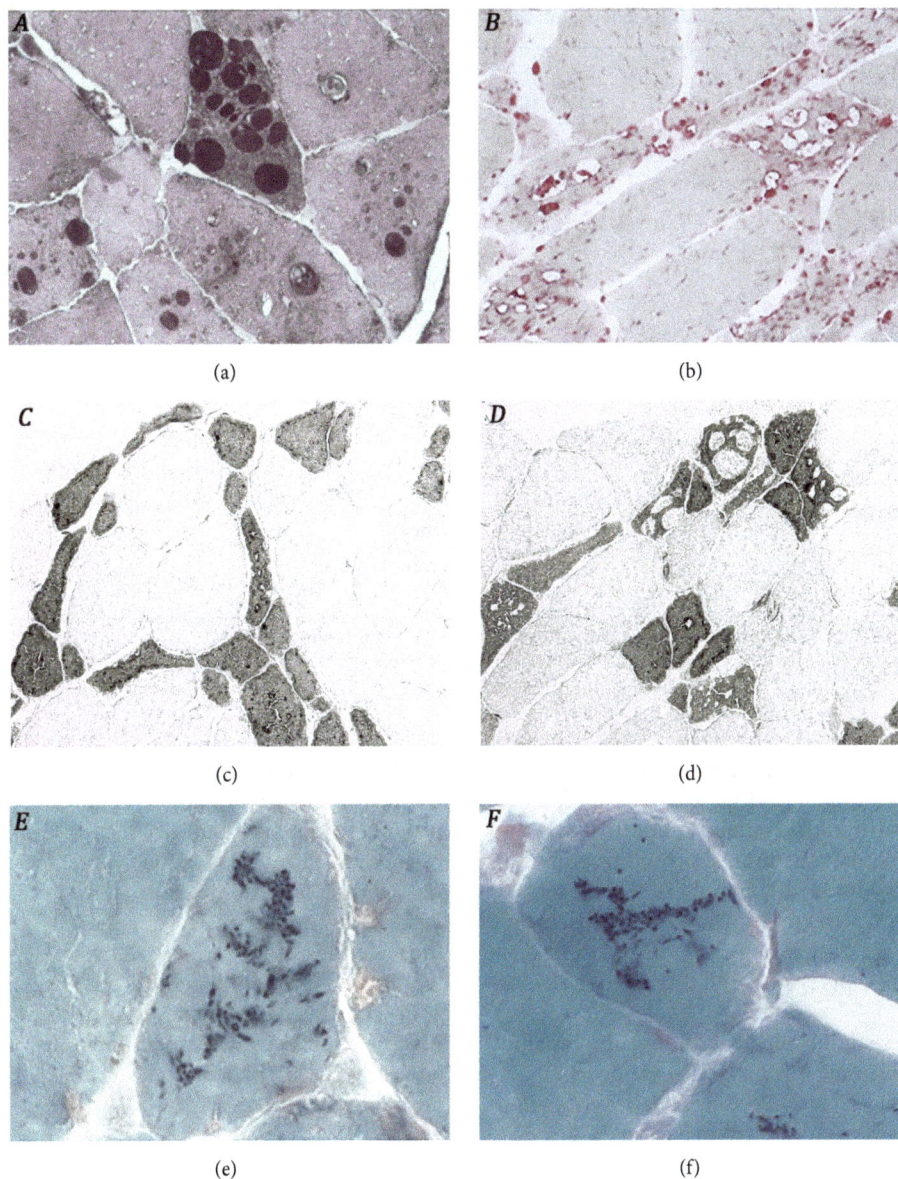

FIGURE 2: Light microscopy of the *left vastus lateralis* ((a), resin; (b)-(f), cryostat). (a) Vacuoles filled with polysaccharide material (PAS, x 40); (b) vacuoles stained positively for acid phosphatase reaction (x 20); (c) ATPase histochemistry at pH 4.3 revealed selective atrophy of type 1 fibers (x 40); (d) vacuoles are present predominantly in type 1 fibers (x 40); (e)-(f) atrophic fibers containing numerous nemaline bodies (Gomori trichrome, x 100).

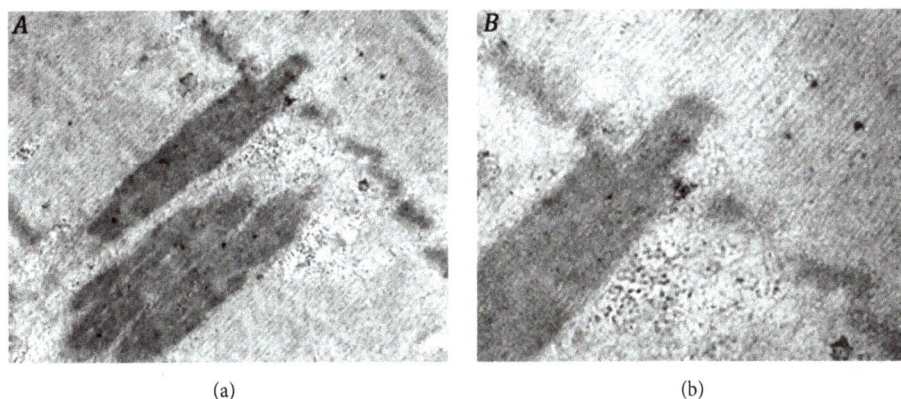

FIGURE 3: By EM, nemaline bodies are oriented consistently with the longitudinal axis of the fibers and they are composed of myofibrillar material in apparent continuity with Z-bands ((a), x 28.000; (b), x 45.000).

TABLE 1: Genetic and acquired etiologies of NB myopathy.

Etiologies of NB Myopathy	NB in other neuromuscular disorders
AD: *NEB, ACTA1, TPM3, TPM2*	**Myopathy**
	Idiopathic inflammatory myopathies
	Acute alcoholic myopathy
	Myotonic dystrophy
AR: *ACTA1, TPM3, TPM2, TNNT1, CFL2, KBTBD13, KLHL40,*	Sarcoglycanopathies
KLHL41, LMOD3, MYPN, MYO18B	Mitochondrial myopathy
	GYG1 polyglucosan body myopathy
	Late-onset Pompe disease
Acquired	**Neuropathy**
MGUS	Spinal muscular atrophy
HIV- associated myopathy	Amyotrophic lateral sclerosis
	Charcot-Marie-Tooth disease
	Other
	Hypothyroidism
	Chronic renal failure

Keys: *genes* are written in *italic* font; AD, autosomal dominant; AR, autosomal recessive; NB, nemaline body; MGUS, monoclonal gammopathy of undetermined significance.

selectively affected in the present case. To our knowledge, this is the first report of NB in Pompe disease.

Nemaline bodies, or rods, contain Z-line material and thin filament material (alpha-actinin, actin and tropomyosin with or without desmin at the periphery). They can be visualized on light microscopy by the Gomori trichrome stain, appearing as dark blue structures localized in the sarcoplasm, predominantly in regions with disrupted sarcomere structure.

NBs are characteristic histological findings in nemaline body myopathy, a congenital myopathy determined by mutations in different genes (Table 1). They are usually seen in both type 1 and type 2 muscle fibers, except in patients with *TPM3* mutations, where they are limited to type 1 fibers [4].

However, NBs have been described as nonspecific alterations in many different conditions, either acquired or genetically determined (Table 1), and they probably represent a common response of muscle fibers to a given pathologic situation. The term Sporadic Late Onset Nemaline Myopathy (SLONM) has been recently proposed to describe patients with a late-onset myopathy, no family history, and NB as the main histological feature [5]. It includes different etiologies among which the most common is monoclonal gammopathy of undetermined significance (MGUS) [6]. Myopathy related to HIV, idiopathic inflammatory myopathy, and neurogenic conditions such as ALS, diabetic polyneuropathy, and vasculitis have also been associated with NB [7]. As to glycogen storage disease, NBs have been described only in one case of polyglucosan body myopathy with mutation in the Glycogenin-1 gene [8].

In our case, the most common causes of NB myopathy, either hereditary or acquired, were ruled out by molecular-genetic testing of *ACTA1* and *NEB* genes, screening for HIV infection and MGUS. Nonetheless, at present we cannot rule out with certainty the possibility of mutations in genes less frequently involved in NB myopathy (i.e., *TPM3*) that could produce a "double-trouble" effect, at least on the genetic and histopathological ground. However, the sporadic and late-onset presentation of the disease and the clinical phenotype lacking dysmorphisms in our patient are not suggestive of those entities.

In conclusion, NBs represent a novel histological finding in GAA deficiency myopathy. We believe that the observation of diffused NB in an otherwise nondiagnostic biopsy from an adult myopathic patient may suggest including LOPED in a panel of possible etiologies.

Conflicts of Interest

The authors state that they have no conflicts of interest (COI).

References

[1] O. Musumeci, G. la Marca, M. Spada, S. Mondello, C. Danesino, GP. Comi et al., "LOPED study: looking for an early diagnosis in a late-onset Pompe disease high-risk population," *Journal of Neurology Neurosurgery & Psychiatry*, vol. 87, no. 1, p. 11, 2016.

[2] C. Terracciano, E. Rastelli, and R. Massa, "Periodic acid-Schiff staining on resin muscle sections: Improvement in the histological diagnosis of late-onset Pompe disease," *Muscle & Nerve*, vol. 45, no. 4, pp. 611-612, 2012.

[3] N. Gayathri, T. C. Yasha, A. Vani, A. B. Taly, A. Nalini, and S. K. Shankar, "Late onset glycogen storage disease type II with "reducing body"-like inclusions," *Clinical Neuropathology*, vol. 29, no. 1, pp. 36–40, 2010.

[4] H. Jungbluth, S. Treves, F. Zorzato et al., "Congenital myopathies: Disorders of excitation-contraction coupling and muscle contraction," *Nature Reviews Neurology*, vol. 14, no. 3, pp. 151–167, 2018.

[5] L. J. Schnitzler, T. Schreckenbach, A. Nadaj-Pakleza et al., "Sporadic late-onset nemaline myopathy: Clinico-pathological characteristics and review of 76 cases," *Orphanet Journal of Rare Diseases*, vol. 12, no. 1, 2017.

[6] A. Uruha and O. Benveniste, "Sporadic late-onset nemaline myopathy with monoclonal gammopathy of undetermined significance," *Current Opinion in Neurology*, vol. 30, no. 5, pp. 457–463, 2017.

[7] A. Hashiguchi, K. Kodama, I. Higuchi, and H. Takashima, "Clinical background of 94 adult patients who recognized nemalin rods in muscle tissue," *Journal of Neuromuscular Diseases*, vol. 5, p. S209, 2018.

[8] G. Tasca, F. Fattori, M. Monforte et al., "Start codon mutation of GYG1 causing late-onset polyglucosan body myopathy with nemaline rods," *Journal of Neurology*, vol. 263, no. 10, pp. 2133–2135, 2016.

28

Imaging Evidence for Cerebral Hyperperfusion Syndrome after Intravenous Tissue Plasminogen Activator for Acute Ischemic Stroke

Yi Zhang,[1] Abhay Kumar,[1] John B. Tezel,[2] and Yihua Zhou[2]

[1]*Department of Neurology, Saint Louis University, Saint Louis, MO 63110, USA*
[2]*Department of Radiology, Saint Louis University, Saint Louis, MO 63110, USA*

Correspondence should be addressed to Yihua Zhou; yzhou31@slu.edu

Academic Editor: Isabella Laura Simone

Background. Cerebral hyperperfusion syndrome (CHS), a rare complication after cerebral revascularization, is a well-described phenomenon after carotid endarterectomy or carotid artery stenting. However, the imaging evidence of CHS after intravenous tissue plasminogen activator (iv tPA) for acute ischemic stroke (AIS) has not been reported. *Case Report.* Four patients were determined to have manifestations of CHS with clinical deterioration after treatment with iv tPA, including one patient who developed seizure, one patient who had a deviation of the eyes toward lesion with worsened mental status, and two patients who developed worsened hemiparesis. In all four patients, postthrombolysis head CT examinations were negative for hemorrhage; CT angiogram showed patent cervical and intracranial arterial vasculature; CT perfusion imaging revealed hyperperfusion with increased relative cerebral blood flow and relative cerebral blood volume and decreased mean transit time along with decreased time to peak in the clinically related artery territory. Vascular dilation was also noted in three of these four cases. *Conclusions.* CHS should be considered in patients with clinical deterioration after iv tPA and imaging negative for hemorrhage. Cerebral angiogram and perfusion studies can be useful in diagnosing CHS thereby helping with further management.

1. Introduction

Cerebral hyperperfusion syndrome (CHS) is a rare but expected complication after carotid endarterectomy or carotid artery stenting. Incidence of CHS is 1–3% after carotid endarterectomy [1]. CHS after iv tPA in patients with acute ischemic stroke (AIS) has also been recognized [2, 3]. However, radiographic evidence of CHS has not been described. We present this case series with imaging evidence of cerebral hyperperfusion after iv tPA treatment for AIS.

2. Case Report

We reviewed a total of 772 CT perfusion (CTP) studies performed in our hospital from July 2009 to October 2015 to identify AIS patients who developed CHS after intravenous thrombolysis treatment. CTP hyperperfusion was characterized by increased relative cerebral blood flow (rCBF) and relative cerebral blood volume (rCBV) and decreased mean transit time (MTT) along with decreased time to peak (TTP) in the clinically related artery territory. Cerebral hyperperfusion syndrome was characterized by focal neurological deficit or seizures developing after cerebral revascularization. Revascularization was confirmed by CT angiogram (CTA). The study was approved by our Institutional Review Board.

We identified four cases of CHS after iv tPA for AIS (Table 1).

Case 1. A 61-year-old Caucasian male with history of chronic lymphocytic leukemia in remission and recurrent sinusitis was found in his garage with right-sided weakness. Examination at the local hospital 2 hours after the onset of the symptoms was significant for aphasia and right hemiplegia. Computed tomography of the head suggested a hyperdense left middle cerebral artery (MCA). He was given iv tPA three hours after onset of the symptoms and then transferred to our hospital for further management. His blood pressure was 157/82 mmHg. En route, the patient developed one

TABLE 1: Four cases of cerebral hyperperfusion syndrome after intravenous tPA for acute ischemic stroke.

	Age	Sex	Stroke symptoms	PMH	NIHSS (onset)	tPA dose	CHS symptoms	NIHSS (D/C)	Infarct area
Case 1	61	M	Aphasia, right hemiplegia	CLL	9	90 mg	Seizure	2	Cortical
Case 2	82	M	Dysarthria, right hemiplegia	Prostate cancer. HTN, Afib	9	70 mg	Worsening hemiplegia	7	Basal ganglia
Case 3	92	M	Aphasia, right hemiplegia, confusion	Colon cancer, Afib	23	74 mg	Worsening hemiplegia	Deceased	Cortical
Case 4	65	F	Aphasia, right hemiplegia	HTN, DVT, colitis	20	90 mg	Eyes deviation, confusion	10	Cortical

PMH: past medical history; NIHSS: NIH stroke scale; CHS: cerebral hyperperfusion syndrome; D/C: at discharge time; M: male; F: female; CLL: chronic lymphocytic leukemia; HTN: hypertension; Afib: atrial fibrillation; DVT: deep vein thrombosis.

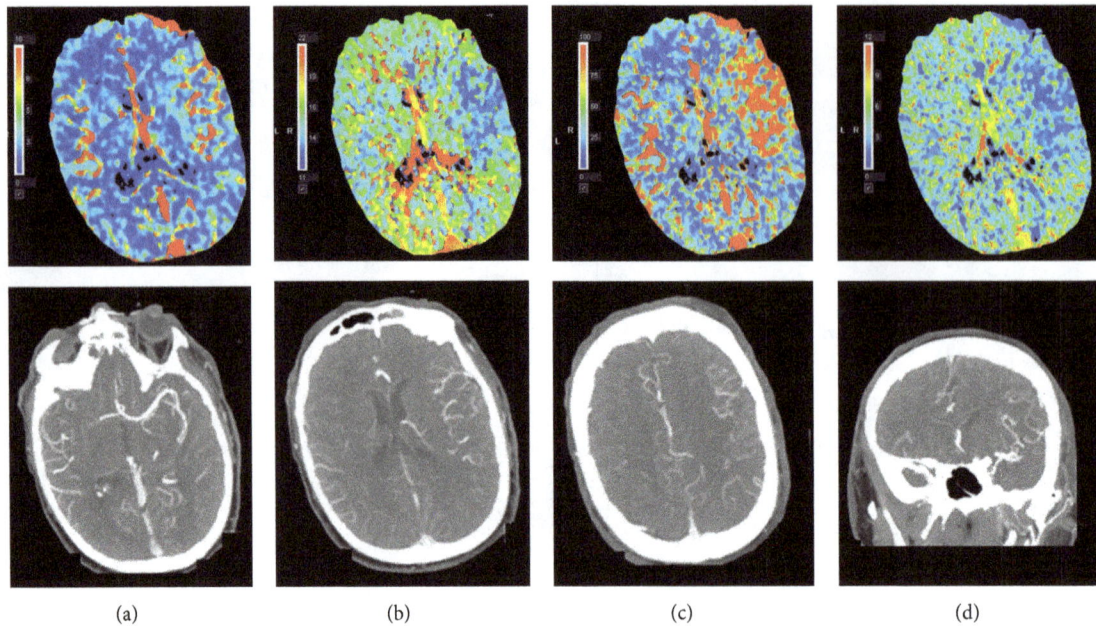

FIGURE 1: Hyperperfusion on computed tomography perfusion and the dilation of the left middle cerebral artery and its branches on CT angiogram after iv tPA treatment: (a) increased cerebral blood volume; (b) shortened time to peak; (c) increased cerebral blood flow; (d) shortened mean transit time.

seizure-like episode with sudden onset jerking movements of all extremities. Upon arrival, he was mute, confused, and agitated; however he was able to move the four extremities symmetrically. His National Institutes of Health Stroke Scale (NIHSS) was 9. The patient underwent CTA and CTP in anticipation of mechanical thrombectomy upon arrival. Instead, CTA showed patent cervical and intracranial arterial vasculature and a dilated left MCA while CTP revealed an increased rCBF and rCBV in the left middle cerebral artery (MCA) territory as well as a decreased MTT and TTP (Figure 1). MRI of the brain performed the following day demonstrated a large acute MCA territory infarct (Figure 2). Further workup revealed evidence of vegetation on the anterior and posterior mitral valve leaflets, likely the source of emboli. The patient was empirically treated with antibiotics for infective endocarditis. He was discharged to a rehabilitation facility on hospital day 6 with NIHSS 2. At the 3-month follow-up visit, the patient's right-sided weakness had resolved although aphasia persisted.

Case 2. An 82-year-old Caucasian male with history of prostate cancer status after prostatectomy, hypertension, and atrial fibrillation developed sudden onset right upper extremity weakness and dysarthria. His warfarin was discontinued a week before for a right knee partial arthroplasty done two days prior to stroke onset. NIHSS was 9 at the local emergency department for which he received iv tPA and was then transferred to our hospital. The patient's blood pressure was 133/62 mmHg. His dysarthria resolved after iv tPA although his right upper extremity strength got worse on hospital day 2. A stat CTA showed no evidence of vessel occlusion but demonstrated dilated left MCA branches. CTP revealed hyperperfusion of the left MCA territory while

noncontrast CT showed a left basal ganglia infarct. The patient also had urinary tract infection at admission, which was treated with antibiotics. The patient remained stable thereafter and improved with an NIHSS of 7 at the time of discharge.

Case 3. A 92-year-old male with history of atrial fibrillation and colon cancer developed right-sided weakness, global aphasia, and confusion. His NIHSS was 23. The patient received iv tPA. The patient's right-sided weakness worsened immediately following the infusion. His blood pressure was 143/76 mmHg. He underwent CTA and CTP, which demonstrated increased cerebral blood perfusion involving the left MCA territory. Noncontrast CT head 24 hours after thrombolysis showed infarction of a cortical area of the left parietal lobe. The patient had bright red blood per rectum one time. His vital signs and hemoglobin had been normal until hospital day 2 when he developed acute myocardial infarction. The family decided on palliative care, considering the patient's preexisting illness and age. The patient was deceased on hospital day 9.

Case 4. A 65-year-old female with history of hypertension, deep venous thrombosis, and colitis developed right-sided weakness and expressive aphasia. She was brought to the local hospital. She was awake and could not respond appropriately. Her NIHSS was 20. Stat CT head revealed a hyperdense left MCA. The patient received iv tPA and subsequently was transferred to our hospital. Her blood pressure was 136/79 mmHg. En route, the patient developed a deviation of the eyes toward the left. She became less arousable. The patient became mute upon arrival. A stat CTA showed patent cervical and intracranial arterial vasculature and a dilated left

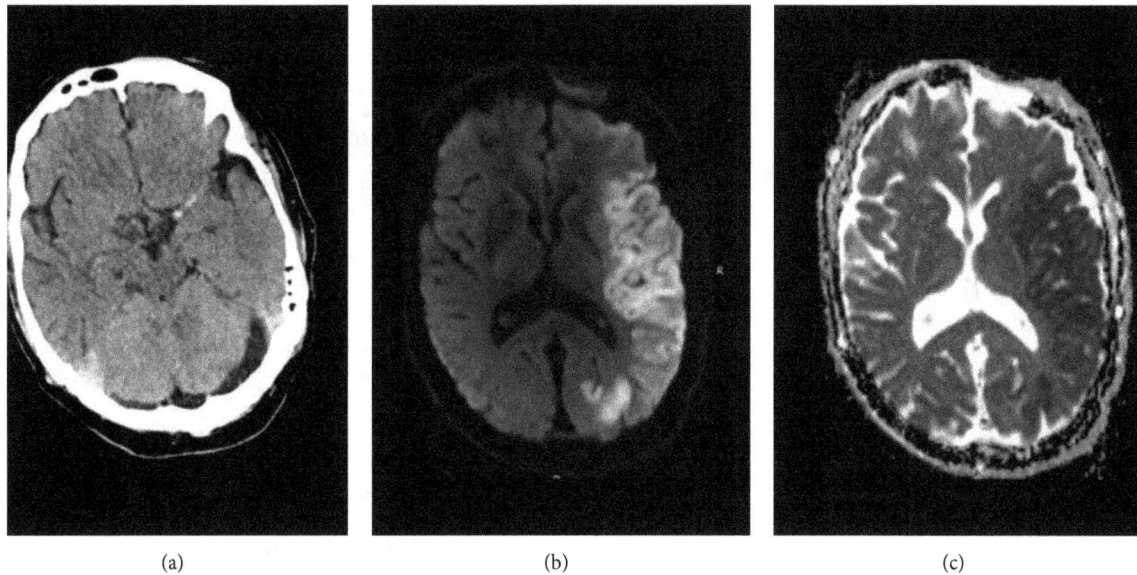

(a)   (b)   (c)

FIGURE 2: Hyperdense middle cerebral artery on the initial CT prior to intravenous tissue plasminogen activator (a). Diffusion-weighted magnetic resonance imaging (b). Apparent diffusion coefficient (c) confirms acute infarction in the left MCA territory.

MCA branch. CTP revealed large area of hyperperfusion on the left hemisphere. Follow-up MRI of the brain performed the following day demonstrated a large acute left MCA territory infarct, which matched the large hyperperfusion area seen on the CTP. During the hospitalization, strength on the right side improved significantly, although global aphasia remained. The patient was discharged to an acute rehabilitation facility at day 5 with NIHSS 10.

3. Discussion

In this case series, we present 4 cases of CHS with radiographic evidence after iv tPA treatment for AIS. CTA and CTP examinations after iv tPA treatment demonstrated recanalization and dilation (in three of the four cases) of the affected intracranial arteries as well as increased perfusion to the regions of the infarcted brain. Therefore, in patients with clinical deterioration after iv tPA treatment of acute ischemic stroke, cerebral CTA and CTP examinations may be helpful to diagnose cerebral hyperperfusion syndrome and provide evidence to guide further management.

Cerebral hyperperfusion syndrome is a rare complication following rapid revascularization. The likely pathophysiology is impaired cerebral autoregulation leading to increased cerebral blood flow, above the metabolic demands of brain tissue [4]. However, knowledge of CHS remains limited. Preexisting disease, such as chronic hypoperfusion from artery stenosis, infection, and chronic inflammatory disease, as well as expression of genes might affect cerebral myogenic, metabolic, or neurogenic regulation. Deficits are usually cortical which may be new or may represent worsening of a preexisting neurological deficit. In the study, three of the four cases had cortical infarction. Seizures may present as focal or generalized, depending on the affected cortical area [5]. One case had generalized seizure.

Cerebral hyperperfusion syndrome is a clinical syndrome of reperfusion injury which can occur in numerous ways including activation of endothelium, excess production of oxygen free radicals, inflammatory responses and leukocyte recruitment, increase in cytokine production, and edema formation [6]. There is disruption of the blood-brain barrier (BBB) through the release of neutrophil-derived oxidants and proteolytic enzymes. Two of the four cases in this study had active infectious disease during thrombolysis. One case had chronic colitis. Hyperperfusion initializes an inflammatory cascade, resulting in the deterioration of salvageable penumbra [7]. Infection appears to be an important trigger that precedes ischemic strokes and can bring about irreversible injury through a range of potential mechanisms. Preexisting infection in our patients may be a contributing factor for the development of CHS.

Interestingly, three of the four cases in the study had history of cancer, which may have contributed to impaired cerebral autoregulation. Tumor endothelial cells often lose their normal barrier function. Changes in endothelial shape result in intercellular gaps or holes that leak fluid, blood, and fibrin into the surrounding tissue [8]. The vascular endothelium is a dynamic cellular "organ" that controls passage of nutrients into tissues, maintains the flow of blood, and regulates the trafficking of leukocytes. Tumor blood vessels have irregular diameters, are fragile and leaky, and have abnormal blood flow [9]. The pathophysiology of cerebral autoregulation in patients with cancer history needs further investigation.

Our case series is limited by the lack of angiographic and perfusion studies prior to thrombolysis, although the presence of hyperdense MCA sign (as in Cases 1 and 4), sudden onset of focal neurological deficits, and high NIHSS suggest large vessel involvement. We were also not able to assess cerebral autoregulation based on the autoregulation index to monitor cerebral blood flow regulation. This would require a more specialized setting to do so. All four cases presented with a left hemisphere stroke. This might be due to reporting bias. A patient with a right hemisphere stroke commonly has neglect, which might mask the clinical deterioration.

A main concern for clinical deterioration following tPA administration has been hemorrhagic transformation which can be evaluated with a noncontrasted head CT. One study showed that early neurological deterioration without clear mechanism affected 7% of the patients with acute stroke [10]. We believe some of these cases may be due to CHS, which is currently underrecognized and may also be delayed in onset as what happened in Case 2. The true incidence of CHS may thus be underreported as well given lack of angiographic and perfusion studies in the post-tPA administration setting. Therefore, when clinical deterioration following iv tPA cannot be simply explained by other obvious reasons such as hemorrhage, CHS should be considered. In addition, early clinical deterioration (or deterioration after improvement) can occur in ischemic stroke patients who have not received iv tPA treatment, which could be attributed to a number of reasons, including hemorrhagic transformation, internal herniation due to mass effect, and ventricular entrapment. However, as early spontaneous thrombolysis can occur, early clinical deterioration can potentially be due to CHS, when other causes are not apparent.

4. Conclusion

The report provides imaging evidence of hyperperfusion in patients with CHS after iv tPA for acute cerebral infarction. Therefore, cerebral CTA and CTP studies should be considered to confirm the presence of cerebral hyperperfusion in patients with clinical deterioration after tPA treatment for acute stroke.

Competing Interests

The authors declare that there are no competing interests regarding this paper.

References

[1] M. Lieb, U. Shah, and G. L. Hines, "Cerebral hyperperfusion syndrome after carotid intervention: a review," *Cardiology in Review*, vol. 20, no. 2, pp. 84–89, 2012.

[2] C.-I. Lau, L.-M. Lien, and W.-H. Chen, "Brainstem hyperperfusion syndrome after intravenous thrombolysis: a case report," *Journal of Neuroimaging*, vol. 21, no. 3, pp. 277–279, 2011.

[3] R. Backhaus, S. Boy, K. Fuchs, B. Ulrich, G. Schuierer, and F. Schlachetzki, "Hyperperfusion syndrome after MCA embolectomy—a rare complication?" *American Journal of Case Reports*, vol. 14, pp. 513–517, 2013.

[4] O. B. Paulson, S. Strandgaard, and L. Edvinsson, "Cerebral autoregulation," *Cerebrovascular and Brain Metabolism Reviews*, vol. 2, no. 2, pp. 161–192, 1990.

[5] T. M. Sundt Jr., F. W. Sharbrough, D. G. Piepgras, T. P. Kearns, J. M. Messick Jr., and W. M. O'Fallon, "Correlation of cerebral blood flow and electroencephalographic changes during carotid endarterectomy: with results of surgery and hemodynamics of cerebral ischemia," *Mayo Clinic Proceedings*, vol. 56, no. 9, pp. 533–543, 1981.

[6] R. Khatri, A. M. McKinney, B. Swenson, and V. Janardhan, "Blood-brain barrier, reperfusion injury, and hemorrhagic transformation in acute ischemic stroke," *Neurology*, vol. 79, no. 13, pp. S52–S57, 2012.

[7] H. C. Emsley and S. J. Hopkins, "Acute ischaemic stroke and infection: recent and emerging concepts," *The Lancet Neurology*, vol. 7, no. 4, pp. 341–353, 2008.

[8] H. Hashizume, P. Baluk, S. Morikawa et al., "Openings between defective endothelial cells explain tumor vessel leakiness," *American Journal of Pathology*, vol. 156, no. 4, pp. 1363–1380, 2000.

[9] A. C. Dudley, "Tumor endothelial cells," *Cold Spring Harbor Perspectives in Medicine*, vol. 2, no. 3, Article ID a006536, 2012.

[10] P. Seners, G. Turc, M. Tisserand et al., "Unexplained early neurological deterioration after intravenous thrombolysis: incidence, predictors, and associated factors," *Stroke*, vol. 45, no. 7, pp. 2004–2009, 2014.

29

Cerebral Venous Sinus Thrombosis in a Patient with Ulcerative Colitis Flare

L. M. Conners ⓘ,[1] R. Ahad,[2] P. H. Janda,[1] and Z. Mudasir[1]

[1]Department of Neurology, Valley Hospital Medical Center, Las Vegas, NV, USA
[2]Pediatric Neurology, University of Las Vegas School of Medicine, Las Vegas, NV, USA

Correspondence should be addressed to L. M. Conners; lisa.conners.neuro@gmail.com

Academic Editor: Shahid Nimjee

Inflammatory bowel disease is characterized by a chronic inflammatory state and is therefore associated with abnormalities in coagulation and a hypercoagulable state. Cerebral venous sinus thrombosis is a rare complication of inflammatory bowel disease yet contributes significant morbidity and mortality to those affected. Early diagnosis is critical, as a delay in diagnosis portends a worse prognosis. This paper seeks to highlight the increased risk of venous sinus thrombosis in patients with inflammatory bowel disease. We start by discussing the case of a seventeen-year-old female who presented with ulcerative colitis flare and developed new-onset seizures, found to be caused by a large venous sinus thrombosis.

1. Introduction

Inflammatory bowel disease has been shown to be associated with abnormalities in coagulation and a hypercoagulable state [1–3]. The relationship between inflammatory bowel disease and thromboembolism was first described in 1936 by Bargen et al. [4] Since then, several studies have supported the association [5]. The most common sites of these thromboses are in the lower extremity and pulmonary venous systems [4]; however, cerebral venous sinus thrombosis is an accepted rare complication of inflammatory bowel disease (IBD) [2]. Because symptoms of cerebral venous sinus thrombosis (CVT) are oftentimes vague and commonplace, clinicians must heed this relationship in the back of their minds to prevent a delayed diagnosis and possible tragic outcome.

2. Case Report

A seventeen-year-old African-American female with mood disorder, infrequent migraine without aura, GERD, and ulcerative colitis presented to the emergency department with four weeks of abdominal pain, hematochezia, and an unintentional 28-pound weight loss over those four weeks. She had been poorly compliant with her medications and follow-up. MRI of the abdomen was notable for diffuse mucosal enhancement of the colon, which contained numerous air fluid levels, consistent with ulcerative colitis exacerbation. Colonoscopy showed multiple ulcerations of the transverse and distal colon. She was hospitalized for three weeks and failed medical management with two rounds of infliximab. Additionally, she required blood transfusions due to intractable bloody diarrhea. Ultimately, the decision was made to proceed with total colectomy and ileostomy, which she tolerated without incident.

Notably, on her fourth day of hospitalization, she was found down in her bathroom. She was disoriented and complained of a headache. Initial head CT without contrast noted a small subdural hematoma overlying the high bilateral frontal lobes and along the falx. She was transferred to the pediatric ICU, where she subsequently suffered three witnessed tonic-clonic seizures over a twenty-four-hour period. She was treated acutely with lorazepam and loaded on both Keppra and fosphenytoin, and her seizures stopped. The following morning, her repeat CT of the head noted hyperdensity of the superior sagittal, right transverse, and right sigmoid sinuses, raising the suspicion of a venous sinus thrombosis. MRI, MRA, and MRV were therefore obtained. MRA was unremarkable. Her MRI and MRV are shown below in Figures 1 and 2, respectively.

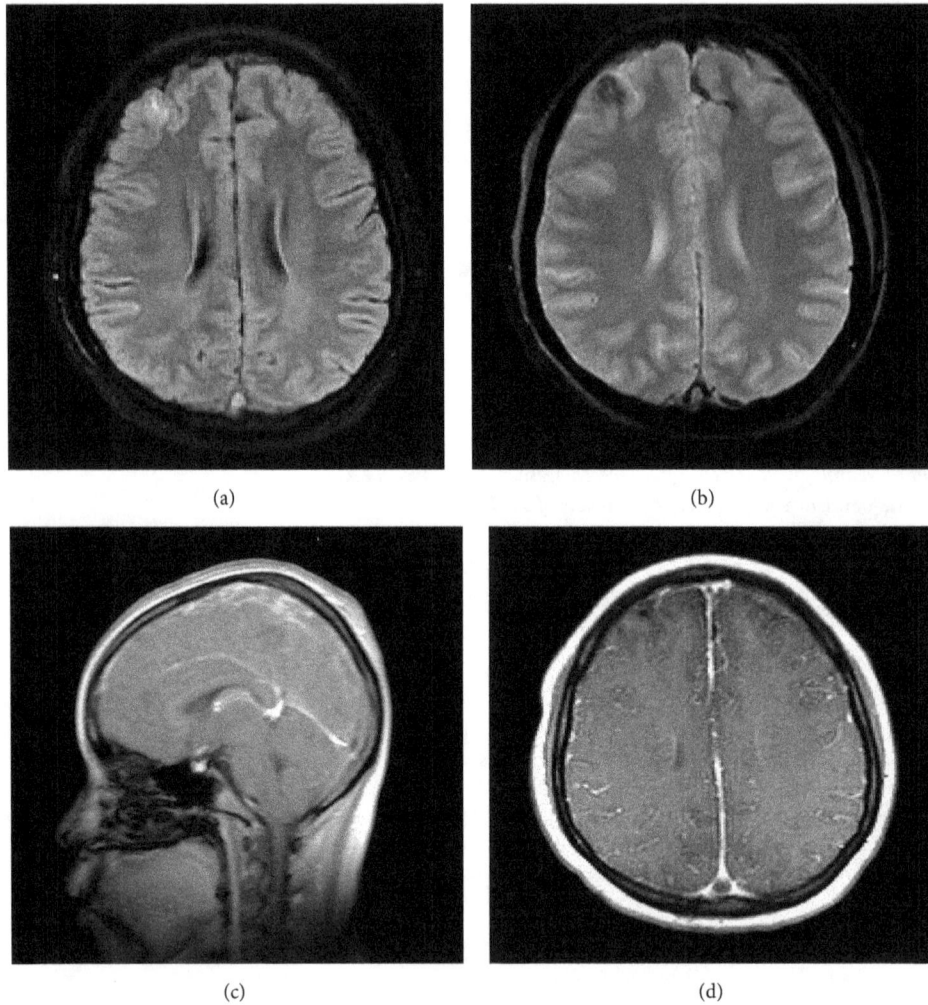

FIGURE 1: Initial MRI brain of our patient with and without contrast showed right frontal hyperintensity on FLAIR (a) with corresponding area on gradient echo (b), suggestive of a small intraparenchymal hemorrhage. GRE also showed decreased signal of two frontal cortical veins (b). Sagittal T1 imaging (c) revealed heterogeneous signal of the superior sagittal sinus. Postcontrast images were remarkable for a filling defect with direct visualization of the thrombus (d) in the superior sagittal sinus.

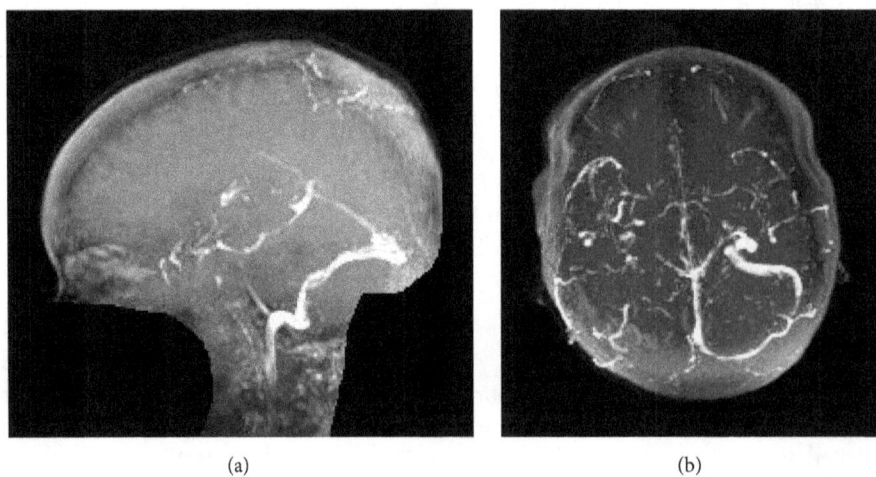

FIGURE 2: MRV of the head without contrast revealed a lack of flow in the superior sagittal sinus (a), as well as right transverse and sigmoid sinuses (b).

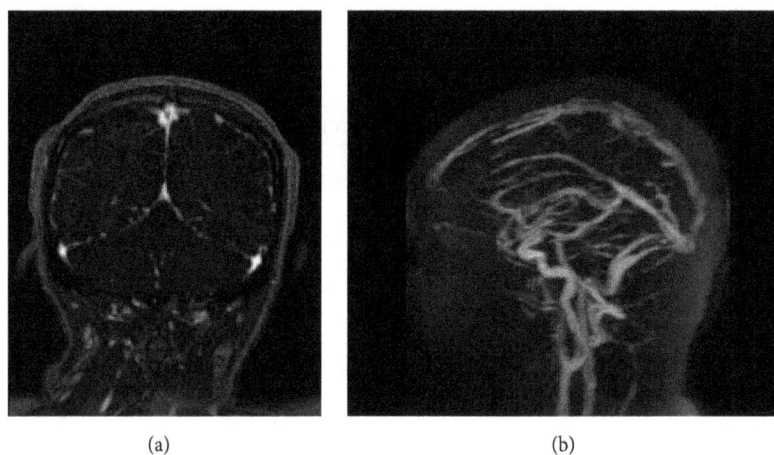

(a)   (b)

FIGURE 3: Follow-up MRV of the head 5 months after diagnosis noted minimal residual thrombus in the superior sagittal sinus (a), with resolution of the thrombus in the right sigmoid, and transverse sinuses (b).

She was started on therapeutic Lovenox with goal Factor Xa level 0.6 since she was anemic from the ulcerative colitis flare. A hypercoagulable panel was negative for protein C deficiency, protein S deficiency, Factor V Leiden, antithrombin deficiency, factor II mutation, and antiphospholipid antibody panel. She was not taking medications prior to hospitalization. She denied a smoking history. Her only known risk factor was ulcerative colitis.

The patient was seen by pediatric neurology while being in the PICU, and her EEG was notable for bifrontal sharps with occasional right temporal sharp complexes. Since her seizures stopped within twenty-four hours, fosphenytoin was discontinued after its load. She was continued on Keppra. Repeat imaging one week later showed significantly improved flow in all three involved sinuses and resolution of the right frontal intraparenchymal and bifrontal subdural hemorrhages.

She was hospitalized for nearly one month for management of the ulcerative colitis flare, which ultimately required total colectomy and ileostomy. At follow-up, she was doing well. She was continued on Keppra and Lovenox. At that time repeat MRV was notable only for a small residual thrombus in the superior sagittal sinus, as seen in Figure 3.

3. Discussion

Cerebral venous sinus thrombosis is an uncommon disease, with incidence between 0.22 and 1.32 patients per 100,000 annually [7, 8]. The prevalence is higher in females than males (approx. 2.5 : 1) [8] (except in children or older adults [9, 10]) and significantly higher in pregnant and postpartum women, 11.6 per 100,000 deliveries [11]. Between 1998 and 2001, Ferro et al. followed 624 adult patients with CVT and noted predisposing factors (Table 1) [6]. Over half had been taking oral contraceptives [6]. Twenty-one percent coincided with pregnancy or the postpartum period [6]. One-third had a hypercoagulable blood disease [6]. 1.6 percent had inflammatory bowel disease [6]. Other risk factors for venous

sinus thrombosis include smoking, malignancy, dehydration, substance abuse, infection, and head trauma. Multiple risk factors were found in almost half of the patients [6]. Nearly thirteen percent of patients did not have any clear risk factors [6].

The risk of venous thromboembolism in the lower extremity or pulmonary system for patients with IBD is threefold that of the general population, even after correction for known prothrombotic factors [4]. Cerebral, portal, retinal, and mesenteric veins may occasionally be affected as well [4]. Patients with IBD also suffer thrombotic events at a younger age [4]. The mechanisms of thrombosis in IBD are complex and incompletely understood [4]. Giannotta et al. sought to uncover the mechanism responsible and, instead, found over a dozen differences in the serum of IBD patients, each of which may independently predispose to venous thromboembolism (VTE) [4]. Table 2 summarizes some of those differences.

The presentation of CVT can be highly variable [12]; however, it usually manifests in one of three patterns, symptoms of intracranial hypertension [13], focal neurological symptoms [12], or encephalopathy [12]. Notably, headache is the most common symptom reported in venous sinus thrombosis, with 89% of patients reporting it [10]. The headache is usually gradual [14] and localized, although it often does not lateralize [15–17]. However, when the headache presents as a manifestation of increased intracranial pressure, it is described as diffuse [6]. Monoparesis or hemiparesis is described in 37% of cases [10]. Thirty-nine percent of patient with CVT have seizure upon presentation, and another six percent have seizure within the next few weeks [10]. Seizures are especially common with supratentorial parenchymal brain lesions and sagittal sinus or cortical vein thrombosis [10].

Head CT without contrast is the initial imaging modality for patients with acute neurological symptoms [6]. Patients with venous sinus thrombosis will have an abnormal head CT without contrast about 30% of the time [6]. Classically, it may show hyperdensity of a cortical vein or dural venous

TABLE 1: Risk dactors for CVT [6].

Condition	Prevalence, %[*]	Consistency[1†]	Strength of association[2†] OR (95% CI)	Biological plausability[3†]	Temporality[4†]	Biological gradient[5†]
Prothrombotic conditions	34.1					
Antithrombin III deficiency		Yes	NA	Yes	Yes	Yes[‡]
Protein C deficiency		Yes	11.1 (1.9–66.0)	Yes	Yes	Yes[‡]
Protein S deficiency		Yes	12.5 (1.5–107.3)	Yes	Yes	Yes[‡]
Antiphospholipid and		Yes	8.8 (1.3–57.4)[*]	Yes	Yes	Yes[‡]
anticardiolipin antibodies	5.9	Yes		Yes	Yes	Yes[‡]
Resistance to activated protein C and and factor V Leiden		Yes	3.4 (2.3–5.1)	Yes	Yes	Yes[‡]
Mutation G20210A of Factor II		Yes	9.3 (5.9–14.7)	Yes	Yes	Yes[‡]
Hyperhomocysteinemia		Yes	4.6 (1.6–12.0)	Yes	Yes	Yes[‡]
Pregnancy and puerperium	21	Yes	NA	Yes	Yes	NA
Oral Contraceptives	54.3	Yes	5.6 (4.0–7.9)	Yes	Yes	Yes
Drugs						
Androgen, danazol, lithium, vitamin A, IV immunoglobulin, ecstasy	7.5		NA	Yes	Yes	NA
Cancer related	7.4	Yes	NA	Yes	Yes	NA
Local compression						
Hypercoagulable						
Antineoplastic drugs (tamoxifen, L-asparaginase)						
Infection	12.3		NA	Yes	Yes	NA
Parameningeal infections (ear, sinus, mouth, face, and neck)		Yes				
Mechanical precipitants	4.5	Yes	NA	Yes	Yes	NA
Complication of epidural blood patch						
Spontaneous intracranial hypotension						
Lumbar puncture						
Other hematologic disorders	12	Yes	NA	Yes	Yes	NA
Paroxysmal nocturnal hemoglobinuria						
Iron deficiency anemia		Yes		Yes	Yes	NA
Nephrotic syndrome	0.6					
Polycythemia, thrombocytopenia	2.8					
Systemic diseases	7.2	Yes	NA	Yes	Yes	NA
Systemic lupus erythematous	1					
Baçet disease	1					
Inflammatory bowel disease	1.6					
Thyroid disease	1.7					
Sarcoidosis	0.2					
Other	1.7					
None Identified	12.5		NA	NA	NA	NA

CVT: cerebral venous thrombosis; OR: odds ratio; CI: confidence interval; NA: nonapplicable/nonavailable; IV: intravenous. [*]Prevalence as per Ferro et al. Percentages for CVT associated with oral contraceptives or pregnancy/puerperium are reported among 381 women ≤ 50 years of age. [†]Cause-and-effect relationship determined as follows: (1) consistency of association: has the association been repeatedly observed by different investigators (yes/no)? (2) Strength of association: how strong is the effect (relative risk or OR)? (3) Biological plausibility: does the association make sense, and can it be explained pathophysiologically (yes/no)? (4) Temporality: does exposure precede adverse outcome (yes/no)? (5) Biological gradient: does a dose-response relationship exist (yes/no)? Evidence of a strong and consistent association, evidence of biological plausibility, a notable risk of recurrent events, and detection of a biological gradient are suggestive of causation rather than association by chance alone. Modified from Grimes and Schulz.

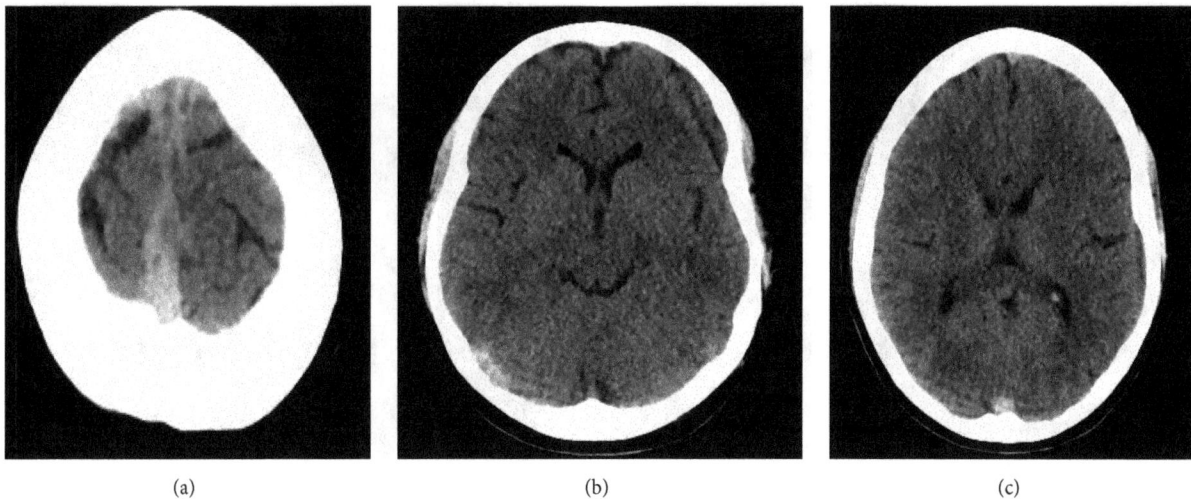

(a) (b) (c)

FIGURE 4: Initial head CT without contrast in our patient described above noted a falcine with bifrontal subdural hematoma at the vertex (a). Note the hyperdense right transverse sinus (b) and "filled delta sign" (c).

TABLE 2: Abnormalities in coagulation, anticoagulation, and fibrinolytic system in IBD patients [4].

Coagulation factors	Fibrinolytic factors	Plasma coagulation inhibitors
↑ fibrinogen	↓ tPA	↓ AT III
↑ prothrombin	↑ PAI-1	↓ TFPI
↑ factors: Va, VIIa, VIIIa, Xa, XIa, XIIa	↑ TAFI	Conflicting data about PS and PC
↑ prothrombin factors 1 + 2		
↑ thrombin-antithrombin III complex (TAT)		
↑ fibrinopeptides A and B		
↑ microparticles		
↓ factor XIII		

sinus (Figures 4(b) and 4(c)) [6]. If the thrombus lies in the superior sagittal sinus, one might see the "filled delta sign" (Figure 4(c)) on noncontrasted CT, which appears as a hyperdense triangle at the superior sagittal sinus on axial view [6]. On contrast-enhanced CT, one might see the well-known "empty delta sign," which would instead show a central hypodensity (due to slow or absent flow) surrounded by contrast enhancement of the sinus [6]. CT may also show edema or infarct, especially abutting a venous sinus or crossing arterial boundaries and may be accompanied by hemorrhage [6]. Approximately 30% of patients with CVT present with intracranial hemorrhage [6]. A prodromal headache, bilateral parenchymal abnormalities, or a hypercoagulable state should also prompt suspicion [6].

In general, MRI is more sensitive than CT for venous sinus thrombosis [6]. Definitive diagnosis by MRI is made by direct visualization of the thrombus within the venous sinus (Figure 5(a)) [6]. In the first week, the thrombus frequently appears as isointense to parenchyma on T1 and hypointense on T2 [6]. After one week, the thrombus contains methemoglobin and will be hyperintense on T1 and T2, producing hyperintense venous sinuses and/or veins (Figure 5(b)) [6]. Absence of flow void with alteration of signal intensity in the dural sinuses and/or veins should prompt high suspicion [6]. Contrasted MRI can be especially helpful as it can provide direct visualization of the thrombus when it shows a central isointense lesion in a venous sinus with surrounding enhancement (Figure 5(a)) and is the MRI equivalent of the "empty delta sign" on CT [6]. DWI may show infarct, and GRE may show hemorrhage or thrombosed veins (Figure 5(c)) [6].

MRV is commonly used to aid in the diagnosis in CVT, especially in those for whom radiation or iodine contrast are contraindicated [6]. The most commonly used MRV techniques are time-of-flight and contrast-enhanced [6]. Thrombosis is suggested by lack of flow in the respected venous sinuses [6], as seen in Figure 6. Note that results may be confounded by anomalous venous anatomy, so diagnosis should be made in conjunction with other imaging modalities such as MRI (ideally contrasted) to provide direct visualization of the thrombus [6].

CT venography (CTV) can provide a rapid and reliable diagnosis of CVT [6], as in Figure 7. CTV is at least equivalent to MRV but is limited in a few regards [6]. It may be compounded by bone artifact if the thrombus is adjacent to bone [6]. Pregnant patients represent a large percentage of venous sinus thrombosis patients and should not undergo radiation unless the benefits outweigh risks. CTV is also limited by those who cannot tolerate its contrast due to allergy or poor renal function.

Anomalous venous anatomy, sinus hypoplasia, asymmetrical sinus drainage, and normal sinus filling defects due to prominent arachnoid granulations or intrasinus septa may suggest thrombosis, yet the definitive diagnosis of venous sinus thrombosis rests on direct visualization of the thrombus [6]. In the few patients for whom the above techniques fail

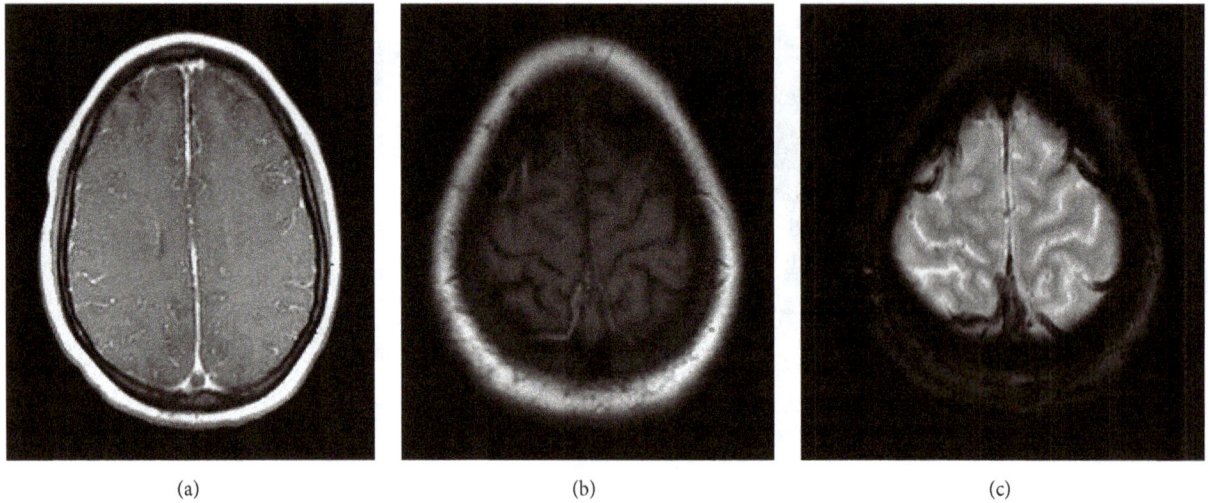

(a)   (b)   (c)

Figure 5: MRI brain with and without contrast showed the MRI equivalent of the "empty delta sign" (a) on postcontrast T1 images. Note the hyperintense cortical veins on T1 (b), which correspond with hemosiderin deposits on GRE (c).

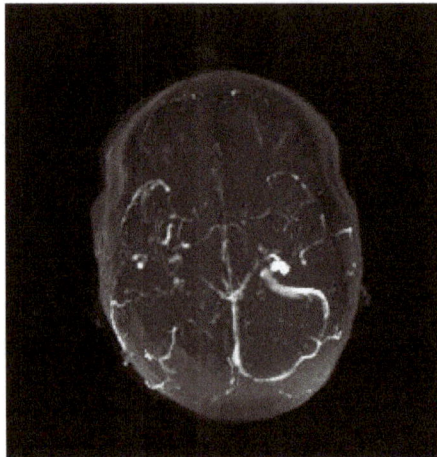

Figure 6: MRV demonstrates absence of flow in the superior sagittal, right transverse, and right sigmoid sinuses in our patient.

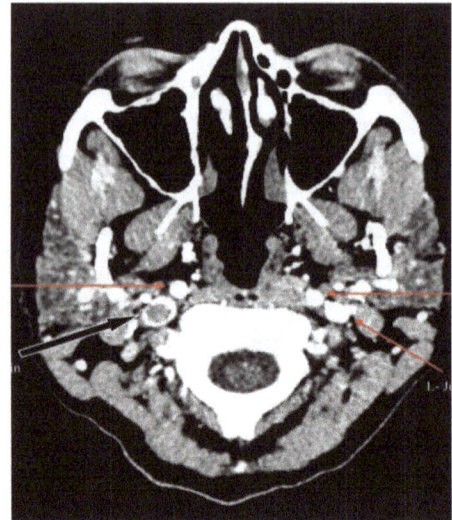

Figure 7: Computed tomographic venogram shows direct visualization of thrombus within the right internal jugular vein in another patient, marked by black arrow [6]. Red arrows mark normal flow voids. Reprinted from [6].

to provide a confident diagnosis, cerebral angiography and direct cerebral venography can be used [6]. On cerebral angiography, findings would include the nonvisualization of one or more sinuses, venous congestion with dilated cortical, scalp, or facial veins, enlargement of typically diminutive veins from collateral drainage, or reversal of venous flow [6]. The venous phase of cerebral angiography would show a filling defect in the thrombosed cerebral vein or sinus [6]. Direct cerebral venography by injecting contrast directly into the sinuses or cerebral veins via the internal jugular artery is usually done only in the setting of endovascular therapeutic procedures [6]. One would see a filling defect or complete nonfilling [6].

4. Conclusion

Evidence-based medicine supports IBD to be an independent risk factor for venous sinus thrombosis, as numerous studies

have demonstrated a correlation [3]. The mechanism for this is multifactorial and incompletely understood [4]. Most healthcare professionals are not aware of this correlation and may not know how to quickly and confidently identify venous sinus thrombosis on various imaging modalities. This paper seeks to highlight the relationship, as a delay in diagnosis of CVT portends a worse prognosis in these young, at-risk patients.

Conflicts of Interest

The authors declare that there are no conflicts of interest regarding the publication of this paper.

References

[1] F. Alqahtani, Y. Farag, A. Aljebreen et al., "Thromboembolic events in patients with inflammatory bowel disease," *Saudi Journal of Gastroenterology*, vol. 22, no. 6, pp. 423–427, 2016.

[2] E. M. DeFilippis, E. Barfield, D. Leifer et al., "Cerebral venous thrombosis in inflammatory bowel disease," *Journal of Digestive Diseases*, 2, no. 16, pp. 104–108, 2015.

[3] J. M. Ferro, P. Canhão, J. Stam et al., "Delay in the diagnosis of cerebral vein and dural sinus thrombosis," *Stroke*, vol. 40, no. 9, pp. 3133–3138, 2009.

[4] M. Giannotta, G. Tapete, G. Emmi, E. Silvestri, and M. Milla, "Thrombosis in inflammatory bowel diseases: what's the link?," *Thrombosis Journal*, vol. 13, no. 1, article 14, 2015.

[5] A. H. Katsanos, K. H. Katsanos, M. Kosmidou, S. Giannopoulus, A. P. Kyritsis, and E. V. Tsianos, "Cerebral sinus venous thrombosis in inflammatory bowel diseases," *Quarterly Journal of Medicine*, vol. 106, pp. 401–413, 2013.

[6] G. Saposnik, F. Barinagarrementeria, R. D. Brown et al., "Diagnosis and management of cerebral venous thrombosis," *Stroke*, Article ID STR-0b013e31820a8364, 2011.

[7] J. M. Ferro, M. Correia, C. Pontes, M. V. Baptista, and F. Pita, "Cerebral vein and dural sinus thrombosis in Portugal: 1980–1998," *Cerebrovascular Diseases*, vol. 11, no. 3, pp. 177–182, 2001.

[8] J. M. Coutinho, S. M. Zuurbier, M. Aramideh, and J. Stam, "The incidence of cerebral venous thrombosis," *Stroke*, vol. 43, no. 12, pp. 3375–3377, 2012.

[9] G. deVeber, M. Andrew, C. Adams et al., "Cerebral sinovenous thrombosis in children," *The New England Journal of Medicine*, vol. 345, no. 6, pp. 417–423, 2001.

[10] J. M. Ferro, P. Canhão, J. Stam, M.-G. Bousser, and F. Barinagarrementeria, "Prognosis of cerebral vein and dural sinus thrombosis," *Stroke*, vol. 35, no. 3, pp. 664–670, 2004.

[11] D. J. Lanska and R. J. Kryscio, "Risk factors for peripartum and postpartum stroke and intracranial venous thrombosis," *Stroke*, vol. 31, no. 6, pp. 1274–1282, 2000.

[12] M. G. Bousser and R. R. Russell, *Cerebral Venous Thrombosis*, WB Saunders, London, UK, 1997.

[13] V. Biousse, A. Ameri, F. Chedru, and M. G. Bousser, "Isolated raised intracranial pressure as the only sign of cerebral venous thrombosis," *Neurology*, vol. 50, no. 4, pp. A13–A14, 1998.

[14] J. Stam, "Current concepts: thrombosis of the cerebral veins and sinuses," *The New England Journal of Medicine*, vol. 352, no. 17, pp. 1791–1798, 2005.

[15] E. Agostoni, "Headache in cerebral venous thrombosis," *Neurological Sciences*, vol. 25, no. 3, pp. 206–210, 2004.

[16] A. Ameri and M. G. Bousser, "Headache in cerebral venous thrombosis: a study of 110 cases," *Cephalalgia*, vol. 13, 13, article 110, 1993.

[17] M. G. Lopes, J. Ferro, C. Pontes, and V. Investigators, "Headache and cerebral venous thrombosis," *Cephalalgia*, vol. 20, article 292, 2000.

30

Long-Lasting Symptomatic Cerebral Hyperperfusion Syndrome following Superficial Temporal Artery-Middle Cerebral Artery Bypass in a Patient with Stenosis of Middle Cerebral Artery

Shinji Shimato (ID), **Toshihisa Nishizawa, Takashi Yamanouchi, Takashi Mamiya, Kojiro Ishikawa, and Kyozo Kato**

Department of Neurosurgery, Kariya Toyota General Hospital, 5-15 Sumiyoshi-cho, Kariya City, Aichi 448-8505, Japan

Correspondence should be addressed to Shinji Shimato; shinji.shimato@gmail.com

Academic Editor: Norman S. Litofsky

Cerebral hyperperfusion syndrome (CHPS) is a complication that can occur after cerebral revascularization surgeries such as superficial temporal artery- (STA-) middle cerebral artery (MCA) anastomosis, and it can lead to neurological deteriorations. CHPS is usually temporary and disappears within two weeks. The authors present a case in which speech disturbance due to CHPS lasted unexpectedly long and three months was taken for full recovery. A 40-year-old woman, with a history of medication of quetiapine, dopamine 2 receptor antagonist as an antipsychotics for depression, underwent STA-MCA anastomosis for symptomatic left MCA stenosis. On the second day after surgery, the patient exhibited mild speech disturbance which deteriorated into complete motor aphasia and persisted for one month. SPECT showed the increase of cerebral blood flow (CBF) in left cerebrum, verifying the diagnosis of CHPS. Although CBF increase disappeared one month after surgery, speech disturbance continued for additionally two months with a slow improvement. This case represents a rare clinical course of CHPS. The presumable mechanisms of the prolongation of CHPS are discussed, and the medication of quetiapine might be one possible cause by its effect on cerebral vessels as dopamine 2 receptor antagonist, posing the caution against antipsychotics in cerebrovascular surgeries.

1. Introduction

Superficial temporal artery (STA) to middle cerebral artery (MCA) anastomosis is a surgical procedure of direct revascularization to improve cerebral blood flow and potentially prevent brain infarction for patients with stenoocclusive cerebrovascular diseases [1]. While this surgical procedure has the advantage of rapid improvement of impaired cerebral blood flow (CBF), there is a potential risk for postoperative cerebral hyperperfusion syndrome (CHPS) [2, 3].

Cerebral hyperperfusion state is defined as a major increase cerebral blood flow (CBF) following surgical repair that is well above the metabolic demands of the brain tissue, and it can be detected using single-photon emission computed tomography (SPECT) [4]. When hyperperfusion reaches symptomatic state, CHPS is characterized by unilateral headache, facial, and ocular pain, seizures, and focal neurological signs [4, 5]. With regard to the time course of

CHPS, the symptoms usually start during the acute stage after bypass surgery [6–8], and the duration is 1-2 weeks in most cases [6, 8, 9].

We report a case of a patient who suffered from speech disturbance for more than three months due to CHPS after the surgery of STA-MCA anastomosis for symptomatic left MCA stenosis. The characteristics of this case and the mechanism of the long duration of CHPS are discussed.

2. Case Report

A 39-year-old woman, who had been taking medication of quetiapine as an antipsychotics for depression, experienced mild dysarthria and visited the department of neurology in our hospital. Her symptom was diagnosed as drug-induced lip dyskinesia, which disappeared in a week. Screening head magnetic resonance imaging (MRI) at this time revealed stenosis of the left MCA with no brain parenchymal lesions

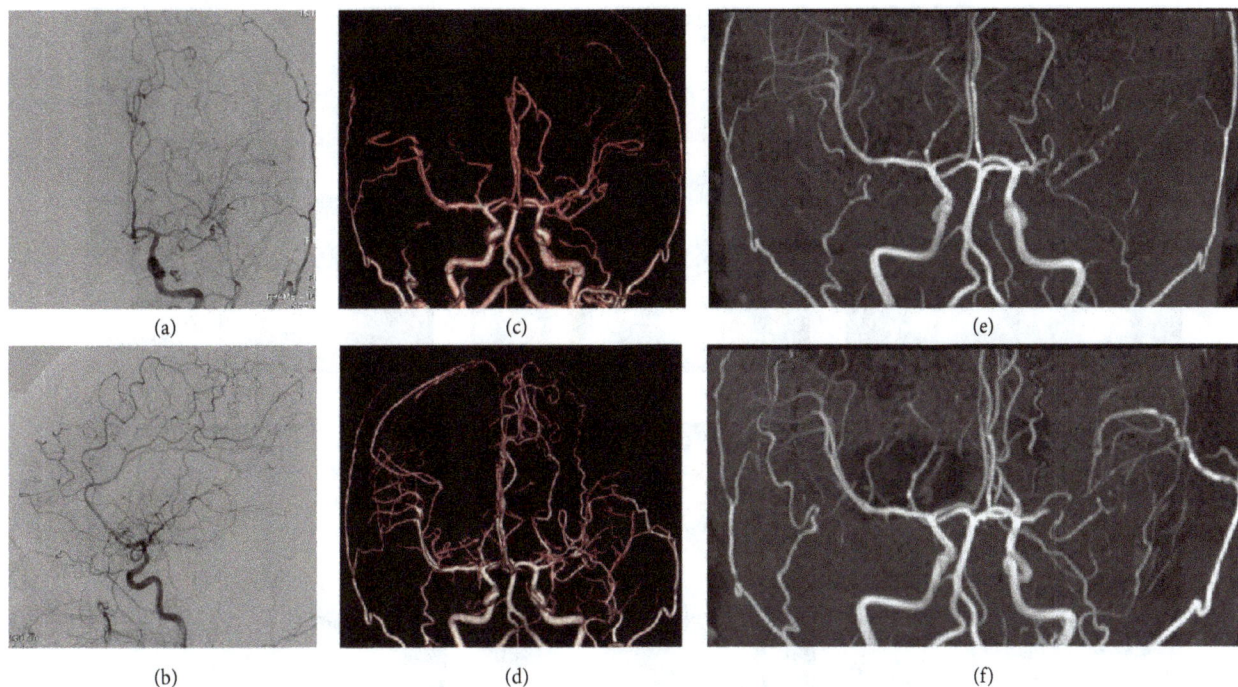

FIGURE 1: Pre- and postoperative cerebrovascular examinations. (a) and (b) Preoperative digital subtraction angiography showing narrowing in the M1 portion of MCA. (c) Preoperative 3D-CT angiography showing narrowing in the M1 portion of MCA. (d) Postoperative 3D-CT angiography showing the patency of STA-MCA anastomosis. (e) Preoperative magnetic resonance angiography (MRA) showing stenosis of M1 portion of left middle cerebral artery (MCA) and poor visualization of peripheral MCA. (f) Postoperative MRA showing the patency of STA-MCA anastomosis and improvement of blood flow in peripheral MCA.

(Figure 1(e)), why she was consulted to our department. We performed angiography, confirming moderate M1 portion stenosis (Figures 1(a) and 1(b)). SPECT showed no apparent laterality in CBF, thereby we decided to observe her with no treatment.

Seven months later, the patient experienced mild weakness and numbness in her right hand and visited our department. Although MRI showed no apparent ischemic change in her brain, arterial spin labelling (ASL) of MRI detected the decrease of CBF in the left cerebrum (Figure 2(a)), which was thought to well correspond for her symptoms. She was admitted and treated with an antiplatelet agent. Two weeks later, she still complained of numbness in her right hand; thereby, we decided to perform left STA-MCA anastomosis to prevent deterioration of her symptoms. Preoperative SPECT showed no apparent laterality in CBF (Figure 2(c)). On operation, left temporal craniotomy was performed, and the parietal branch of the STA was anastomosed with the M4 portion on the temporal lobe (Figures 1(d) and 1(f)). The intraoperative course was uneventful, and the patient recovered from anesthesia without any new neurological symptoms

Postoperatively, her speech was normal until postoperative day 1 (POD1). On POD2, she exhibited mild speech disturbance, which worsened day by day finally resulting in complete motor aphasia on POD6. Her comprehension was kept normal. On POD3, generalized convulsion occurred, which ceased quickly by diazepam, and levetiracetam was

initiated. On the same day, she presented with mild weakness of right upper extremity, which improved gradually and disappeared on POD7. MRI and CT showed no ischemic or hemorrhagic changes, but ASL and SPECT revealed remarkable increase of CBF in the left cerebrum (Figures 2(b) and 2(d)), by which the symptoms were diagnosed as CHPS. Despite the treatment with strict blood pressure and the administration of edaravone and minocycline, complete motor aphasia remained unchanged on POD21. MRI showed no abnormality except slightly hypointense changes on T2 weighted images and FLAIR (Figure 2(e)). At this point, the patient was discharged partly because of the request from the patient, and we continued to follow her in outpatient visit. One month after the surgery, the patient started to utter words that were not fluent, when SPECT and MRI showed normalization (Figure 2(f)). Thereafter, the improvement of her speech was slow, and totally more than three months was taken for full recovery after the surgery.

3. Discussion

Cerebral hyperperfusion syndrome (CHPS) following cerebral revascularization is well recognized particularly in the context of carotid endarterectomy (CEA) and carotid artery stenting (CAS) [4, 10]. STA-MCA anastomosis, which can be indicated for atherosclerotic diseases as well as moyamoya disease [1, 11], is another surgical procedure in which CHPS can occur [2, 3]. The incidence of postoperative CHPS varies

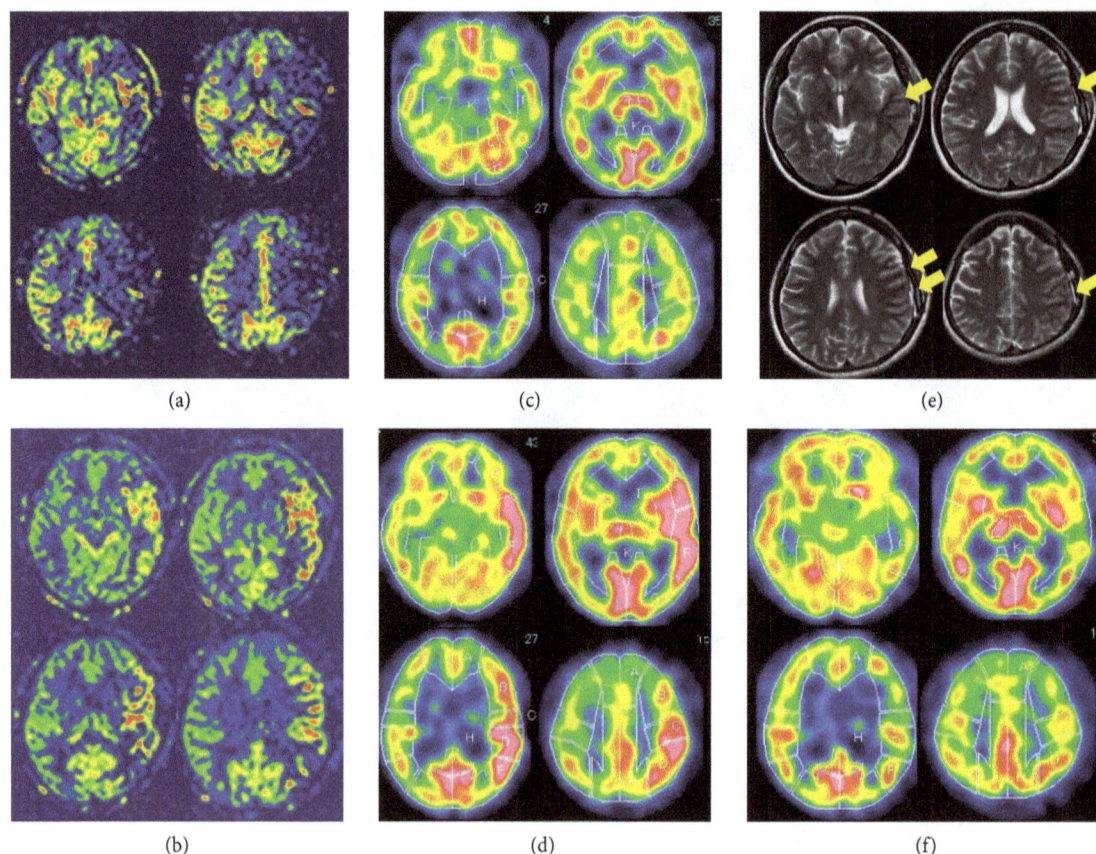

FIGURE 2: Pre- and postoperative neuroradiologic examinations. (a) Arterial spin labelling (ASL) of MRI showing decrease of CBF in the left brain when the patient presented with right hand weakness and numbness; (b) ASL on postoperative day (POD) 5 showing an increase of CBF in the left cerebrum; (c) preoperative single-photon emission computed tomography (SPECT) showing no apparent laterality in CBF. (d) SPECT on POD12 showing remarkable increase of CBF in the left cerebrum; (e) MRI T2WI on POD16 showing slightly hypointense change in the subcortex of the left cerebrum (arrows). (f) SPECT on POD33 showing normalization of CBF.

according to the surgical procedures or background of the patients, and it has been reported to occur in up to 50% of patients after STA-MCA anastomosis [2, 3, 10]. Resultant neurological deficits may be permanent and severe if intracranial hemorrhage occurs due to CHPS [12]. Otherwise, hyperperfusion is usually a temporary status that disappears within one week after surgery, and the symptoms are expected to disappear within 1-2 weeks in most cases [6, 8, 9].

In the present case, the initial presentation of CHPS appears typical in terms of the symptoms as well as the pattern of hyperperfusion on SPECT, because the area of hyperperfusion is frequently in localized brain cortex after STA-MCA anastomosis [6–8], and the focal neurologic signs in accordance with the anatomical location of the site of anastomosis are the most frequent symptoms in STA-MCA bypass surgery [6]. Then, hyperperfusion state detected on ASL or SPECT as well as complete motor aphasia continued for more than three weeks, which was longer than usually seen. More unexpectedly, the improvement of speech was slow even after the normalization of CBF on SPECT, requiring additionally more than two months for full recovery. The cytogenic edema could be a possible cause for persisting neurological deficits in patients with severe hyperperfusion

[13]. In our case, although slightly hypointense change on MRI-T2 and FLAIR images was observed in the subcortex area of the left cerebrum, no changes indicating edema or stroke were seen at all. Epilepsy was denied as well by the fact that no seizures occurred after the initiation of levetiracetam and she was alert all the time. Therefore, we assume that her prolonged symptoms were the sequela of CHPS, and the full recovery of her symptoms could support it.

There are two cases showing long duration of CHPS after STA-MCA bypass reported in the literature, both of which were the patients with moyamoya disease [6, 14]. In one case by Takemoto et al., a 59-year-old female patient experienced 5 weeks duration of aphasia and right hemiparesis [14], and the period of hyperperfusion detected on SPECT was three weeks, which is similar to that in our case. In another case shown in the study of 27 consecutive patients by Fujimura et al. [6], a 37-year-old male suffered from 30-day duration of aphasia and sensory disturbance. In their case, SPECT was taken only on POD2 and 7, and the actual duration of hyperperfusion on SPECT is unknown. The total duration of symptoms due to CHPS in our case is the longest in the literature, and this is the first case in atherosclerotic diseases, to our knowledge.

Although underlying mechanisms for hyperperfusion remain undetermined, possible pathophysiology for CHPS has been suggested to be the impaired autoregulation, endothelial dysfunction mediated by free radicals, breakdown of the baroreceptor reflex, and breakdown of blood-brain-barrier (BBB), which results from a rapid increase in cerebral blood flow [15, 16]. The impaired autoregulation is thought to be the central mechanism because the reduction of preoperative CBF and cerebral vascular reserve capacity (CVRC), which lead to impaired autoregulation, are known as the significant risk factors for hyperperfusion [13, 15]. In the case reported by Takemoto et al. mentioned above, regional differences in the functional recovery of cerebrovascular reactivity were suggested to the possible cause, based on the observation that the area of hyperperfusion shifted from basal ganglia to the cortex surrounding the anastomosis for three weeks [14]. In our case, speech disturbance persisted long while paresis of right upper extremity disappeared on POD7 although relatively large area covering motor area for right upper extremity was affected. Subtle differences between regions in the functional recovery of cerebrovascular reactivity might have led to such discrepancy in the length of the symptoms, which image studies could not detect. Preoperative measurement of CBF with acetazolamide in addition to that at the resting state is demonstrated to be helpful to predict the development of CHPS [17], and it might have shown some evidences revealing impaired autoregulation with regional differences.

Positron emission tomography (PET) is another tool to detect hyperperfusion in different aspects than MRI or SPECT can detect, and the decrease of oxygen extraction fraction (OEF) and the tendency of high cerebral blood volume (CBV) are reported to be the factors observed on PET in patients who developed CHPS [18]. In particular, prolonged recovery of CBV values is suggested to have a key role in the development of hyperperfusion and the associated clinical symptoms [18]. Therefore, in our case, impaired oxygen metabolism or increased CBV might have persisted long even after the normalization of CBF.

Considering that the symptoms persisted extremely long despite all possible treatments including strict control of blood pressure and the administration of edaravone and minocycline [19–21], there might have been some particular factors in this patient. Here, in view of the daily medication of quetiapine that the patient had been taking for depression, we suggest one hypothesis that quetiapine, which has an antagonistic action on dopamine 2 receptor, might have affected cerebral vessels and prolonged hyperperfusion, based on the previous reports regarding the effect of dopamine 2 receptor antagonist (D2 antagonist) on cerebral vessels [22–24]. Ion et al. reported in a postmortem study for Schizophrenia patients that D2 antagonist may affect the neurovascular unit and small structural microvascular changes [22]. Another study with adult rats by Gepdiremen et al. showed that wall thickness of basilar artery decreased significantly due to vasoconstriction when haloperidol, D2 antagonist, was given [23]. In addition, similar antipsychotics are reported to be likely to incur cytotoxic effects and apoptosis of BBB endothelia with an impairment of barrier functionality [24].

In our case, the cerebral vessels had presumably been exposed to D2 antagonist for a long time; thus, they might have sustained the impairment of vasoconstriction or BBB, leading to prolonged dilatation of the vessels or impaired oxygen metabolism following the increase of CBF after STA-MCA bypass surgery. In this regard, we should mention that we restarted the daily medication of quetiapine immediately after the surgery and continued it throughout the course. The hypothesis mentioned above could not be verified, and no cases with any brain diseases have been reported in which antipsychotics is suggested to affect cerebral blood flow, to our knowledge. Therefore, the degree of the influence of quetiapine on CHPS in this case could not be extrapolated. However, our case with such rare relationship could pose the alarm regarding the management of antipsychotics for cerebral revascularization surgeries.

This case represented a rare clinical course of CHPS. Factors causing long duration could not be determined, but we suggest a possibility of the involvement of antipsychotics by its effect on cerebral vessels as D2 antagonist. Further studies are needed to elucidate the mechanisms of CHPS and to establish the optimal treatment strategy for better prognosis.

Conflicts of Interest

There are no conflicts of interest about this study.

References

[1] C. Muroi, N. Khan, D. Bellut, M. Fujioka, and Y. Yonekawa, "Extracranial-intracranial bypass in atherosclerotic cerebrovascular disease: Report of a single centre experience," *British Journal of Neurosurgery*, vol. 25, no. 3, pp. 357–362, 2011.

[2] J. E. Kim and J. S. Jeon, "An update on the diagnosis and treatment of adult Moyamoya disease taking into consideration controversial issues," *Neurological Research*, vol. 36, no. 5, pp. 407–416, 2014.

[3] J. W. Hwang, H. M. Yang, H. Lee et al., "Predictive factors of symptomatic cerebral hyperperfusion after superficial temporal artery-middle cerebral artery anastomosis in adult patients with moyamoya disease," *British Journal of Anaesthesia*, vol. 110, no. 5, pp. 773–779, 2013.

[4] D. G. Piepgras, M. K. Morgan, T. M. Sundt Jr., T. Yanagihara, and L. M. Mussman, "Intracerebral hemorrhage after carotid endarterectomy," *Journal of Neurosurgery*, vol. 68, no. 4, pp. 532–536, 1988.

[5] R. A. Solomon, C. M. Loftus, D. O. Quest, and J. W. Correll, "Incidence and etiology of intracerebral hemorrhage following carotid endarterectomy," *Journal of Neurosurgery*, vol. 64, no. 1, pp. 29–34, 1986.

[6] M. Fujimura, T. Kaneta, S. Mugikura, H. Shimizu, and T. Tominaga, "Temporary neurologic deterioration due to cerebral hyperpeffusion after superficial temporal artery-middle cerebral artery anastomosis in patients with adult-onset moyamoya disease," *World Neurosurgery*, vol. 67, no. 3, pp. 273–282, 2007.

[7] M. Fujimura, T. Kaneta, H. Shimizu, and T. Tominaga, "Symptomatic hyperperfusion after superficial temporal artery - Middle cerebral artery anastomosis in a child with moyamoya

disease," *Child's Nervous System*, vol. 23, no. 10, pp. 1195–1198, 2007.

[8] M. Fujimura, H. Shimizu, T. Inoue, S. Mugikura, A. Saito, and T. Tominaga, "Significance of focal cerebral hyperperfusion as a cause of transient neurologic deterioration after extracranial-intracranial bypass for moyamoya disease: Comparative study with non-moyamoya patients using n-isopropyl-p-[123I]iodoamphetamine single-photon emission computed tomography," *Neurosurgery*, vol. 68, no. 4, pp. 957–965, 2011.

[9] T. Ishikawa, K. Houkin, H. Kamiyama, and H. Abe, "Effects of surgical revascularization on outcome of patients with pediatric moyamoya disease," *Stroke*, vol. 28, no. 6, pp. 1170–1173, 1997.

[10] K. Ogasawara, N. Sakai, T. Kuroiwa et al., "Intracranial hemorrhage associated with cerebral hyperperfusion syndrome following carotid endarterectomy and carotid artery stenting: retrospective review of 4494 patients," *Journal of Neurosurgery*, vol. 107, no. 6, pp. 1130–1136, 2007.

[11] S. Miyamoto, "Study Design for a Prospective Randomized Trial of Extracranial-Intracranial Bypass Surgery for Adults with Moyamoya Disease and Hemorrhagic Onset: The Japan Adult Moyamoya Trial Group," *Neurologia medico-chirurgica*, vol. 44, no. 4, pp. 218-219, 2004.

[12] F. Matano, Y. Murai, T. Mizunari, K. Adachi, S. Kobayashi, and A. Morita, "Intracerebral Hemorrhage Caused by Cerebral Hyperperfusion after Superficial Temporal Artery to Middle Cerebral Artery Bypass for Atherosclerotic Occlusive Cerebrovascular Disease," *NMC Case Report Journal*, vol. 4, no. 1, pp. 27–32, 2017.

[13] K. Ogasawara, H. Yukawa, M. Kobayashi et al., "Prediction and monitoring of cerebral hyperperfusion after carotid endarterectomy by using single-photon emission computerized tomography scanning," *Journal of Neurosurgery*, vol. 99, no. 3, pp. 504–510, 2003.

[14] M. Morioka, Y. Hasegawa, T. Kawano et al., "Prolonged and regionally progressive symptomatic cerebral hyperperfusion syndrome after superficial temporal artery-middle cerebral artery anastomosis in a patient with moyamoya disease," *Surgical Neurology International*, vol. 3, no. 1, p. 106, 2012.

[15] W. N. K. A. Van Mook, R. J. M. W. Rennenberg, G. W. Schurink et al., "Cerebral hyperperfusion syndrome," *The Lancet Neurology*, vol. 4, no. 12, pp. 877–888, 2005.

[16] S. Ivens, S. Gabriel, G. Greenberg, A. Friedman, and I. Shelef, "Blood-brain barrier breakdown as a novel mechanism underlying cerebral hyperperfusion syndrome," *Journal of Neurology*, vol. 257, no. 4, pp. 615–620, 2010.

[17] S. Oshida, K. Ogasawara, H. Saura et al., "Does preoperative measurement of cerebral blood flow with acetazolamide challenge in addition to preoperative measurement of cerebral blood flow at the resting state increase the predictive accuracy of development of cerebral hyperperfusion after carotid endarterectomy? Results from 500 cases with brain perfusion single-photon emission computed tomography study," *Neurologia medico-chirurgica*, vol. 55, no. 2, pp. 141–148, 2015.

[18] Y. Kaku, K. Iihara, N. Nakajima et al., "Cerebral blood flow and metabolism of hyperperfusion after cerebral revascularization in patients with moyamoya disease," *Journal of Cerebral Blood Flow & Metabolism*, vol. 32, no. 11, pp. 2066-2075, 2012.

[19] O. Z. Chi, J. Grayson, S. Barsoum, X. Liu, A. Dinani, and H. R. Weiss, "Effects of dexmedetomidine on microregional O2 balance during reperfusion after focal cerebral ischemia," *Journal of Stroke and Cerebrovascular Diseases*, vol. 24, no. 1, pp. 163–170, 2015.

[20] H. Uchino, N. Nakayama, K. Kazumata, S. Kuroda, and K. Houkin, "Edaravone reduces hyperperfusion-related neurological deficits in adult moyamoya disease: Historical control study," *Stroke*, vol. 47, no. 7, pp. 1930–1932, 2016.

[21] M. Fujimura, K. Niizuma, T. Inoue et al., "Minocycline prevents focal neurological deterioration due to cerebral hyperperfusion after extracranial-intracranial bypass for moyamoya disease," *Neurosurgery*, vol. 74, no. 2, pp. 163–170, 2014.

[22] I. Udristoiu, I. Marinescu, MC. Pirlog et al., "The microvascular alterations in frontal cortex during treatment with antipsychotics: a post-mortem study," *Romanian Journal of Morphology and Embryology*, vol. 57, pp. 501–506, 2016.

[23] A. Gepdiremen, N. Aydin, Z. Halici et al., "Chronic treatment of haloperidol causes vasoconstriction on basilar arteries of rats, dose dependently," *Pharmacological Research*, vol. 50, no. 6, pp. 569–574, 2004.

[24] E. Elmorsy, L. M. Elzalabany, H. M. Elsheikha, and P. A. Smith, "Adverse effects of antipsychotics on micro-vascular endothelial cells of the human blood-brain barrier," *Brain Research*, vol. 1583, no. 1, pp. 255–268, 2014.

31

Cognitive Impairments Preceding and Outlasting Autoimmune Limbic Encephalitis

Robert Gross,[1] Jennifer Davis,[2] Julie Roth,[3] and Henry Querfurth[3]

[1]*Department of Neurology, Icahn School of Medicine at Mount Sinai, New York, NY 10029, USA*
[2]*Department of Psychiatry, Rhode Island Hospital, Brown University School of Medicine, Providence, RI 02903, USA*
[3]*Department of Neurology, Rhode Island Hospital, Brown University School of Medicine, Providence, RI 02903, USA*

Correspondence should be addressed to Robert Gross; robert.gross@mssm.edu

Academic Editor: Mathias Toft

Mild cognitive impairment (MCI) can be the initial manifestation of autoimmune limbic encephalitis (ALE), a disorder that at times presents a diagnostic challenge. In addition to memory impairment, clinical features that might suggest this disorder include personality changes, agitation, insomnia, alterations of consciousness, and seizures. Once recognized, ALE typically responds to treatment with immune therapies, but long-term cognitive deficits may remain. We report two cases of patients with MCI who were ultimately diagnosed with ALE with antibodies against the voltage gated potassium channel complex. Months after apparent resolution of their encephalitides, both underwent neuropsychological testing, which demonstrated persistent cognitive deficits, primarily in the domains of memory and executive function, for cases 1 and 2, respectively. A brief review of the literature is included.

1. Introduction

Mild cognitive impairment (MCI) has a prevalence of 16–20% in over 65 population [1–3]. 6% constitute amnestic MCI with a high likelihood to advance to Alzheimer's disease [2]. MCI is a heterogeneous entity and includes some patients on an indolent path to a nonneurodegenerative and potentially treatable encephalopathy, as well as those with lingering deficits from such a disease process presenting in the recovery phase. If the illness evolves rapidly, a variant of AD may still be considered; however, the presence of atypical signs should raise suspicion for an infectious, paraneoplastic, or autoimmune etiology. 51% of ALE patients may be seronegative [4].

Here we report two cases of antivoltage gated potassium channel complex (VGKCC) encephalitis that initially presented as MCI with atypical features. Both had early nonconvulsive spells ascribed to limbic or dystonic seizures. After remission, both were left with MCI corresponding to amnestic or dysexecutive syndromes.

2. Case 1

A 71-year-old woman first presented to us for progressive memory complaints over one year in the context of the loss of a loved one and stress in the family. Past medical history included anxiety, lumbago, psoriasis, and multiple drug sensitivities including to a steroid injection. She had a high school education and worked as a telecommunication operator until retiring at age 65. Initially she would become confused with directions, missed appointments, and had occasional word finding difficulty but then had increasing problems with calculations and penmanship. She had forgotten her daughter's recent pregnancy. She began to have infrequent incidents consisting of rising paresthesiae, during which she was seen to tense her body, clench her teeth, become flushed, and look afraid. They resembled "panic attacks." These events were associated with amnesia for the event and were followed by confusion. She had also been having myoclonic jerks, though these had subsided by the time of

(a)

(b)

(c)

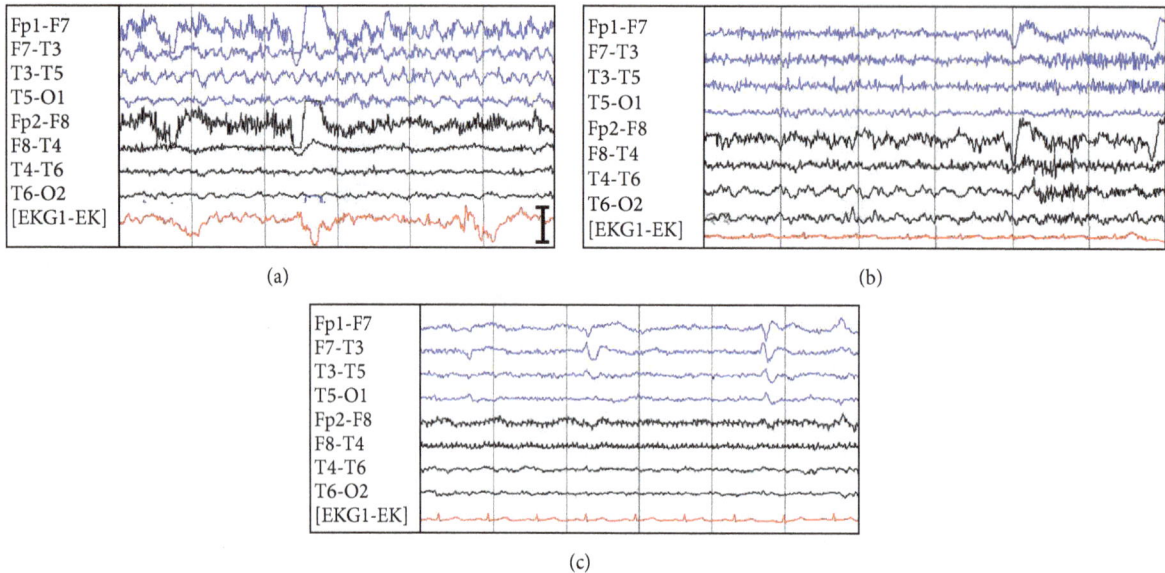

FIGURE 1: Sample 24 hr video EEG tracings from case 1. Push button activation processes and video recorded panic/fear attacks corresponding to left (a) alternating with right (b) temporal lobe activations and electrographic seizures. (c) The interictal record showing periodic left anterior sharp wave epileptiform discharges. 1 Hz time intervals, $2\,\mu$V/mm sensitivity, and bar 100 μV.

her initial presentation. A first neurologist started her on levetiracetam for suspected seizures, but this was discontinued after causing delirium. A second neurologist recorded a Mini Mental Status Score (MMSE) of 29/30, a Montreal Cognitive Assessment (MOCA) of 24 (1/5 verbal recall), diagnosed depression/anxiety, and initiated donepezil. This too was discontinued soon thereafter for ineffectiveness.

On our initial evaluation, her Clinical Dementia Rating (CDR) was 0.5 and MMSE was 28 (1/3 delayed verbal recall). Formal neuropsychological testing showed a largely intact cognitive profile with the exception of inefficient learning and impaired recall of verbal information. The Dementia Rating Scale (DRS) score was 139. The Beck Inventory was 8, not suggestive of active depression. MRI brain showed moderate global cerebral atrophy, though not specifically in the mesial temporal lobes, and small vessel ischemic changes. Fluorodeoxyglucose positron emission tomography (FDG PET) of the brain showed no areas of abnormal metabolism. She was diagnosed with MCI, amnestic type, and started on galantamine. There was clinical stabilization.

A little over a year from her presentation, she developed increasing anxiety, new auditory hallucinations, sleep disturbance, compulsive behaviors, and attacks resembling panic. Escitalopram and alprazolam were prescribed, subsequently changed to sertraline and lorazepam, and quetiapine was added. Memory complaints resurfaced: an MMSE was 27 (0/3 recall). Galantamine was discontinued due to diarrhea, cramps, and weight loss, and she was started on rivastigmine, to which memantine was added.

Over the next 3 months increasing anxiety led to a brief psychiatric evaluation in the ED. Mild hyponatremia (131 meq/L) was noted. A routine electroencephalogram (EEG) around this time showed bitemporal sharp waves. By 18 months after presentation, mental status had sharply

deteriorated with a larger number of stereotyped panic-fear attacks. 48-hour ambulatory EEG showed interictal periodic sharp and slow wave discharges in bilateral temporal lobes, and bitemporal electrographic seizures correlated to these clinical events, hereafter referred to as seizures (Figure 1). She was promptly started on phenytoin and lamotrigine and admitted to the hospital.

MMSE during this hospitalization was 15/30. Noncontrast head CT showed global atrophy but no acute findings. Cerebrospinal fluid (CSF) showed 1 nucleated cell, protein 32 mg/dL, glucose 63 mg/dL, and negative infectious studies. CSF 14-3-3 was mildly elevated at 2.6 ng/mL (normal < 1.5). Cytology was negative. CSF $A\beta_{(1-42)}$ was 148 pg/mL (reduced), and CSF total tau was 223 pg/mL (elevated) for an $A\beta$42-tau index of 0.29, but CSF phospho-tau (44 pg/mL) was not elevated, an inconclusive pattern. Calcium and thyroid stimulating hormone (TSH) were normal. Send-out testing subsequently returned borderline elevated for anti-VGKCC titers (498 pmol/L) and strongly positive for anti-leucine-rich glioma inactivated 1 protein (LGI1) antibodies by immunocytochemistry. She was diagnosed with LGI1 LE and readmitted for a 5-day course of intravenous immunoglobulin (IVIg).

After a 2-3-week period of recovery (MMSE = 27), she relapsed and was readmitted for wandering, emotional lability, agitation, and suicidal ideation. A second course of IVIg was supplemented with 4 days of high dose IV methylprednisolone. Shortly after finishing, she began to show signs of improvement. Epileptic fits stopped, and agitation and psychosis subsided. MMSE improved to 28, but insight remained impaired, and labile behavior persisted. 24 hr EEG revealed no further evidence of epileptiform activity. In rehabilitation, lamotrigine was discontinued due to rash, and she was discharged home on quetiapine, phenytoin, and low-dose lorazepam.

TABLE 1: Summary of posttreatment neuropsychological testing of both patients. Case 1 is 6 months and case 2 is 2 years following last hospitalization.

Test	Case 1		Case 2	
	Raw score	Normed score	Raw score	Normed score
Global Cognition				
MMSE	30	Intact	30	Intact
Dementia Rating Scale	133	$T = 43$	139	$T = 53$
Attention				
Coding	56	$T = 53$	51	$T = 50$
Trails A (seconds)	27″	$T = 59$	40″	$T = 41$
Executive functions				
Trails B (seconds)	92″	$T = 49$	**136″**	**T = 35**
FAS	45	$T = 58$	**26**	**T = 37**
Animals	12	$T = 40$	20	$T = 54$
Rey Figure (organization)	5	$T = 50$	5	$T = 45$
Language				
Boston Naming Test	50	$T = 47$	60	$T = 63$
Visuospatial skills				
Rey Copy	**13**	**T = 35**	**18**	**T = 60**
Judgment of Line Orientation	11	$T = 47$	13	$T = 55$
Memory				
Verbal memory (HVLT-R)				
Total learning trials 1–3	5, 6, 7	$T = 40$	10, 10, 11	$T = 65$
Delayed recall	**0**	**T = 19**	**11**	**T = 60**
Recognition (Hits-FP)	9	$T = 43$	11	$T = 54$
Visual memory (BVMT-R)				
Total learning trials 1–3	3, 4, 11	$T = 45$	2, 8, 7	$T = 43$
Delayed recall	9	$T = 55$	8	$T = 50$
Recognition (Hits-FP)	5	>16th percentile	5	>16th percentile
Mood				
Beck Depression Inventory	1	WNL	12	WNL

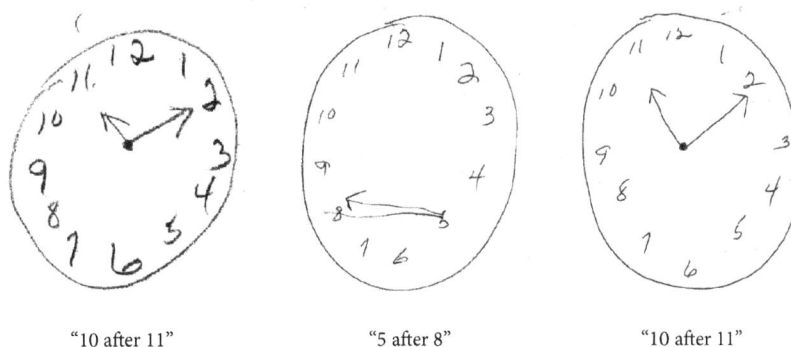

"10 after 11"　　　　"5 after 8"　　　　"10 after 11"

FIGURE 2: From left to right, clock drawing in 13 months, 32 months, and 38 months from symptom onset.

Repeat neuropsychological testing 1 month after discharge, compared to her previous baseline, demonstrated declines in working memory, psychomotor speed and executive function, and persistently impaired verbal memory. By 24 months after presentation, a third neuropsychological evaluation showed that while many of these changes had reversed, she continued to have difficulty in verbal memory and visuospatial skills (Table 1), albeit normalization of clock draw (Figure 2).

3. Case 2

A 72-year-old man first presented to us for evaluation of a one-month history of abnormal movements of his limbs and face associated with alteration of awareness and subsequent amnesia for the events. Past medical history was notable for recurrent bronchitis, dyslipidemia, abdominal and thoracic aortic aneurysms, and essential tremor. He had been on oral steroids intermittently over several years for bronchitis and

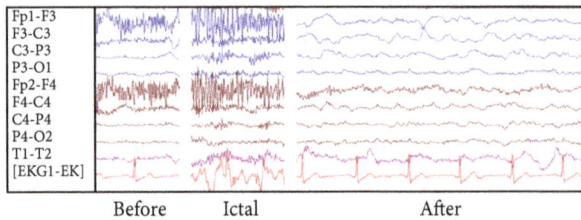

FIGURE 3: Sample tracing from 24 hr VEEG of case 2. Push button activation and video recorded faciobrachial dystonic seizures; pre-ictal, ictal (largely muscle artifact), and postictal recording samples, the latter displaying left greater than right side slowing in the theta and delta range, thereafter becoming symmetric (not shown) (bar 100 μV).

was on a tapering schedule when the abnormal movements began. They consisted of stereotyped myoclonic jerking and dystonic posturing of the right more than left upper extremity and face. He exhibited hand clenching, index finger or thumb extension, shoulder elevation, and facial contortion. The attacks occurred several times a day, lasting from a few seconds up to a minute each, and were becoming more frequent, occurring every 15–20 minutes and at night. During them, he would be less responsive and thereafter lethargic. He occasionally expressed the delusion of the TV transmitting commands to his wrist. His family reported behavioral changes over the previous month: his personality became more subdued. They also noticed short term memory and word finding difficulties. He had no previous history of seizures or mood disorders. The neurological and medical reviews of symptoms were unrevealing.

He had presented to a different hospital 2 weeks earlier and had undergone evaluation, including an MRI brain (1.5 T) with gadolinium, MRA head and neck, and routine EEG, all unremarkable. A neurologist diagnosed partial motor seizures and treated him with valproic acid at first, sequentially adding levetiracetam and zonisamide, with little benefit. Another neurologist obtained a Kokmen mental status screen score of 36/38. He was then admitted to university hospital for 48-hour video EEG (VEEG).

On initial examination, he was alert and oriented to place and date and followed commands. Speech and language were normal. He endorsed ideas of reference but was not overtly psychotic. His affect was flattened and he was mildly sluggish but was able to read and name the months backwards. Word recall was 1-2/3 at 10 minutes. There was bilateral postural tremor, but the remainder of the elemental neurological exam was normal.

Over the first 48 hours on VEEG, numerous brief, right greater than left stereotyped episodes were captured, all without associated distinct epileptiform discharges, though many had an electrographic correlate consisting of left temporal bursts of midtheta rhythms seen immediately following the push button events (Figure 3). Valproic acid and zonisamide were discontinued, and phenytoin was added. Lumbar puncture was traumatic and had 1053 RBCs and 9 nucleated cells in the first tube, 42 RBCs and 5 nucleated cells in the fourth tube, protein 50 mg/dL, and glucose 69 mg/dL. He was started

empirically on acyclovir, which was stopped after 3 doses when PCR for HSV 1 and HSV 2 returned negative.

Hospital course was complicated by acute kidney injury and pulmonary edema with respiratory failure resulting in brief intubation and stay in the Medical ICU. Several days after extubation and transfer back to the ward, he was noted to have impairments in insight, problem solving, attention to multistep commands, and short term memory. He became labile and impulsive and went through a brief period of threatening visual hallucinosis. Encephalopathy workup revealed mildly elevated titers of anti-thyroid peroxidase (TPO) and anti-thyroglobulin (TG) antibodies (137.8 IU/mL and 73.1 IU/mL, resp.); he was tentatively diagnosed with Hashimoto encephalopathy and treated with IV methylpred-nisolone for 5 days. The movement spells grew less frequent, were of shorter duration, and appeared less dramatic with the addition of clonazepam and then haloperidol to his regimen.

MRI brain (3T) with gadolinium was again unremarkable. An extensive infectious workup was similarly unrevealing, including for tickborne and viral pathogens. CSF 14-3-3 was negative. Serum ceruloplasmin and TSH were normal. Urine delta ALA and serum porphobilinogen were normal. Hospital course was further complicated by mild hyponatremia (130 meq/L) and a small retroperitoneal bleed that was conservatively managed. He was discharged home after a 10-day stay on phenytoin 150 mg twice daily and low doses of clonazepam, haloperidol, and prednisone.

After discharge, autoimmune encephalitis panel returned with elevated titers of anti-VGKCC autoantibodies at 572 pmol/L. Other autoantibodies (Hu, Ma1, CV2, Amphiph-ysin, NMDA, and GAD65) were absent (specific anti-LGI1 testing was not yet available). He underwent a workup for underlying malignancy with CT chest, abdomen, and pelvis, which was negative. Haloperidol was discontinued. His former personality had returned, and he remained seizure-free at last follow-up on low doses of phenytoin and prednisone. Neuropsychological testing 2 years after discharge revealed lasting impairments in executive function (divided attention and fluency) and low-average psychomotor speed. Notably, memory testing proved normal (Table 1).

4. Discussion

These two cases share several similar features. Both patients developed insidious memory loss and behavioral changes over months qualifying initially as MCI or cognitive impairment/decline, no dementia (CIND). Complex partial and dystonic seizures occurred in case 1 and case 2, respectively. Furthermore, both developed hyponatremia. At the peak of their illnesses, both became confused and had hallucinations. Both underwent extensive workups before the correct diagnosis was revealed. Both had variable responses to symptomatic treatments, including anticonvulsants, but improved dramatically with immunotherapies. Finally, there were persistent cognitive deficits in both patients long after apparent resolution of their ALE.

Clinically, VGKCC LE overlaps with other ALE cases. Case 2 highlights the fact that steroid-responsive encephalopathy associated with autoimmune thyroiditis

(SREAT or Hashimoto's encephalopathy [HE]) is among the top differential diagnoses to consider. Confusion, myoclonus, hallucinations, psychosis, and seizures are found in both [5–7], though hyponatremia is commonly seen with VGKCC LE, while stroke-like events, such as episodes of transient aphasia, frequently occur in HE [8]. Anti-TPO and anti-TG antibodies are often present in cases of VGKCC LE and are found in 10–15% of the general population [9], so their presence should be considered nonspecific. Neuroimaging and CSF evaluations are not sensitive: MRI shows high signal in the medial temporal lobes in about half to 80% cases of VGKCC LE, and CSF is often normal [6, 7, 9–12].

Serum autoantibodies against the VGKCC have been associated with acquired neuromyotonia (Isaac's syndrome), Morvan syndrome, epilepsy, and ALE [11]. Most autoantibodies are not directed against the VGKC subunits Kv1.1, 1.2, and 1.6, but rather against associated proteins LGI1 and contactin-associated protein-2 (CASPR2). LGI1 is the most common target of pathogenic autoantibodies in VGKCC LE [6, 12]. A neuronal protein associated with Kv1.1 in presynaptic terminals of the central nervous system, LGI1, is secreted and serves as a cell surface ligand for the ADAM22 and ADAM23 transmembrane proteins. It is strongly expressed in the hippocampus; autopsies of LGI1 LE have demonstrated CD45 and CD8+ T cell lymphocytic and CD68+ microglial infiltrates and hippocampal neuronal loss, the latter predominantly in the CA4 layer [13, 14]. Genetic mutations in *LGI1* are seen in autosomal dominant lateral temporal epilepsy [15] and in autosomal dominant partial epilepsy with auditory features [16]. It has been demonstrated that autoantibodies to LGI1 disrupt the ligand-receptor interaction of LGI1 with ADAM22 or ADAM23, which leads to reduction in synaptic AMPA receptors [17].

The second case featured faciobrachial dystonic seizures (FBDS), which is highly correlated with LGI1 LE [10, 16]. These consist of brief dystonic movements of the face and ipsilateral arm and leg, usually involving alteration of consciousness, sometimes alternating sides, and occurring up to 360 times per day. The EEG may show frank ictal epileptiform potentials or, as with case 2, a suggestive electrographic correlate, or it may be unrevealing. FDG PET studies have demonstrated altered glucose metabolism in the temporal lobes and basal ganglia of patients with FBDS [18, 19].

There is no distinctive neuropsychological profile in VGKCC LE. While subacute cognitive impairment is the most common manifestation, with severe short term memory loss found in most cases, verbal or visual memory may be spared in a small subset [20]. A cohort of 19 patients with LGI1 LE underwent neuropsychological testing both at the height of the illness and at posttreatment follow-up (median interval between testing 254 days) [21]. The investigators found broad, profound cognitive impairment during the acute phase of illness and functional recovery in many cognitive domains after treatment, though anterograde amnesia persisted in about one-third of their patients. Notably, executive function tended to improve into normal ranges after recovery. These results are in accord with what we observed in our first patient. However, a nonamnestic, dysexecutive type MCI was the outcome of the other, perhaps reflecting more lasting

basal ganglia-frontal dysfunction in patients with FBDS presentations. Our cases may be contrasted with another ALE syndrome that associated with AMPA-R antibodies. Those cases present more acutely with either frank confusion or fulminant encephalitis or as an isolated anterograde amnesia or mesiotemporal seizure but not apparently MCI [22].

Treatment of LGI1 LE consists of immunotherapies: steroids, plasmapheresis, and IVIg. There are no randomized controlled trials demonstrating superiority of one approach over another, though, in case series, patients tend to respond well to immune treatments and poorly to anticonvulsants [6, 7, 9, 12], again, similar to what we observed. Relapses can occur infrequently, especially as steroids are being titrated down [6], as case 2 experienced.

These cases underscore the difficulty associated with diagnosing LGI1 LE and confirm earlier findings that cognitive deficits may persist months to years after treatment [20]. When evaluating MCI, one should especially be vigilant for concomitant neuropsychiatric or epileptic disorders.

Conflict of Interests

The authors declare that there is no conflict of interests regarding the publication of this paper.

Authors' Contribution

Robert Gross and Henry Querfurth contributed equally to the writing of the paper. Jennifer Davis performed the neuropsychological testing. Julie Roth interpreted the EEGs.

References

[1] R. Roberts and D. S. Knopman, "Classification and epidemiology of MCI," *Clinics in Geriatric Medicine*, vol. 29, no. 4, pp. 753–772, 2013.

[2] O. L. Lopez, W. J. Jagust, S. T. DeKosky et al., "Prevalence and classification of mild cognitive impairment in the cardiovascular health study cognition study: part 1," *Archives of Neurology*, vol. 60, no. 10, pp. 1385–1389, 2013.

[3] J. E. Graham, K. Rockwood, B. L. Beattie et al., "Prevalence and severity of cognitive impairment with and without dementia in an elderly population," *The Lancet*, vol. 349, no. 9068, pp. 1793–1796, 1997.

[4] L. Bataller, K. A. Kleopa, G. F. Wu, J. E. Rossi, M. R. Rosenfeld, and J. Dalmau, "Autoimmune limbic encephalitis in 39 patients: immunophenotypes and outcomes," *Journal of Neurology, Neurosurgery and Psychiatry*, vol. 78, no. 4, pp. 381–385, 2007.

[5] P. Castillo, B. Woodruff, R. Caselli et al., "Steroid-responsive encephalopathy associated with autoimmune thyroiditis," *Archives of Neurology*, vol. 63, no. 2, pp. 197–202, 2006.

[6] M. Lai, M. G. M. Huijbers, E. Lancaster et al., "Investigation of LGI1 as the antigen in limbic encephalitis previously attributed to potassium channels: a case series," *The Lancet Neurology*, vol. 9, no. 8, 2010.

[7] K. M. Tan, V. A. Lennon, C. J. Klein, B. F. Boeve, and S. J. Pittock, "Clinical spectrum of voltage-gated potassium channel autoimmunity," *Neurology*, vol. 70, no. 20, pp. 1883–1890, 2008.

[8] N. Schiess and C. A. Pardo, "Hashimoto's encephalopathy," *Annals of the New York Academy of Sciences*, vol. 1142, pp. 254–265, 2008.

[9] F. Asztely and E. Kumlien, "The diagnosis and treatment of limbic encephalitis," *Acta Neurologica Scandinavica*, vol. 126, no. 6, pp. 365–375, 2012.

[10] S. R. Irani, A. W. Michell, B. Lang et al., "Faciobrachial dystonic seizures precede Lgi1 antibody limbic encephalitis," *Annals of Neurology*, vol. 69, no. 5, pp. 892–900, 2011.

[11] S. R. Irani, S. Alexander, P. Waters et al., "Antibodies to Kv1 potassium channel-complex proteins leucine-rich, glioma inactivated 1 protein and contactin-associated protein-2 in limbic encephalitis, Morvan's syndrome and acquired neuromyotonia," *Brain*, vol. 133, no. 9, pp. 2734–2748, 2010.

[12] A. Vincent, S. R. Irani, and B. Lang, "Potentially pathogenic autoantibodies associated with epilepsy and encephalitis in children and adults," *Epilepsia*, vol. 52, supplement 8, pp. 8–11, 2011.

[13] N. L. Khan, M. A. Jeffree, C. Good, W. Macleod, and S. Al-Sarraj, "Histopathology of VGKC antibody-associated limbic encephalitis," *Neurology*, vol. 72, no. 19, pp. 1703–1705, 2009.

[14] J. Schultze-Amberger, D. Pehl, and W. Stenzel, "LGI-1-positive limbic encephalitis: a clinicopathological study," *Journal of Neurology*, vol. 259, no. 11, pp. 2478–2480, 2012.

[15] J. M. Morante-Redolat, A. Gorostidi-Pagola, S. Piquer-Sirerol et al., "Mutations in the LGI1/Epitempin gene on 10q24 cause autosomal dominant lateral temporal epilepsy," *Human Molecular Genetics*, vol. 11, no. 9, pp. 1119–1128, 2002.

[16] R. Ottman, M. R. Winawer, S. Kalachikov et al., "*LGI1* mutations in autosomal dominant partial epilepsy with auditory features," *Neurology*, vol. 62, no. 7, pp. 1120–1126, 2004.

[17] T. Ohkawa, Y. Fukata, M. Yamasaki et al., "Autoantibodies to epilepsy-related LGI1 in limbic encephalitis neutralize LGI1-ADAM22 interaction and reduce synaptic AMPA receptors," *Journal of Neuroscience*, vol. 33, no. 46, pp. 18161–18174, 2013.

[18] A. Kunze, R. Drescher, K. Kaiser, M. Freesmeyer, O. W. Witte, and H. Axer, "Serial FDG PET/CT in autoimmune encephalitis with faciobrachial dystonic seizures," *Clinical Nuclear Medicine*, vol. 39, pp. e436–e438, 2014.

[19] J. Y. Yoo and L. J. Hirsch, "Limbic encephalitis associated with anti-voltage-gated potassium channel complex antibodies mimicking Creutzfeldt-Jakob disease," *JAMA Neurology*, vol. 71, no. 1, pp. 79–82, 2014.

[20] A. Vincent, C. Buckley, J. M. Schott et al., "Potassium channel antibody-associated encephalopathy: a potentially immunotherapy-responsive form of limbic encephalitis," *Brain*, vol. 127, no. 3, pp. 701–712, 2004.

[21] C. R. Butler, T. D. Miller, M. S. Kaur et al., "Persistent anterograde amnesia following limbic encephalitis associated with antibodies to the voltage-gated potassium channel complex," *Journal of Neurology, Neurosurgery and Psychiatry*, vol. 85, no. 4, pp. 387–391, 2014.

[22] B. Joubert, P. Kerschen, A. Zekeridou et al., "Clinical spectrum of encephalitis associated with antibodies against the α-amino-3-hydroxy-5-methyl-4-isoxazolepropionic acid receptor: case series and review of the literature," *JAMA Neurology*, vol. 72, no. 10, pp. 1163–1169, 2015.

32

Chronic Encapsulated Expanding Thalamic Hematoma Associated with Obstructive Hydrocephalus following Radiosurgery for a Cerebral Arteriovenous Malformation

Jun Takei,[1] Toshihide Tanaka,[1] Yohei Yamamoto,[1] Akihiko Teshigawara,[1] Satoru Tochigi,[1] Yuzuru Hasegawa,[1] and Yuichi Murayama[2]

[1]*Department of Neurosurgery, Jikei University School of Medicine Kashiwa Hospital, 163-1 Kashiwa-shita, Kashiwa, Chiba 277-8567, Japan*
[2]*Department of Neurosurgery, Jikei University School of Medicine, 3-25-8 Nishi-Shinbashi, Minato-ku, Tokyo 105-8461, Japan*

Correspondence should be addressed to Toshihide Tanaka; ttanaka@jikei.ac.jp

Academic Editor: Chin-Chang Huang

Chronic encapsulated intracerebral hematoma is a unique type of intracerebral hematoma accompanied by a capsule that is abundant in fragile microvasculature occasionally causing delayed regrowth. A 37-year-old man who had undergone radiosurgery for an arteriovenous malformation (AVM) causing intracerebral hematoma in the left parietal lobe presented with headache, vomiting, and progressive truncal ataxia due to a cystic lesion that had been noted in the left thalamus, leading to progressive obstructive hydrocephalus. He underwent left frontal craniotomy via a transsylvian fissure approach, and the serous hematoma was aspirated. The hematoma capsule was easy to drain and was partially removed. Pathological findings demonstrated angiomatous fibroblastic granulation tissue with extensive macrophage invasion. The concentration of vascular endothelial growth factor (VEGF) was high in the hematoma (12012 pg/mL). The etiology and pathogenesis of encapsulated hematoma are unclear, but the gross appearance and pathological findings are similar to those of chronic subdural hematoma. Based on the high concentration of VEGF in the hematoma, expansion of the encapsulated hematoma might have been caused by the promotion of vascular permeability of newly formed microvasculature in the capsule.

1. Introduction

Stereotactic radiosurgery (SRS) has become a therapeutic alternative for the treatment of cerebral arteriovenous malformations (AVMs). However, several delayed complications following SRS for AVMs including parenchymal hemorrhage, radiation necrosis, and cyst formation have been reported [1]. Among them, chronic encapsulated intracerebral hematoma is a rare cerebrovascular disease [1–8]. This type of hematoma expands slowly and behaves as a space-occupying lesion, sometimes resulting in obstructive hydrocephalus, uniquely located in the thalamus.

The thickened hematoma capsule possesses abundant microvasculature and can bleed easily when removed surgically, whereas the hematoma itself is serous and is usually easily aspirated. Therefore, the gross appearance and histological findings are similar to chronic subdural hematoma.

Vascular endothelial growth factor (VEGF), also known as vascular permeability factor (VPF), which promotes vascular permeability resulting in extravasation, is thought to be involved in the pathogenesis of chronic subdural hematoma [9, 10]. The role of VEGF in neovascularization and vascular hyperpermeability has been documented, confirming previous studies in which it has been stated that inflammation is responsible for angiogenesis of the hematoma capsule [9, 11, 12].

Surgical resection is the treatment of choice for improving neurological symptoms. Several different modalities of surgery have been suggested, including craniotomy, burr hole irrigation, and, in situations where the hematoma cavity is located near the ventricles causing obstructive hydrocephalus, endoscopic aspiration of the hematoma with fenestration.

2. Case Report

A 37-year-old man presented with headache, vomiting, and progressive truncal ataxia. He had undergone radiosurgery and surgical extirpation for an arteriovenous malformation (AVM) causing intracerebral hematoma in the left parietal lobe 15 years prior to presentation. Since then, he had already been experiencing motor aphasia and right spastic hemiparesis. Eleven years after the radiosurgery for AVM, a cystic lesion with iso-low-density was noted in the left thalamus on computed tomography (CT) (Figure 1(a)). Initially, he was followed conservatively as he had no new neurological symptoms. The lesion was followed every other year and eventually revealed that the isodense cystic mass had grown gradually and was accompanied by progressive obstructive hydrocephalus (Figures 1(b) and 1(c)). Magnetic resonance imaging (MRI) showed a cystic lesion with a septum that appeared iso- and hyperintense on T1- and T2-weighted imaging, respectively (Figures 1(d)–1(f)).

Four years after initial CT, the patient underwent left frontal craniotomy via a trans-Sylvian fissure approach. The Sylvian fissure was dissected, and the lesion was identified. The cyst wall was incised and old serous hematoma was recognized. After aspiration of the hematoma, an elastic, hard, brownish-yellow cystic wall was partially removed because the hematoma capsule bled easily and hemostasis was very difficult to achieve, and then the foramen of Monro was identified. After the cerebrospinal fluid was drained, the swelling of the cerebral tissue resolved.

Histological findings revealed that the hematoma wall consisted of an outer layer of dense collagenous tissue (Figures 2(a) and 2(c)) and an inner layer of angiomatous fibroblastic granulation tissue with extensive macrophage infiltration (Figure 2(b)).

Postoperatively, the patient's condition improved. Postoperative CT and MRI showed that the hematoma had been evacuated, and the hydrocephalus had improved (Figures 1(g) and 1(h)).

The concentration of VEGF quantified by ELISA (enzyme-linked immunosorbent assay) was 12012 pg/mL in the surgically excised hematoma. Neither further progression nor recollection of the hematoma was observed. He was transferred for further rehabilitation.

Follow-up CT scan one year after surgery demonstrated neither recurrence of the hematoma nor progressive hydrocephalus (Figure 1(i)).

3. Discussion

Chronic encapsulated intracerebral hematoma is a unique type of intracerebral hematoma first described by Hirch et al. and characterized by the presence of a fibrotic capsule [13]. Vascular anomalies such as AVM, cavernous angioma microaneurysm, and venous angioma are frequently seen. Thus, the pathogenesis of chronic encapsulated intracerebral

hematoma is probably "self-destruction" or thrombosis during hemorrhagic episodes [14–16].

In recent years, chronic encapsulated hematoma has also been found to be associated with stereotactic radiosurgery for AVMs. Since Kurita et al. described an encapsulated intracerebral hematoma that developed after radiosurgery during the course of obliterating AVMs [1], 12 cases have been reported, including the present case (Table 1) [1–8]. Most of the lesions are located in the basal ganglia. Larger nidus volume and higher radiation dose may be a risk factor for delayed cyst formation [17]. The mean interval between radiosurgery for AVMs and surgical extirpation of chronic encapsulated hematoma was 6.5 years. Patient's average age was 34 years. In the series of encapsulated hematoma cases, most were accompanied by perifocal edema (Table 1).

Kurita et al. assumed that the cause of hematoma was probably repetitive bleeding from the fragile vessels contained in the thick hematoma capsule [1]. Chronic encapsulated intracerebral hematoma sometimes grows progressively while forming the capsule. However, the mechanism of the formation of chronic encapsulated hematoma still needs to be fully elucidated.

In contrast to previous reports, in the present case, CT demonstrated a low-density cystic lesion, indicating encapsulated hematoma in the chronic stage and progression of liquefied chronic hematoma. The AVM and encapsulated hematoma were situated apart from one another, and a residual nidus was not observed during surgery.

Potential mechanisms were considered for the development of a capsule after radiosurgery for AVMs histopathological findings demonstrated extensive microvasculature and suggested neovascularization in the densely collagenous capsule. Radiation necrosis was seen sporadically within the capsule as was active organization from fresh thrombus into hemosiderin within the fibrous tissue.

Bleeding and exudation from these fragile, newly formed vessels may have expanded the lesion in a fashion similar to chronic subdural hematoma.

Among the factors modulating angiogenesis, VEGF is one of the most likely candidates for a specific regulator that may promote the growth of this type of hematoma. VEGF, also known as VPF, is a potent mitogen for vascular endothelial cells and also promotes vascular permeability via the formation of vesiculovacuolar organelles in the cytoplasm of vascular endothelial cells [11, 12]. VEGF is thought to cause hypervascular tumor formation with expanding perifocal edema. In the same manner, a hematoma with a hypervascular capsule and perifocal edema might be caused by VEGF. The high concentration and expression of VEGF in the hematoma in the present case, similar to the previous report [6], as well as the microvascular endothelial proliferation in the hematoma capsule seen on immunohistochemical findings [5], suggest that angiogenesis and vascular permeability induced by VEGF might accelerate expansion of the hematoma.

Chronic encapsulated intracerebral hematoma often causes progressive neurological deficits due to mass effect. Two surgical approaches are typically considered: one is craniotomy via a trans-Sylvian route, and the other is an

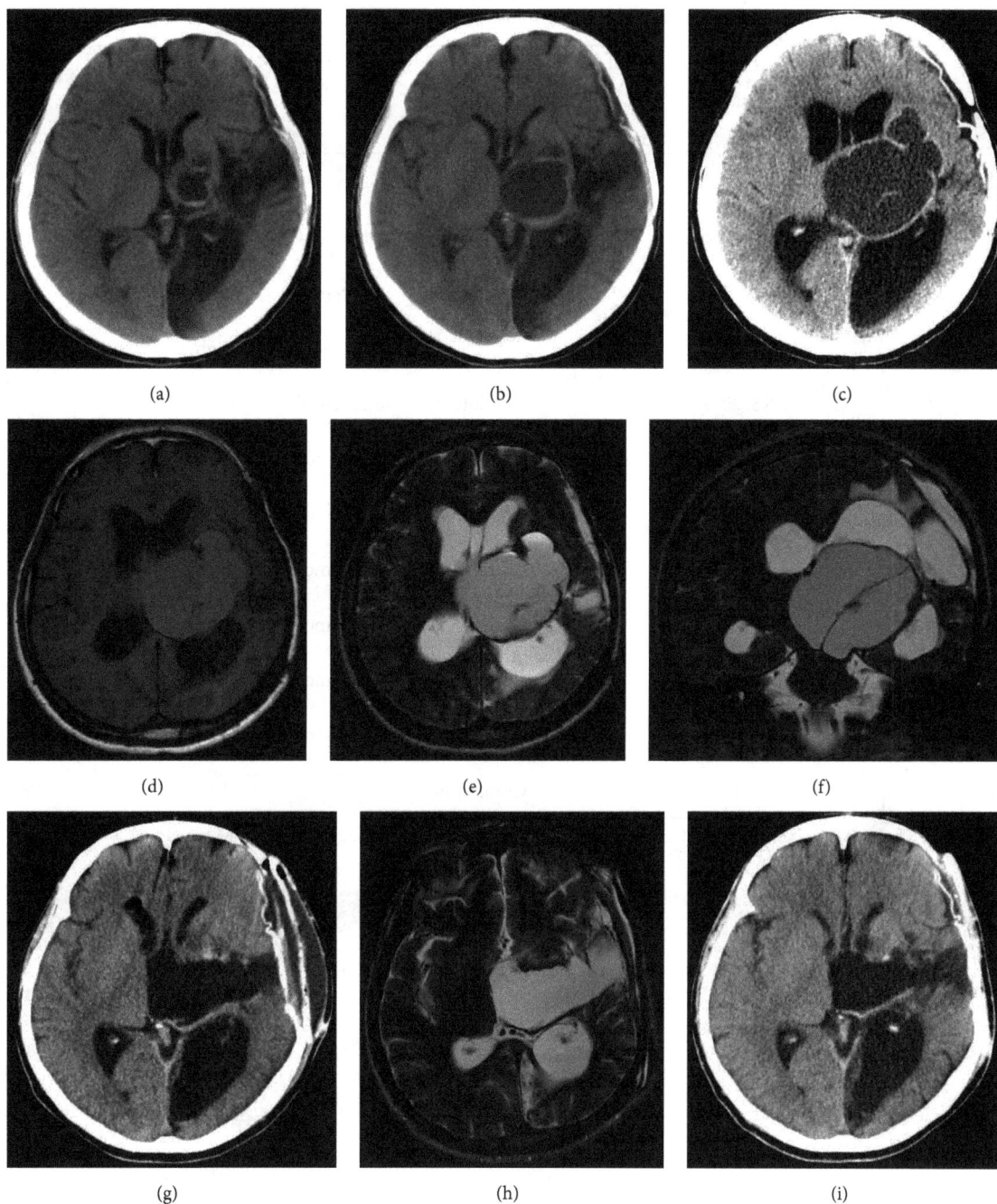

FIGURE 1: (a) Preoperative initial computed tomography (CT) 11 years after radiosurgery for an arteriovenous malformation in the left parietal lobe showing the cyst in the left thalamus. (b) Two years later, CT reveals that the size of the cyst is increased without hydrocephalus. (c) Four years later, CT reveals that the multilobular cyst is larger and accompanied by obstructive hydrocephalus. Preoperative magnetic resonance imaging (MRI) showing a cystic lesion in the left thalamus appearing isointense on T1-weighted imaging (d) and hyperintense on T2-weighted axial (e) and coronal (f) imaging as well as association with obstructive hydrocephalus. Note thickened cyst wall and septum in the middle of the cyst. Postoperative CT (g) and MRI (h) show shrinkage of the hematoma cavity and improvement of hydrocephalus. CT scan one year after surgery demonstrates neither recurrence of the hematoma nor progressive hydrocephalus (i).

endoscopic approach with aspiration of the hematoma and cyst fenestration. As shown in Table 1, most cases have been treated by craniotomy. Only one case was treated by stereotactic aspiration of the hematoma followed by implantation of an Ommaya reservoir [6]. Since the chronic encapsulated intracerebral hematoma in our case had a tough membrane, separating the hematoma from the normal brain parenchyma was easy, as previously described [18]. We selected craniotomy; however, the capsule was very fragile and difficult to separate from the thalamus and bled easily. We

TABLE 1: Patients with chronic encapsulated intracerebral hematoma (CEIH) following radiosurgery for arteriovenous malformation.

Case number	Age	Sex	Location	Radiosurgery	Interval from radiosurgery to surgery (years)	Treatment of CEIH	Hematoma capsule	CT density	Edema	References
1	19	M	Rt. basal ganglia	GKS, 20 Gy	2	Craniotomy	Total removal	High	+	Kurita et al. 1996 [1]
2	51	M	Rt. basal ganglia	GKS, 22.5 Gy	6	Craniotomy	Total removal	High	+	Maruyama et al. 2006 [3]
3	47	M	Rt. caudate	GKS, 25 Gy	9	Craniotomy	Total removal	ND	+	Motegi et al. 2008 [4]
4	15	F	Rt. basal ganglia	LINAC, 15 Gy	7	Stereotactic aspiration	Not removed	High	−	Takeuchi et al. 2009 [6]
5	23	M	Rt. basal ganglia	GKS, 20 Gy	2	Craniotomy	Total removal	High	+	Nakamizo et al. 2011 [5]
6	57	M	Rt. basal ganglia	GKS, 22.5 Gy	5	Craniotomy	Total removal	High	+	Nakamizo et al. 2011 [5]
7	15	F	Rt. basal ganglia	GKS, 18 Gy	3	Craniotomy	Total removal	High	+	Nakamizo et al. 2011 [5]
8	55	M	Rt. frontal	LINAC, 20 Gy	11	Craniotomy	Total removal	ND	+	Nakamizo et al. 2011 [5]
9	49	M	Lt. basal ganglia	LINAC, 18 Gy	4	Craniotomy	Total removal	ND	+	Takeuchi et al. 2011 [7]
10	20	M	Rt. frontal	ND	10	Craniotomy	Total removal	ND	+	Lee et al. 2011 [2]
11	20	F	Lt. cerebellar	GKS, 20 Gy	4	Craniotomy	Total removal	High	+	Watanabe et al. 2014 [8]
12	37	M	Lt. thalamus	ND	15	Craniotomy	Partial removal	Iso	+	Present case

F: female; M: male; Lt.: left; Rt.: right; GKS: gamma knife surgery; LINAC: linear accelerator radiosurgery; ND: not described.

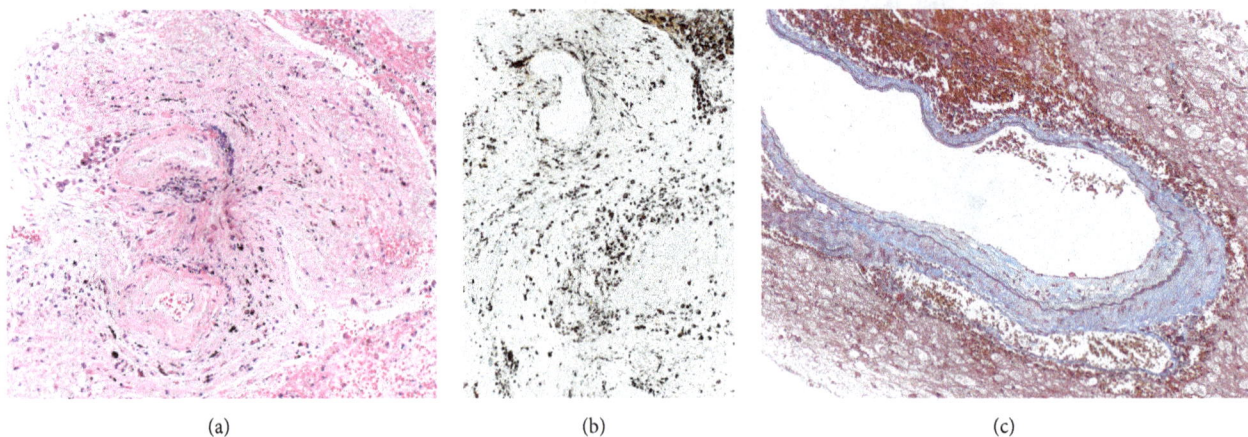

(a)   (b)   (c)

FIGURE 2: (a) Histological findings reveal hematoma capsule consisting of a dense collagenous layer with extensive invasion of macrophages, hematoxylin and eosin, ×40. (b) Immunohistochemical findings showing numerous CD68-positive cells in the cyst wall, original magnification ×40. (c) Vessel wall is thickened and internal elastica lamina is intact, revealing no residual nidus in the incised cyst wall, Masson, ×100.

were therefore only able to partially remove the hematoma capsule. Hemostasis was achieved by inserting cotton and thin-sliced Gelfoam soaked with fibrin glue. The hematoma was aspirated completely, whereas the capsule was only partially removed, which provided communication between the lateral ventricle and the third ventricle because the lesion was located in the thalamus and had led to obstructive hydrocephalus. For the reasons described above, in terms of hemostasis from the capsule of the hematoma, craniotomy was considered to be better than an endoscopic approach.

We believe that when the cystic hematoma revealed slow progression causing obstructive hydrocephalus, the patient should have undergone surgical resection earlier in order to obtain easier access and a more adequate working space. Moreover, closer long-term follow-up should be required for monitoring of the residual hematoma capsule. Radical resection of the capsule containing abundant neovasculature is obviously necessary to treat this type of hematoma; however, partial resection of the capsule is an alternative, especially in the case of a hematoma located in the thalamus accompanied by obstructive hydrocephalus.

Conflict of Interests

None of the authors have any conflict of interests to declare.

References

[1] H. Kurita, T. Sasaki, S. Kawamoto et al., "Chronic encapsulated expanding hematoma in association with gamma knife stereotactic radiosurgery for a cerebral arteriovenous malformation: case report," *Journal of Neurosurgery*, vol. 84, no. 5, pp. 874–878, 1996.

[2] C.-C. Lee, D. H.-C. Pan, D. M.-T. Ho et al., "Chronic encapsulated expanding hematoma after gamma knife stereotactic radiosurgery for cerebral arteriovenous malformation," *Clinical Neurology and Neurosurgery*, vol. 113, no. 8, pp. 668–671, 2011.

[3] K. Maruyama, M. Shin, M. Tago et al., "Management and outcome of hemorrhage after gamma knife surgery for arteriovenous malformations of the brain," *Journal of neurosurgery*, vol. 105, pp. 52–57, 2006.

[4] H. Motegi, S. Kuroda, N. Ishii et al., "De novo formation of cavernoma after radiosurgery for adult cerebral arteriovenous malformation—case report," *Neurologia Medico-Chirurgica*, vol. 48, no. 9, pp. 397–400, 2008.

[5] A. Nakamizo, S. O. Suzuki, N. Saito et al., "Clinicopathological study on chronic encapsulated expanding hematoma associated with incompletely obliterated AVM after stereotactic radiosurgery," *Acta Neurochirurgica*, vol. 153, no. 4, pp. 883–893, 2011.

[6] S. Takeuchi, Y. Takasato, H. Masaoka et al., "Development of chronic encapsulated intracerebral hematoma after radiosurgery for a cerebral arteriovenous malformation," *Acta Neurochirurgica*, vol. 151, no. 11, pp. 1513–1515, 2009.

[7] S. Takeuchi, Y. Takasato, and H. Masaoka, "Chronic encapsulated intracerebral hematoma formation after radiosurgery for cerebral arteriovenous malformation," *Neurology India*, vol. 59, no. 4, pp. 624–626, 2011.

[8] T. Watanabe, H. Nagamine, and S. Ishiuchi, "Progression of cerebellar chronic encapsulated expanding hematoma during late pregnancy after gamma knife radiosurgery for arteriovenous malformation," *Surgical Neurology International*, vol. 5, supplement 16, pp. S575–S579, 2014.

[9] A. Hohenstein, R. Erber, L. Schilling, and R. Weigel, "Increased mRNA expression of VEGF within the hematoma and imbalance of angiopoietin-1 and -2 mRNA within the neomembranes of chronic subdural hematoma," *Journal of Neurotrauma*, vol. 22, no. 5, pp. 518–528, 2005.

[10] J. Vaquero, M. Zurita, and R. Cincu, "Vascular endothelial growth-permeability factor in granulation tissue of chronic subdural haematomas," *Acta Neurochirurgica*, vol. 144, no. 4, pp. 343–347, 2002.

[11] A. M. Dvorak, S. Kohn, E. S. Morgan, P. Fox, J. A. Nagy, and H. F. Dvorak, "The vesiculo-vacuolar organelle (VVO): a distinct endothelial cell structure that provides a transcellular pathway for macromolecular extravasation," *Journal of Leukocyte Biology*, vol. 59, no. 1, pp. 100–115, 1996.

[12] H. F. Dvorak, L. F. Brown, M. Detmar, and A. M. Dvorak, "Vascular permeability factor/vascular endothelial growth factor, microvascular hyperpermeability, and angiogenesis," *American Journal of Pathology*, vol. 146, no. 5, pp. 1029–1039, 1995.

[13] L. F. Hirsh, H. B. Spector, and B. M. Bogdanoff, "Chronic encapsulated intracerebral hematoma," *Neurosurgery*, vol. 9, no. 2, pp. 169–172, 1981.

[14] E. Fiumara, M. Gambacorta, V. D'Angelo, M. Ferrara, and C. Corona, "Chronic encapsulated intracerebral haematoma: pathogenetic and diagnostic considerations," *Journal of Neurology Neurosurgery and Psychiatry*, vol. 52, no. 11, pp. 1296–1299, 1989.

[15] E. Pozzati, G. Giuliani, G. Gaist, G. Piazza, and G. Vergoni, "Chronic expanding intracerebral hematoma," *Journal of Neurosurgery*, vol. 65, no. 5, pp. 611–614, 1986.

[16] H. Sakaida, M. Sakakura, H. Tochio, K. Nakao, A. Taniguchi, and T. Yabana, "Chronic encapsulated intracerebral hematoma associated with angiographically occult arteriovenous malformation—case report," *Neurologia Medico-Chirurgica*, vol. 33, no. 9, pp. 638–642, 1993.

[17] M. Izawa, M. Hayashi, M. Chernov et al., "Long-term complications after gamma knife surgery for arteriovenous malformations," *Journal of Neurosurgery*, vol. 102, no. 1, pp. 34–37, 2005.

[18] A. Nishiyama, H. Toi, H. Takai et al., "Chronic encapsulated intracerebral hematoma: three cases reports and a literature review," *Surgical Neurology International*, vol. 5, no. 1, article 88, 2014.

33

An Unusual Case of Asystole Occurring during Deep Brain Stimulation Surgery

Ha Son Nguyen,[1] Harvey Woehlck,[2] and Peter Pahapill[1,3]

[1]Neurosurgery, Medical College of Wisconsin, Milwaukee, WI 53226, USA
[2]Anesthesiology, Medical College of Wisconsin, Milwaukee, WI 53226, USA
[3]Neurosurgery, Clement J. Zablocki VA Medical Center, Milwaukee, WI 53295, USA

Correspondence should be addressed to Ha Son Nguyen; hsnguyen@mcw.edu

Academic Editor: Abbass Amirjamshidi

Background. Symptomatic bradycardia and hypotension in neurosurgery can produce severe consequences if not managed appropriately. The literature is scarce regarding its occurrence during deep brain stimulation (DBS) surgery. *Case Presentation.* A 67-year-old female presented for left DBS lead placement for essential tremors. During lead implantation, heart rate and blood pressure dropped rapidly; the patient became unresponsive and asystolic. Chest compressions were initiated and epinephrine was given. Within 30 seconds, the patient became hemodynamically stable and conscious. A head CT demonstrated no acute findings. After deliberation, a decision was made to complete the procedure. Assuming the etiology of the episode was the Bezold-Jarisch reflex (BJR), appropriate accommodations were made. The procedure was completed uneventfully. *Conclusion.* The episode was consistent with a manifestation of the BJR. The patient had a history of neurocardiogenic syncope and a relatively low-volume state, factors prone to the BJR. Overall, lead implantation can still occur safely if preventive measures are employed.

1. Background

Deep brain stimulation (DBS) has become a widely accepted therapy for adjustable, reversible modulation of brain function. Rare, but notable, intraoperative complications include critical hemodynamic instability, particularly symptomatic bradycardia and hypotension, which has been associated with venous air embolism [1]. To the authors' knowledge, there has been no occurrence linked to the Bezold-Jarisch reflex (BJR), a cardioinhibitory reflex that has been associated with states of hypovolemia. Herein, the authors describe a patient who exhibited acute, dramatic asystole during DBS surgery. The episode was consistent with the BJR. After appropriate measures were pursued, the patient underwent an uneventful implantation of her electrode.

2. Case Report

2.1. Initial Presentation. A 67-year-old right-handed female with a history of neurocardiogenic syncope, irritable bowel syndrome, and hypothyroidism had been suffering from essential tremors for 25 years. Notably, she also had an extensive family history of neurocardiogenic syncope. Exam revealed bilateral upper extremity grade 2/4 intention tremors. Baseline vital signs included height 167 cm, weight 46 kg, blood pressure 90–100s/50–60s, and heart rate 60–90s.

2.2. Initial DBS Implantation. She underwent a Leksell frame-based placement of a left VIM DBS with microrecording, resulting in a significant lesion effect and intraoperative tremor arrest with macrostimulation. Immediately, postoperatively, the patient demonstrated mild difficulty with coordination and speech production, as well as an odd sensation in the right hand. A CT head demonstrated a small hemorrhage at the tip of the lead (Figure 1). At the first programming session, her initial postoperative symptoms, including her lesion effect, had resolved and she demonstrated no benefits from stimulation. An MRI brain confirmed a small resolving hematoma at the tip of the lead (Figures 2(a) and 2(b)); consequently, further programming was held off until the hematoma resolved. A month later, DBS programming again

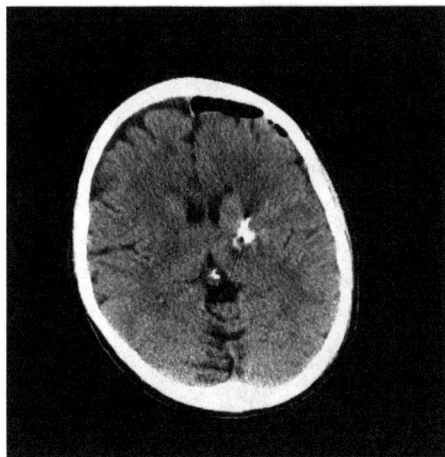

FIGURE 1: CT head demonstrated a small hemorrhage at the tip of the lead.

demonstrated no benefits. Revision surgery was recommended.

2.3. Initial Revision Attempt. During application of the Leksell stereotactic frame, the patient felt nauseated and promptly became unresponsive. Vital signs were stable. The frame was removed and the patient was placed supinely. Within minutes, she was back to neurologic baseline. A CT head demonstrated no acute findings. The case was cancelled, and the patient was admitted for further evaluation. Workup included medicine, neurology, psychiatry, and cardiology consultations. No structural heart disease or malignant arrhythmias were identified. Further history revealed several recent fainting episodes. The present episode was attributed to neurocardiogenic syncope. She was also evaluated for a potential psychiatric component given the fact that this occurred a few days away from what would have been her late husband's birthday and a few weeks from the one-year anniversary of his death. A diagnosis of major depressive disorder related to grief was made and a trial of mirtazapine was started. She reported improvement in mood, appetite, and sleep.

2.4. Revision Surgery. Three months later, frame placement ensued without issues. The previous burr hole was exposed. After microelectrode mapping, the DBS electrode was placed. Prior to test macrostimulation through the DBS lead, the patient complained of severe nausea. HR decreased quickly from 80–90s to 20–30s and blood pressure from 120s/60s to 60s/30s. The patient became unresponsive and asystolic; respiratory rate remained stable at 10–16. Chest compressions were initiated immediately by the movement disorder neurologist and administration of epinephrine 0.1 mg IV occurred. Subsequently, within 30 seconds, the patient demonstrated return of hemodynamic stability and became responsive, answering simple questions. HR was in the 90s to 100s, and BP was 90s/50s. The procedure was stopped. The DBS electrode and stereotactic arc, but not frame, were removed and

the incision was closed. A stat CT head did not demonstrate any abnormality.

Extensive discussions occurred with the patient, the anesthesia team, the neurology team, and the patient's family. The decision was made to bring her immediately back to the operating room and complete the procedure by implanting the DBS electrode as planned. Believing the episode was due to the BJR, the patient was treated with glycopyrrolate and a 20 mL/kg normal saline bolus. There was no recurrence of bradycardia, hypotension, or asystole. Test stimulation through the implanted DBS electrode revealed tremor arrest. There were no postoperative concerns and the patient was discharged the following morning. The patient was seen at 2 weeks' follow-up for adjustment of her DBS settings, which was left at C(+)0(−), 2.2 v, 60 uS, and 150 Hz with tremor arrest and no side effects. At 14 months, she continued to do well and was considering placement of a right DBS electrode to control her remaining left-sided tremors.

3. Discussion

We believe the described episode was consistent with the BJR reflex. This reflex is a cardioinhibitory reflex that has been associated with states of hypovolemia [2]. Its afferent limb is facilitated by cardiac receptors via nonmyelinated type C vagal fibers [3]. An initial response to hypovolemia is sensed in the carotid sinus baroreceptors, causing a compensatory phase with increased heart rate, vasoconstriction, and contractility [3]. However, with an empty hypercontractile ventricle, stimulation of the intramyocardial C fibers can potentiate a sudden withdrawal of sympathetic outflow, increasing vagal tone, which can trigger bradycardia and hypotension [3]. The reflex has been described during spinal anesthesia, due to the decrease in preload, and during shoulder arthroscopic surgery interscalene brachial plexus block, due to venous blood pooling associated with the sitting position. A debatable predisposing factor has been the use of exogenous epinephrine (as a local anesthetic), which may prompt beta-adrenergic effects that increase cardiac contractility, triggering reflex arterial vasodilation and bradycardia [4, 5]. Treatment options include immediate fluid resuscitation, vagolytics (atropine and glycopyrrolate) [6, 7], and early use of IV epinephrine [2]. Other reported therapeutic medications include ondansetron [7], metoprolol [8], and ephedrine [6]. Altering the patient's position to a supine position can also help hemodynamics [9].

Our patient was predisposed to the BJR: (1) she had a history of vasovagal (neurocardiogenic?) syncope, (2) she possessed a thin body frame, which likely put her in a sensitive volume state, (3) she received limited intravenous fluids perioperatively to avoid hypertension, and (4) she was in a beach chair position for surgery, causing venous pooling. Hypovolemia (relative or absolute) could increase the risk of vasodepressor and bradycardic responses [2]. Likewise, short- and long-acting local anesthetic with epinephrine were utilized for the procedure.

Other etiologies of symptomatic bradycardia and hypotension in cranial neurosurgery include venous air embolism and the trigeminal cardiac reflex (TCR) (Table 1). Air

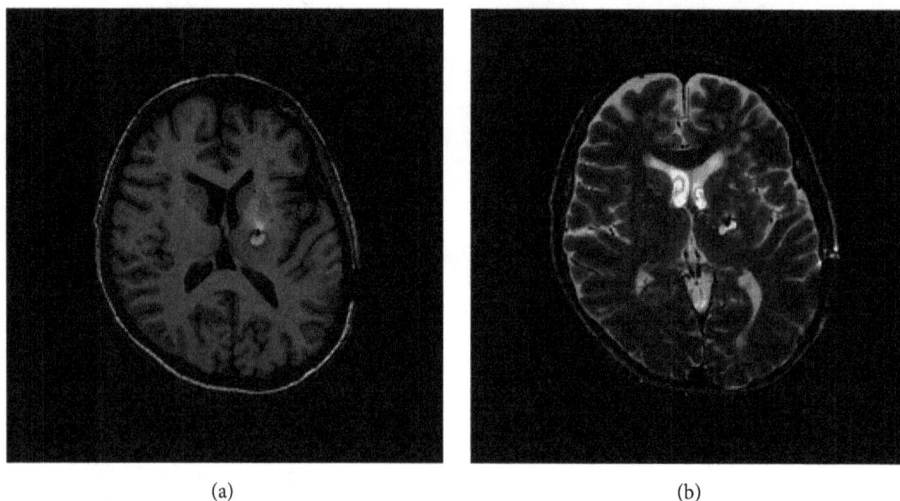

(a)   (b)

FIGURE 2: (a) An MRI brain confirmed a small resolving hematoma at the tip of the lead. (b) An MRI brain confirmed a small resolving hematoma at the tip of the lead.

TABLE 1: Comparison of various etiologies of symptomatic bradycardia and hypotension.

	Venous air embolism	Trigeminal cardiac reflex	Bezold-Jarisch reflex
Incidence	Up to 4.5% in DBS surgeries [10]	Up to 18% in neurosurgery series [11]. No known prior reports in DBS surgery	No known prior reports in neurosurgery
Triggers	Trephination	Irritation of trigeminal nerve or sensory branches	Hypovolemia, spinal anesthesia leading to decrease preload
Mechanism	Entrance of air into venous system	Afferent limb, stimulation of the trigeminal nerve or sensory branches	Afferent limb, cardiac receptors via nonmyelinated type C vagal fibers
		Efferent limb, activation of vagal motor nucleus and inhibition of heart and systemic vascular system	Efferent limb, intramyocardial C fibers can potentiate a sudden withdrawal of sympathetic outflow, increasing vagal tone
Presentation	ST-T changes, right heart strain, oxygen desaturation, low end tidal CO_2, coughing, wheezing, chest pain, "swoon," and so forth	Bradycardia, hypotension, apnea, and gastric hypermotility	Bradycardia, hypotension
Predisposing factors	Sitting position, semisitting position	Use of medications (beta blockers, calcium channel blockers, sufentanil, and alfentanil), history of vagal episodes, presence of hypercapnea or hypoxemia, and light anesthesia	History of neurocardiogenic syncope, hypovolemia, medications (local anesthetic with epinephrine), sitting position, decreasing preload, and venous blood pooling
Treatment	Obtaining hemostasis, irrigation of surgical field, leveling patient's head to right atrium in left lateral decubitus, and use of central venous catheter for aspiration of air	Increased depth of anesthesia (i.e., propofol bolus)	Immediate fluid resuscitation, vagolytics (atropine and glycopyrrolate), ondansetron, metoprolol, and ephedrine

embolism typically occurs during trephination, with an episode of coughing followed by a "swoon" in blood pressure [12, 13]. However, in the case presented here, the episode occurred 90 minutes after her previous burr hole was exposed. There was no new trephination, coughing episode, or elevation in respiratory rate to suggest that venous air embolism was the underlying etiology. Moreover, symptoms from venous air embolism would be gradually progressive and improve only after appropriate therapeutic maneuvers were performed. Our patient had a rapid clinical course, which was inconsistent with a venous air embolism.

The TCR involves stimulation of the trigeminal nerve or sensory branches, which leads to activation of the vagal motor nucleus and inhibition of the heart and systemic vascular system [1, 14]. Placement of a stereotactic frame can elicit the TCR if a pin was erroneously placed on the supraorbital nerve [15]. Irritation of the dura mater (i.e., cauterization of the cerebellar tentorium [16], evacuation of a subdural empyema [17], embolization of dural-based vascular pathologies [14, 18], and resection of a falcine meningioma [19]) may also elicit the reflex. Predisposing factors include the use of certain perioperative medications (beta blockers, calcium channel blockers, sufentanil, and alfentanil), a history of high vagal tone, and the presence of hypercapnea or hypoxemia [16, 20–22]. On the other hand, the depth of sedation and anesthesia may play a role in blocking the reflex [22, 23]. Although the patient was not sedated during implantation of the DBS macroelectrode, irritation of the dura was likely minimal during implantation. Table 1 summarizes the key differences between venous air embolism, TCR, and BJR.

4. Conclusions

With neurosurgery, intraoperative symptomatic bradycardia and hypotension can produce severe consequences if not managed appropriately. The hemodynamic instability may be explained by venous air embolism, the TCR, or the BJR. Previous instances during DBS surgery have been ascribed to venous air embolism during trephination. This report describes a precipitous episode with eventual asystole that was likely mediated by the BJR. This has not been documented previously with DBS surgery. The patient's threshold for the BJR was lowered due to her underlying history, coupled with hypovolemia (based on fluid management, body habitus, and beach chair positioning) and the use of epinephrine as a local anesthetic. After appropriate preventive interventions, the surgery was performed uneventfully.

Competing Interests

The authors declare no competing interests.

References

[1] T. Chowdhury, A. Petropolis, and R. B. Cappellani, "Cardiac emergencies in neurosurgical patients," *BioMed Research International*, vol. 2015, Article ID 751320, 14 pages, 2015.

[2] S. M. Kinsella and J. P. Tuckey, "Perioperative bradycardia and asystole: relationship to vasovagal syncope and the Bezold-Jarisch reflex," *British Journal of Anaesthesia*, vol. 86, no. 6, pp. 859–868, 2001.

[3] J. A. Campagna and C. Carter, "Clinical relevance of the Bezold-Jarisch reflex," *Anesthesiology*, vol. 98, no. 5, pp. 1250–1260, 2003.

[4] K. C. Seo, J. S. Park, and W. S. Roh, "Factors contributing to episodes of bradycardia hypotension during shoulder arthroscopic surgery in the sitting position after interscalene block," *Korean Journal of Anesthesiology*, vol. 58, no. 1, pp. 38–44, 2010.

[5] S. Sia, F. Sarro, A. Lepri, and M. Bartoli, "The effect of exogenous epinephrine on the incidence of hypotensive/bradycardic events during shoulder surgery in the sitting position during interscalene block," *Anesthesia and Analgesia*, vol. 97, no. 2, pp. 583–588, 2003.

[6] J. G. D'Alessio, R. S. Weller, and M. Rosenblum, "Activation of the Bezold-Jarisch reflex in the sitting position for shoulder arthroscopy using interscalene block," *Anesthesia and Analgesia*, vol. 80, no. 6, pp. 1158–1162, 1995.

[7] R. M. Martinek, "Witnessed asystole during spinal anesthesia treated with atropine and ondansetron: a case report," *Canadian Journal of Anesthesia*, vol. 51, no. 3, pp. 226–230, 2004.

[8] G. A. Liguori, R. L. Kahn, J. Gordon, M. A. Gordon, and M. K. Urban, "The use of metoprolol and glycopyrrolate to prevent hypotensive/bradycardic events during shoulder arthroscopy in the sitting position under interscalene block," *Anesthesia and Analgesia*, vol. 87, no. 6, pp. 1320–1325, 1998.

[9] Y. H. Kim, D. J. Kim, and W. Y. Kim, "Bezold–Jarisch reflex caused by postural change," *Journal of Anesthesia*, vol. 29, no. 1, p. 158, 2014.

[10] A. K. Hooper, M. S. Okun, K. D. Foote et al., "Venous air embolism in deep brain stimulation," *Stereotactic and Functional Neurosurgery*, vol. 87, no. 1, pp. 25–30, 2009.

[11] F. Lemaitre, T. Chowdhury, and B. Schaller, "The trigeminocardiac reflex—a comparison with the diving reflex in humans," *Archives of Medical Science*, vol. 11, no. 2, pp. 419–426, 2015.

[12] A. J. Fenoy and R. K. Simpson Jr., "Risks of common complications in deep brain stimulation surgery: management and avoidance-clinical article," *Journal of Neurosurgery*, vol. 120, no. 1, pp. 132–139, 2014.

[13] C. Kenney, R. Simpson, C. Hunter et al., "Short-term and long-term safety of deep brain stimulation in the treatment of movement disorders," *Journal of Neurosurgery*, vol. 106, no. 4, pp. 621–625, 2007.

[14] B. Schaller, A. Filis, and M. Buchfelder, "Trigeminocardiac reflex in embolization of intracranial dural arteriovenous fistula," *American Journal of Neuroradiology*, vol. 29, no. 7, article E55, 2008.

[15] P. Stavrinou, N. Foroglou, I. Patsalas, and P. Selviaridis, "Trigeminocardiac reflex and ipsilateral mydriasis during stereotactic brain tumor biopsy: an insight into the anatomical and physiological pathways involved," *Acta Neurochirurgica*, vol. 152, no. 4, pp. 727–728, 2010.

[16] K. Usami, K. Kamada, N. Kunii, H. Tsujihara, Y. Yamada, and N. Saito, "Transient asystole during surgery for posterior fossa meningioma caused by activation of the trigeminocardiac reflex: three case reports," *Neurologia Medico-Chirurgica*, vol. 50, no. 4, pp. 339–342, 2010.

[17] T. Spiriev, N. Sandu, B. Arasho, S. Kondoff, C. Tzekov, and B. Schaller, "A new predisposing factor for trigemino-cardiac reflex during subdural empyema drainage: a case report," *Journal of Medical Case Reports*, vol. 4, article 391, 2010.

[18] X. Lv, Y. Li, C. Jiang, and Z. Wu, "The incidence of trigeminocardiac reflex in endovascular treatment of dural arteriovenous fistula with onyx," *Interventional Neuroradiology*, vol. 16, no. 1, pp. 59–63, 2010.

[19] D. F. Bauer, A. Youkilis, C. Schenck, C. R. Turner, and B. G. Thompson, "The falcine trigeminocardiac reflex: case report and review of the literature," *Surgical Neurology*, vol. 63, no. 2, pp. 143–148, 2005.

[20] A. Amirjamshidi, K. Abbasioun, F. Etezadi, and S. B. Ghasemi, "Trigeminocardiac reflex in neurosurgical practice: report of two new cases," *Surgical Neurology International*, vol. 4, article 126, 2013.

[21] L. M. Cavallo, D. Solari, and F. Esposito, "Trigeminocardiac reflex: a predictable event with unpredictable aspects," *World Neurosurgery*, vol. 76, no. 5, pp. 407–408, 2011.

34

Late Recovery from Severe *Streptococcus pneumoniae* Comatose Meningitis with Concomitant Diffuse Subcortical Cytotoxic Edema and Cortical Hypometabolism

Philippe Hantson [ID][1] **and Thierry Duprez**[2]

[1]*Department of Intensive Care, Cliniques St-Luc, Université Catholique de Louvain, Brussels, Belgium*
[2]*Department of Neuroradiology, Cliniques St-Luc, Université Catholique de Louvain, Brussels, Belgium*

Correspondence should be addressed to Philippe Hantson; philippe.hantson@uclouvain.be

Academic Editor: Massimiliano Filosto

A 75-year-old woman was admitted to ICU with coma following *Streptococcus pneumoniae* meningitis with bacteremia. Her Glasgow Coma Scale (GCS) score fluctuated around 4 to 6 over the next four weeks. There was no evidence of increased intracranial pressure (ICP). Electroencephalogram (EEG) showed only diffuse aspecific slowing. Impaired cerebral blood flow (CBF) autoregulation was suggested at transcranial Doppler (TCD). Repeated brain magnetic resonance imaging (MRI) examination failed to demonstrate venous thrombosis, arterial ischemic stroke, or brain abscesses but revealed diffuse but reversible cortical cytotoxic edema at diffusion-weighted (DW) sequences. The brain FDG-positron emission tomography (FDG-PET) showed diffuse cortical hypometabolism. The patient unexpectedly experienced a complete neuropsychological recovery the next few weeks. The suggested hypothesis to explain this unusual disease course could be a transient alteration of CBF autoregulation due to some degree of diffuse subcortical microangiopathy. A concomitant reduction of brain metabolism probably prevented the progression towards cortical irreversible ischemic damage.

1. Introduction

Streptococcus pneumoniae meningitis still remains a severe condition leading to a high mortality and morbidity rate in spite of optimal intensive care management. Poor issue usually results from delayed ischemic damage due to inflammation and (micro)vascular thrombosis [1–8]. But a few patients experience a good neurological outcome despite an initially severe and even prolonged coma. A careful analysis of such cases could allow insights into the pathophysiology of brain perfusion and metabolic response at the acute phase in patients experiencing recovery.

2. Case Report

A 75-year-old woman (weight: 72 kg) was admitted to the Emergency Department for agitation with an altered consciousness. Patient's medical history was unremarkable, except for arterial hypertension treated by atenolol. Symptoms started acutely a few hours earlier, with a progressive loss of verbal contact. On admission, the Glasgow Coma Score (GCS) score was 9/15 (E4, V1, M4), with moderate neck stiffness. There was no lateralized deficit and pupils were mid-size, reactive, and symmetric. Vital signs were as follows: body temperature of 36.6°C, arterial blood pressure of 180/95 mm Hg, heart rate of 120/min, and respiratory rate of 60/min. A brain computed tomography (CT) without iodinated contrast agent (CA) perfusion before lumbar puncture did not reveal any significant abnormality. Intubation was required because of progressive respiratory distress. The cerebrospinal fluid (CSF) analysis revealed white blood cells (WBC) count at 560/μl, with 99% granulocytes, proteins at 1264 mg/dl, glucose at 3 mg/dl, and lactate at 27 mmol/l.

The CSF and blood cultures grew positive for *Streptococcus pneumoniae* sensitive to penicillin G and ceftriaxone. The minimal inhibitory concentration (MIC) was 0.016 mcg/ml

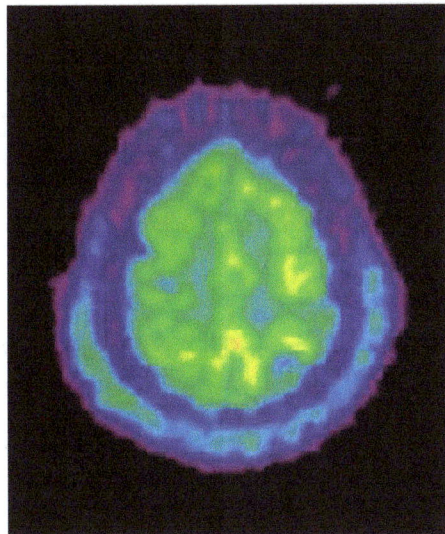

FIGURE 1: Brain ^{18}fluorodeoxyglucose (FDG) positron emission tomography (PET) showing diffuse cortical hypometabolism featured by decreased uptake of the tracer.

for penicillin G and ceftriaxone in the CSF and 0.012 and 0.008 mcg/ml in blood for penicillin G and ceftriaxone, respectively. Treatment combining dexamethasone (10 mg q6h for 4 days) and ceftriaxone (2 g q12h for 14 days) was initiated. CSF analysis was repeated after 10 days and confirmed both a drop in WBC count and eradication of the causative microorganism.

The patient was subsequently referred to the Intensive Care Unit (ICU) because of worsening of GCS score at 6/15 (E1, V1, M4). Despite the lack of evidence of acute hydrocephalus, intracranial pressure (ICP) was monitored by intraventricular catheter and remained within the normal range during the whole ICU stay. The mean arterial blood pressure was around 80 mm Hg. No sedative drugs were required for mechanical ventilation and GCS score remained stable at 6/15. A control brain CA-enhanced CT after 72 hours of therapy failed to reveal brain abscesses, thrombosis, or ischemic lesions. The patient was repeatedly examined by electroencephalogram (EEG) in order to exclude non-convulsive status epilepticus. There was only diffuse slowing with predominance of delta and theta waves, together with some triphasic activity. A brain positron emission tomography (PET) using ^{18}fluorodeoxyglucose (FDG) as tracer was performed on day 13 and was consistent with a diffuse cortical hypometabolism and relatively preserved uptake within grey nuclei (Figure 1). A transcranial Doppler (TCD) examination performed at day 3 suggested that cerebral autoregulation at different levels of mean arterial pressure was abolished. There was no increase in cerebral blood flow velocity (CBFV).

Brain magnetic resonance imaging (MRI) was performed on days 8, 11, and 30. On day 8, while the diffusion-weighted imaging (DWI) and T2/fluid attenuated inversion recovery (FLAIR) sequences were not significantly modified (not shown), there was a marked decrease (300-500 instead of 700.10^{-6} mm^2.sec^{-1}) in the apparent diffusion coefficient

(ADC) diffusely in the subcortical areas, at both the supratentorial and infratentorial levels. This finding was suggestive of cytotoxic edema of U-fibers and immediately adjacent superficial white matter. The picture was relatively unchanged on day 11; magnetic resonance spectroscopy in the areas with low ADC values failed to retrieve any peak of lactate. On day 30, while the patient was still comatose, ADC values in the subcortical territories had returned to normal range and no ischemic damage within overlying cortex had appeared.

The patient remained in deep coma (GCS from 4 to 6/15) for more than four weeks but then started progressively to wake up, with eye opening, and became able to understand verbal command.

She presented two episodes of pneumonia during the ICU stay: a first episode with methicillin-resistant *Staphylococcus aureus* (present at admission screening in the nose and throat sampling) and thereafter a relapse *with Pseudomonas aeruginosa* which had also been initially detected in the throat. Blood cultures remained negative and the patient did not develop septic shock or acute renal failure. However, due to the extension of nosocomial pneumonia, it was necessary to ventilate the patient with 0.5 FiO$_2$ for a long period. Hypoxemia was never observed. Neuromuscular blocking agents were not used during mechanical ventilation. Thus far, in our opinion, the delayed neurological recovery was independent from these infectious complications. The patient stayed in the ICU for a total of 64 days, mainly because of a difficult weaning from the ventilator due to nosocomial pneumonia and critical illness polyneuropathy. At 6-month follow-up, the neuropsychological testing confirmed excellent recovery.

3. Discussion

Cerebrovascular complications are well described during the course of *S. pneumoniae* meningitis [1]. They may extend from cerebral infarction within the first days of the disease to delayed cerebral ischemia that may even occur in patients with an apparently good initial recovery [2–8]. Some reports indicate that vascular complications may occur later on, even months after the meningitis, due to the development of intracranial vascular stenosis [6].

Investigations by TCD in patients with acute bacterial meningitis have shown that patients with lower GCS score at admission had a higher incidence of elevated CBFV (>150 cm/sec) and a higher incidence of ischemic stroke [9]. Arterial vascular narrowing was documented in a significant number of patients, but not all, suggesting that other vascular alterations could occur. The ischemic complications are likely related to the development of a cerebral vasculopathy triggered by the presence of purulent material. In addition to arterial brain vessel narrowing that can be seen at angiography, there is also evidence of widespread microangiopathy involving the primary inflammatory reaction, immune mechanisms, and microthrombosis [10]. The benefit of corticosteroids therapy in *S. pneumoniae* meningitis must not be underestimated [11]. However, it seems difficult to demonstrate that the protective effect of dexamethasone administration is linked to a reduction of ischemic complications [12, 13].

The spectrum of pathological brain MRI was investigated in 136 patients with documented purulent bacterial meningitis (*S. pneumoniae* in 52.6%) [14]. The involvement of cortical parenchyma (20%) and white matter (26.7%) was found in a substantial amount of cases. DWI appeared as a sensitive technique to detect cortical and/or white matter cytotoxic edema. Subcortical low intensity on T2/FLAIR MR images has also been highlighted in a minority of cases of bacterial meningitis [15]. This feature is present at the acute stage and is usually transient. The mechanism beyond this transient subcortical low intensity appears unclear in meningeal diseases. A paramagnetic substance as seen in free radicals could be involved as oxygen free radicals have been implicated as pathologic mediators in experimental models of pneumococcal meningitis [16]. The subcortical low-intensity lesions may have intermediate to low signal intensity on DW images, with the measured ADCs slightly lower than those on the normal white matter. The reason for low ADCs despite poorly modified DW images could be consistent with the accumulation of free radicals in the subcortical white matter rather than with structural lesions [15].

In the present case, central nervous system dysfunction could be related not only to meningitis but also to sepsis [17]. However, the depth and duration of coma were unexpectedly long for sepsis-related encephalopathy. The EEG findings could be consistent with this hypothesis, but they remain unspecific. Regarding MRI, patients with septic shock who develop delirium, coma, seizures, or a focal deficit exhibit evidence of white matter hyperintensities (21%) or ischemic stroke (18%) [18]. White matter hyperintensities may be associated with long-term cognitive impairment. Ischemic stroke is associated with coma, focal neurologic signs, and unfavorable outcomes. Conflicting studies have addressed the influence of sepsis on cerebral blood flow (CBF), and experimental studies have highlighted either increased or decreased CBF. In rats, pneumococcal bacteremia triggered cerebral vasodilation but did not entirely abolish CBF autoregulation in the absence of meningitis [19]. In contrast, CBF autoregulation was lost after intracisternal inoculation of the agent and subsequent meningitis [20]. As our patient suffered systemic hypertension, the theoretical risk for critical hypoperfusion and ischemia was higher during the episodes of low blood pressure. The management of arterial blood pressure was therefore adapted.

4. Conclusion

Despite deep initial and sustained coma, good functional recovery remains possible in some patients suffering from severe *S. pneumoniae* meningitis. In this setting, prolonged coma is not related to the development of diffuse brain abscesses, ischemic damage, vascular thrombosis, or hydrocephalus with increased ICP. Combined brain imaging using MRI and PDG PET could be helpful to assess concomitantly some degree of diffuse but reversible cytotoxic edema (MR diffusion-weighted imaging), more probably due to hypoperfusion together with life-saving diffuse cerebral hypometabolism (FDG-PET) preventing the development of irreversible ischemic damage. This could be considered as a form of reversible microangiopathy, but it remains impossible to affirm that dexamethasone could be helpful in the condition.

Conflicts of Interest

The authors declare that there are no conflicts of interest regarding the publication of this paper.

References

[1] J. Katchanov, P. U. Heuschmann, M. Endres, and J. R. Weber, "Cerebral infarction in bacterial meningitis: Predictive factors and outcome," *Journal of Neurology*, vol. 257, no. 5, pp. 716–720, 2010.

[2] M. Weisfelt, D. Van De Beek, L. Spanjaard, J. B. Reitsma, and J. De Gans, "Clinical features, complications, and outcome in adults with pneumococcal meningitis: A prospective case series," *The Lancet Neurology*, vol. 5, no. 2, pp. 123–129, 2006.

[3] S. Kastenbauer and H.-W. Pfister, "Pneumococcal meningitis in adults: Spectrum of complications and prognostic factors in a series of 87 cases," *Brain*, vol. 126, no. 5, pp. 1015–1025, 2003.

[4] W. Weststrate, A. Hijdra, and J. De Gans, "Brain infarcts in adults with bacterial meningitis [10]," *The Lancet*, vol. 347, no. 8998, p. 399, 1996.

[5] E. S. Schut, M. C. Brouwer, J. De Gans, S. Florquin, D. Troost, and D. Van De Beek, "Delayed cerebral thrombosis after initial good recovery from pneumococcal meningitis," *Neurology*, vol. 73, no. 23, pp. 1988–1995, 2009.

[6] Y. Kato, H. Takeda, T. Dembo, and N. Tanahashi, "Delayed recurrent ischemic stroke after initial good recovery from pneumococcal meningitis," *Internal Medicine*, vol. 51, no. 6, pp. 647–650, 2012.

[7] C. M. Rice, M. Ramamoorthi, S. A. Renowden, P. Heywood, A. L. Whone, and N. J. Scolding, "Cerebral ischaemia in the context of improving, steroid-treated pneumococcal meningitis," *QJM: An International Journal of Medicine*, vol. 105, no. 5, pp. 473–475, 2012.

[8] X. Wittebole, T. Duprez, and P. Hantson, "Delayed cerebral ischaemic injury following apparent recovery from Streptococcus pneumoniae meningitis," *Acta Clinica Belgica: International Journal of Clinical and Laboratory Medicine*, vol. 71, no. 5, pp. 343–346, 2016.

[9] M. Klein, U. Koedel, T. Pfefferkorn, G. Zeller, B. Woehrl, and H. Pfister, "Arterial cerebrovascular complications in 94 adults with acute bacterial meningitis," *Critical Care*, vol. 15, no. 6, p. R281, 2011.

[10] M. D. I. Vergouwen, E. S. Schut, D. Troost, and D. Van De Beek, "Diffuse cerebral intravascular coagulation and cerebral infarction in pneumococcal meningitis," *Neurocritical Care*, vol. 13, no. 2, pp. 217–227, 2010.

[11] M. C. Brouwer, P. McIntyre, K. Prasad, and D. van de Beek, "Corticosteroids for acute bacterial meningitis.," *Cochrane Database of Systematic Reviews*, vol. 6, p. CD004405, 2013.

[12] M. Jit, "The risk of sequelae due to pneumococcal meningitis in high-income countries: A systematic review and meta-analysis," *Infection*, vol. 61, no. 2, pp. 114–124, 2010.

[13] G. Buchholz, U. Koedel, H.-W. Pfister, S. Kastenbauer, and M. Klein, "Dramatic reduction of mortality in pneumococcal meningitis," *Critical Care*, vol. 20, no. 1, 2016.

[14] N. Lummel, M. Koch, M. Klein, H. W. Pfister, H. Brückmann, and J. Linn, "Spectrum and Prevalence of Pathological Intracranial Magnetic Resonance Imaging Findings in Acute Bacterial Meningitis," *Clinical Neuroradiology*, vol. 26, no. 2, pp. 159–167, 2016.

[15] J. H. Lee, D. G. Na, K. H. Choi et al., "Subcortical low intensity on MR images of meningitis, viral encephalitis, and leptomeningeal metastasis," *American Journal of Neuroradiology*, vol. 23, no. 4, pp. 535–542, 2002.

[16] U. Koedel, A. Bernatowicz, R. Paul, K. Frei, A. Fontana, and H. W. Pfister, "Experimental pneumococcal meningitis: cerebrovascular alterations, brain edema, and meningeal inflammation are linked to the production of nitric oxide," *Annals of Neurology*, vol. 37, no. 3, pp. 313–323, 1995.

[17] A. Polito, F. Eischwald, A.-L. L. Maho et al., "Pattern of Brain Injury in the Acute Setting of Human Septic Shock," *Critical Care*, vol. 17, no. 5, 2013.

[18] A. Mazeraud, Q. Pascal, F. Verdonk, N. Heming, F. Chrétien, and T. Sharshar, "Neuroanatomy and Physiology of Brain Dysfunction in Sepsis," *Clinics in Chest Medicine*, vol. 37, no. 2, pp. 333–345, 2016.

[19] M. Pedersen, C. T. Brandt, G. M. Knudsen et al., "The effect of S. pneumoniae bacteremia on cerebral blood flow autoregulation in rats," *Journal of Cerebral Blood Flow & Metabolism*, vol. 28, no. 1, pp. 126–134, 2008.

[20] M. Pedersen, C. T. Brandt, G. M. Knudsen et al., "Cerebral blood flow autoregulation in early experimental S. pneumoniae meningitis," *Journal of Applied Physiology*, vol. 102, no. 1, pp. 72–78, 2007.

35

Bamboo Leaf Sign as a Sensitive Magnetic Resonance Imaging Finding in Spinal Subependymoma

Hiroyuki Toi, Yukari Ogawa, Keita Kinoshita, Satoshi Hirai, Hiroki Takai, Keijiro Hara, Nobuhisa Matsushita, Shunji Matsubara, and Masaaki Uno

Department of Neurosurgery, Kawasaki Medical School, Kurashiki, Okayama, Japan

Correspondence should be addressed to Hiroyuki Toi; ht11251974@yahoo.co.jp

Academic Editor: Isabella Laura Simone

Background and Importance. Subependymoma occurs very rarely in the spinal cord. We report another case of spinal subependymoma along with a review of the literature and discussion of a radiological finding that is useful for preoperative diagnosis of this tumor. *Clinical Presentation.* A 51-year-old man presented with a 2-year history of progressive muscle weakness in the right lower extremity. Sagittal magnetic resonance imaging (MRI) showed spinal cord expansion at the Th7–12 vertebral level. Surgical resection was performed and the tumor was found to involve predominantly subpial growth. Histological diagnosis was subependymoma, classified as Grade I according to criteria of World Health Organization. We made an important discovery of what seems to be a characteristic appearance for spinal subependymoma on sagittal MRI. Swelling of the spinal cord is extremely steep, providing unusually large fusiform dilatation resembling a bamboo leaf. We have termed this characteristic MRI appearance as the "bamboo leaf sign." This characteristic was apparent in 76.2% of cases of spinal subependymoma for which MRI findings were reported. *Conclusion.* The bamboo leaf sign on spinal MRI is useful for differentiating between subependymoma and other intramedullary tumors. Neurosurgeons encountering the bamboo leaf sign on spinal MRI should consider the possibility of subependymoma.

1. Background and Importance

Subependymoma, first described by Scheinker [1] in 1945, is a rare central nervous system tumor, accounting for 0.7% of all intracranial tumors [2]. Subependymoma is a relatively slow-growing benign tumor corresponding histologically to World Health Organization (WHO) Grade I [3]. About 50% of these tumors are clinically silent and only found incidentally at autopsy [3, 4], with the remaining 50% presenting symptomatically during life. This pathology is most frequently identified in the fourth ventricle (50–60%), followed by the lateral ventricles (30–40%) [3–6], and occurs very rarely in the spinal cord. To the best of our knowledge, only 54 cases of spinal subependymomas have been reported in the literature [2, 7–30]. We report here another case of spinal subependymoma with a review of the literature and the new radiological findings, which may be useful for a preoperative diagnosis of this tumor.

2. Clinical Presentation

A 51-year-old man presented with a 2-year history of progressive muscle weakness in the right lower extremity and dysesthesia in both lower extremities. Neurological examination revealed severe loss of all sensory modalities below the L1 dermatomes. Motor examination revealed monoparesis of the right lower limbs, and muscle power assessment showed Grade 1/5 in tibialis anterior, extensor hallucis longus, gastrocnemius, and flexor hallucis longus in Manual Muscle Testing. Deep tendon reflexes in both lower limbs were hyperactive. He presented with slight bladder and rectal disturbance of constipation and inability to urinate.

2.1. Neuroimaging Findings. Sagittal images from T2-weighted imaging (T2WI) (Figure 1(a)) showed cord expansion and a hyperintense signal extending from the Th7 to Th12 vertebral level, surrounding both anterior and posterior aspects of

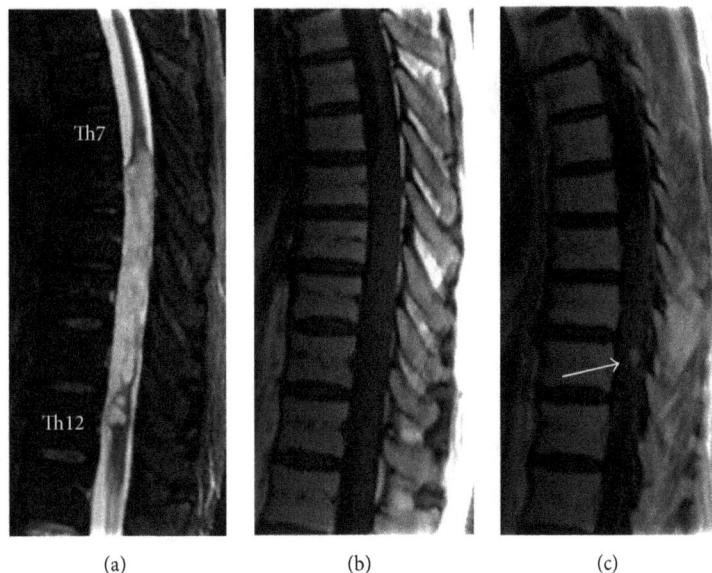

(a)   (b)   (c)

FIGURE 1: (a) Sagittal T2W1 showing cord expansion and hyperintense signal extending from the Th7 level to Th12 level surrounding both anterior and posterior aspects of cord. (b) Sagittal T1W1 showing an isointense mass with no clear-cut demarcation between cord and tumor. (c) Gadolinium contrast-enhanced MRI reveals slight enhancement. This is only a part of the tumor.

the cord. Sagittal images from T1-weighted imaging (T1WI) (Figure 1(b)) revealed an isointense mass lesion with no clear-cut demarcation of the interface between the spinal cord and tumor. A small enhanced portion was seen with gadolinium administration (Figure 1(c)). Axial T2WI showed extension of the tumor along bilateral surfaces of the spinal cord with strong compression (Figure 2). The spinal cord was severely deformed from compression by the tumor. At the marginal portion of the tumor, cord expansion was extremely steep. Imaging findings were considered to favor an intramedullary tumor, and differential diagnoses of ependymoma and astrocytoma were considered.

2.2. Operative Intervention and Findings. A two-stage operation for resection of the tumor was performed. The first surgery included Th7–Th12 laminectomy and removal of half of the tumor. Two weeks postoperatively, a second surgery was performed to remove the residual tumor. The tumor was found to be predominantly subpial, showing an eccentric position with an indistinct plane between the tumor and cord. The tumor was soft, greyish, and avascular and was lying bilaterally alongside the spinal cord. Radical tumor decompression was performed and subtotal resection was achieved.

2.3. Histopathological Findings. The tumor tissue was fixed in 10% neutral-buffered formalin, routinely processed, and embedded in paraffin. Sections of $5\,\mu$m thickness were cut, stained with hematoxylin and eosin, and examined. The tumor comprised cells with fine processes and round-to-ovoid nuclei, arranged in clusters within microcystic backgrounds. No ependymal rosette formation was seen. Morphological features of malignancy, such as cellular anaplasia, necrosis, and increased mitosis, were absent. MIB-I labeling index was very low (0.1%). Based on these features, a

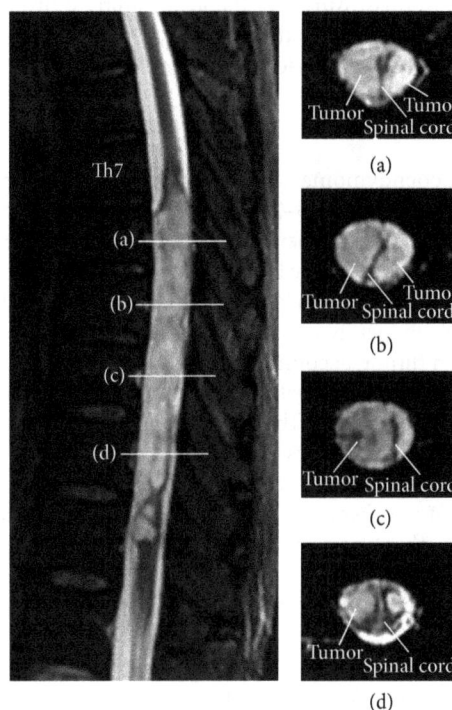

FIGURE 2: Axial T2WI at the Th8–11 level, showing an eccentric intramedullary tumor located bilaterally. Bars indicate levels of axial views for Th8 (a), Th9 (b), Th10 (c), and Th11 (d).

histological diagnosis of subependymoma (WHO Grade I) was made.

2.4. Postoperative Course. Postoperatively, the patient developed paraparesis and severe bladder and rectal disturbance.

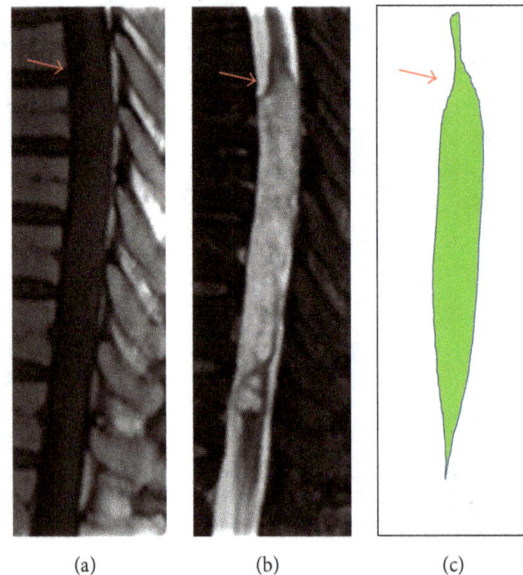

(a)   (b)   (c)

FIGURE 3: Bamboo leaf sign. The figure shows MRI of spinal subependymoma from our case. (a) T1WI. (b) T2WI. Sagittal MRI shows steep swelling of the spinal cord (arrows) and unusually large fusiform dilatation, resembling the shape of a bamboo leaf (c).

Muscle power assessment of the lower limbs showed Grade 2/5. No delayed complications or tumor recurrence occurred during the follow-up period of 24 months.

3. Discussion

Spinal subependymoma is much less frequent than intracranial subependymoma [3–7, 13, 31]. Since the initial description of spinal cord subependymoma by Boykin et al., 54 cases have been reported in the literature [1–48]. Most reports have involved single cases; no large series have been described.

Spinal subependymoma is a slow-growing and noninvasive benign tumor, accounting for 1~2% of all spinal ependymal tumors [32]. This pathology corresponds histologically to WHO Grade I [33]. The age of patients at diagnosis has ranged from 6 to 73 years, with a mean of 43.6 years. A male preponderance has been noted (males : females = 3 : 2) [1–48]. The majority of these tumors have shown an intramedullary location, within the cervical (26 cases), thoracic (22 cases), or lumbar region (2 cases). One patient displayed holocord subependymoma. In 3 cases, location of the tumor was not described [9].

The majority of spinal subependymomas originate from intra-axial tissue. A distinctive feature noted at surgery is the eccentric subpial location of these subependymomas, in contrast with the central location of ependymomas and astrocytomas. A number of reports have described subependymoma exhibiting subpial growth.

This tumor is difficult to differentiate from spinal astrocytoma or ependymoma on the basis of clinical and radiological findings. No pathognomonic features distinctive for subependymoma have previously been reported on MRI. We report for the first time a specific feature of spinal subependymoma on MRI which may help distinguish this tumor from other intramedullary tumors, such as astrocytoma or ependy-

moma. We made an important discovery of a characteristic appearance common to spinal subependymomas on sagittal MRI. Swelling of the spinal cord is extremely steep, taking the form of an unusually large fusiform dilatation resembling a bamboo leaf on sagittal MRI (Figure 3). We have therefore termed this characteristic appearance as the "bamboo leaf sign" (Figure 4). MRI findings have been described for 21 cases reported since 1995 (including the present case), with 16 cases (76.2%) displaying the bamboo leaf sign (Table 1). This sign is the product of the steep swelling of the spinal cord resulting from subpial growth of the tumor (Figure 4).

Spinal astrocytoma and ependymoma do not show the bamboo leaf sign due to their central location in the spinal cord. MRI instead reveals gradual fusiform dilatation of the spinal cord with these tumors. The bamboo leaf sign thus appears useful for differentiating between subependymoma and other intramedullary tumors, although careful differentiation is needed for subpial growing tumors such as hemangioblastomas and intramedullary infection.

4. Conclusion

Due to the rarity of spinal subependymoma, this pathology may be omitted from preoperative differential diagnosis; however, awareness of the existence of these tumors within the spinal cord is necessary. It is important for neurosurgeons and pathologists to recognize and diagnose this entity and to differentiate it from both astrocytoma and ependymoma. The importance of correct diagnosis lies in the fact that these tumors are completely benign, and total resection will achieve complete cures without the need for adjuvant therapy. When total resection is impossible due to a lack of demarcation from the cord or tumor infiltration into the surrounding cord, aggressive treatment should be avoided.

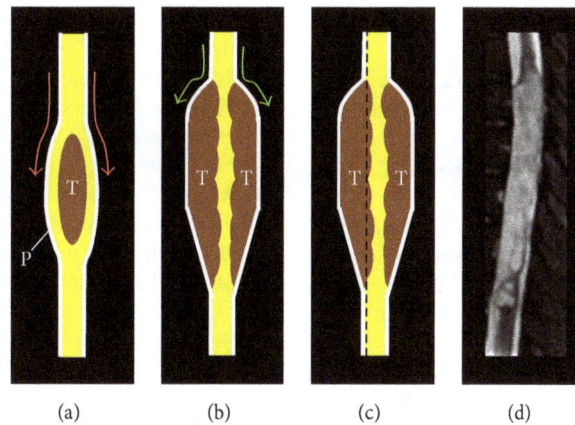

FIGURE 4: Schematic representation of MRI findings for spinal subependymoma demonstrating the bamboo leaf sign. (a) Other intramedullary tumors like ependymoma and astrocytoma show gradual dilatation of the spinal cord. (b) Spinal subependymoma shows steep swelling of the spinal cord due to subpial growth. (c) Blue dashed line shows sagittal section for MRI of the spinal subependymoma. (d) Sagittal T2WI of subependymoma showing bamboo leaf sign. T, tumor; P, pia mater.

TABLE 1: Summary of cases of spinal subependymomas reported since 1995.

Author, year	Number of reported cases	MRI available cases	Tumor location (MRI available cases)	Bamboo leaf sign
Hoeffel et al., 1995	1	1	C1–5	+
Tacconi et al., 1996	1	1	C6-7	+
Jallo et al., 1996	6	3	C6-Th1/C4-Th1/C7-Th1	+/+/−
Dario et al., 2001	1	1	Th9-L1	+
Matsumoto and Nakagaki, 2002	1	1	Th2–7	+
Sarkar et al., 2003	1	1	C3–7	−
Shimada et al., 2003	2	1	Th5–8	+
Kremer et al., 2004	1	1	Th11-L2	+
Fukuzumi et al., 2006	1	1	Th3–7	+
Yadav et al., 2008	1	1	Th5–9	+
Jang et al., 2009	1	1	Th11-12	−
Orakcioglu et al., 2009	2	2	Th10-l2/Th11-L1	+/+
Zenmyo et al., 2010	1	1	C1-2	−
Jabri et al., 2010	1	1	Th10-L1	+
Yamamoto, 2010	4	1	C6-Th5	+
Krishnan et al., 2012	1	1	C3-Th4	+
Iwasaki et al., 2013	1	1	Th11-12	−
Our case, 2013	1	1	Th7–12	+
Total	28	21	C: 8 cases/Th: 13 cases	16 (76.2%)

Even if the tumor remains, long-term prognosis is considered good because of the benign behavior of this pathology. For neurosurgeons encountering the bamboo leaf sign on spinal MRI, the possibility of subependymoma should be kept in mind.

Competing Interests

The authors have no personal financial or institutional interest in any of the drugs, materials, or devices in the article.

References

[1] I. M. Scheinker, "Subependymoma: a newly recognized tumor of subependymal derivation," *Journal of Neurosurgery*, vol. 2, no. 3, pp. 232–240, 1945.

[2] L. Tacconi, F. G. Johnston, and D. G. T. Thomas, "Subependymoma of the cervical cord," *Clinical Neurology and Neurosurgery*, vol. 98, no. 1, pp. 24–26, 1996.

[3] O. D. Wiestler and D. Schiffer, "Subependymoma," in *Pathology & Genetics: Tumours of the Nervous System*, P. Kleihues and

W. K. Cavenee, Eds., pp. 80–81, IARC Press, Lyon, France, 2000.

[4] B. W. Scheithauer, "Symptomatic subependymoma. Report of 21 cases with review of the literature," *Journal of Neurosurgery*, vol. 49, no. 5, pp. 689–696, 1978.

[5] R. Jooma, M. J. Torrens, J. Bradshaw, and B. Brownell, "Subependymomas of the fourth ventricle. Surgical treatment in 12 cases," *Journal of Neurosurgery*, vol. 62, no. 4, pp. 508–512, 1985.

[6] J. W. Ironside, T. H. Moss, D. N. Louis, J. S. Lowe, and R. O. Weller, "Ependymal and choroid plexus tumours," in *Diagnostic Pathology of Nervous System Tumours*, pp. 145–183, Churchill Livingstone, London, UK, 2002.

[7] F. C. Boykin, D. Cowen, C. A. Iannucci, and A. Wolf, "Subependymal glomerate astrocytomas," *Journal of Neuropathology and Experimental Neurology*, vol. 13, no. 1, pp. 30–49, 1954.

[8] F. Slowik, E. Pásztor, and B. Szöllösi, "Subependymal gliomas," *Neurosurgical Review*, vol. 2, no. 2, pp. 79–86, 1979.

[9] F. Pluchino, S. Lodrini, G. Lasio, and A. Allegranza, "Complete removal of holocord subependymoma. Case report," *Acta Neurochirurgica*, vol. 73, no. 3-4, pp. 243–250, 1984.

[10] M. Salcman and R. Mayer, "Intramedullary subependymoma of the cervical spinal cord: case report," *Neurosurgery*, vol. 14, no. 5, pp. 608–611, 1984.

[11] J. Cervos-Navarro, J. Artigas, and A. Perez-Canto, "Clinical and immunohistological findings in subependymomas of the spinal cord," *Verhandlungen der Deutschen Gesellschaft fur Pathologie*, vol. 70, pp. 376–379, 1986.

[12] K. S. Lee, J. N. Angelo, J. M. McWhorter, and C. H. Davis Jr., "Symptomatic subependymoma of the cervical spinal cord. Report of two cases," *Journal of Neurosurgery*, vol. 67, no. 1, pp. 128–131, 1987.

[13] A. Matsumura, A. Hori, and O. Spoerri, "Spinal subependymoma presenting as an extramedullary tumor: case report," *Neurosurgery*, vol. 23, no. 1, pp. 115–117, 1988.

[14] L. Bardella, M. Artico, and F. Nucci, "Intramedullary subependymoma of the cervical spinal cord," *Surgical Neurology*, vol. 29, no. 4, pp. 326–329, 1988.

[15] M. Nagashima, T. Isu, Y. Iwasaki et al., "Intramedullary subependymoma of the cervical spinal cord. Case report," *Neurologia Medico-Chirurgica*, vol. 28, no. 3, pp. 303–308, 1988.

[16] J. Vaquero, R. Martinez, I. Vegazo, and P. Ponton, "Subependymoma of the cervical spinal cord," *Neurosurgery*, vol. 24, pp. 625–627, 1989.

[17] A. Guha, L. Resch, and C. H. Tator, "Subependymoma of the thoracolumbar cord. Case report," *Journal of Neurosurgery*, vol. 71, no. 5, pp. 781–787, 1989.

[18] B. Lach, N. Russell, and B. Benoit, "Atypical subependymoma of the spinal cord: ultrastructural and immunohistochemical studies," *Neurosurgery*, vol. 27, no. 2, pp. 319–325, 1990.

[19] T. A. Bergman and S. J. Haines, "Subependymoma of the cervical spinal cord. A case report of long-term survival," *Minnesota Medicine*, vol. 74, no. 11, pp. 21–24, 1991.

[20] F. H. Tomlinson, B. W. Scheithauer, P. J. Kelly, and G. S. Forbes, "Subependymoma with rhabdomyosarcomatous differentiation: report of a case and literature review," *Neurosurgery*, vol. 28, no. 5, pp. 761–768, 1991.

[21] S. Nakasu, Y. Nakasu, A. Saito, and J. Handa, "Intramedullary subependymoma with neurofibromatosis. Report of two cases," *Neurologia Medico-Chirurgica*, vol. 32, no. 5, pp. 275–280, 1992.

[22] C. A. Pagni, S. Canavero, M. T. Giordana, M. Mascalchi, and G. Arnetoli, "Spinal intramedullary subependymomas: case report

and review of the literature," *Neurosurgery*, vol. 30, no. 1, pp. 115–117, 1992.

[23] M. Salvati, A. Raco, M. Artico, S. Artizzu, and P. Ciappetta, "Subependymoma of the spinal cord. Case report and review of the literature," *Neurosurgical Review*, vol. 15, no. 1, pp. 65–69, 1992.

[24] A. T. H. Casey, H. Marsh, and P. Wilkins, "Subependymoma of the thoracic cord: potential pitfalls in diagnosis," *British Journal of Neurosurgery*, vol. 7, no. 3, pp. 319–322, 1993.

[25] M. Polivka, G. Lot, F. Woimant, A. Lavergne, F. Chedru, and J. Mikol, "Seven cases of subependymoma. Anatomoclinical study and review of the literature," *Archives d'Anatomie et de Cytologie Pathologiques*, vol. 42, pp. 141–148, 1994.

[26] M. B. Roeder, J. R. Jinkins, and C. Bazan, "Subependymoma of filum terminale: MR appearance," *Journal of Computer Assisted Tomography*, vol. 18, no. 1, pp. 129–130, 1994.

[27] C. Hoeffel, M. Boukobza, M. Polivka et al., "MR manifestations of subependymomas," *American Journal of Neuroradiology*, vol. 16, no. 10, pp. 2121–2129, 1995.

[28] G. I. Jallo, D. Zagzag, and F. Epstein, "Intramedullary subependymoma of the spinal cord," *Neurosurgery*, vol. 38, no. 2, pp. 251–257, 1996.

[29] P. Bret, R. Bougeard, G. Saint-Pierre, J. Guyotat, A.-C. Ricci, and C. Confavreux, "Intramedullary subependymoma of the cervical spinal cord. Review of the literature a propos of a case," *Neurochirurgie*, vol. 43, no. 3, pp. 158–163, 1997.

[30] A. Dario, P. Fachinetti, M. Cerati, and A. Dorizzi, "Subependymoma of the spinal cord: case report and review of literature," *Journal of Clinical Neuroscience*, vol. 8, no. 1, pp. 48–50, 2001.

[31] D. Schiffer, A. Chiò, M. T. Giordana et al., "Histologic prognostic factors in ependymoma," *Child's Nervous System*, vol. 7, no. 4, pp. 177–182, 1991.

[32] A. Boström, M. von Lehe, W. Hartmann et al., "Surgery for spinal cord ependymomas: outcome and prognostic factors," *Neurosurgery*, vol. 68, no. 2, pp. 302–309, 2011.

[33] D. N. Louis, H. Ohgaki, O. D. Wiestler, and W. K. Cavenee, *WHO Classification of Tumours of the Central Nervous System*, International Agency for Research on Cancer (IARC), Lyon, France, 4th edition, 2007.

[34] M. Artico, L. Bardella, P. Ciappetta, and A. Raco, "Surgical treatment of subependymomas of the central nervous system. Report of 8 cases and review of the literature," *Acta Neurochirurgica*, vol. 98, no. 1-2, pp. 25–31, 1989.

[35] Y. Fukuzumi, S. Tani, A. Isoshima, H. Nagashima, T. Abe, and J. Fujigasaki, "Spinal cord subependymoma—a case report and review of the literature," *Spinal Surgery*, vol. 20, no. 4, pp. 245–251, 2006.

[36] H.-D. Herrmann, M. Neuss, and D. Winkler, "Intramedullary spinal cord tumors resected with CO2 laser microsurgical technique: recent experience in fifteen patients," *Neurosurgery*, vol. 22, no. 3, pp. 518–522, 1988.

[37] M. Iwasaki, K. Hida, T. Aoyama, and K. Houkin, "Thoracolumbar intramedullary subependymoma with multiple cystic formation: a case report and review," *European Spine Journal*, vol. 22, Supplement 3, pp. S317–S320, 2013.

[38] H. E. Jabri, M. A. Dababo, and A. M. Alkhani, "Subependymoma of the spine," *Neurosciences*, vol. 15, no. 2, pp. 126–128, 2010.

[39] W.-Y. Jang, J.-K. Lee, J.-H. Lee et al., "Intramedullary subependymoma of the thoracic spinal cord," *Journal of Clinical Neuroscience*, vol. 16, no. 6, pp. 851–853, 2009.

[40] P. Kremer, S. Zoubaa, and P. Schramm, "Intramedullary subependymoma of the lower spinal cord," *British Journal of Neurosurgery*, vol. 18, no. 5, pp. 548–551, 2004.

[41] S. S. Krishnan, M. Panigrahi, S. Pendyala, S. I. Rao, and D. R. Varma, "Cervical Subependymoma: a rare case report with possible histogenesis," *Journal of Neurosciences in Rural Practice*, vol. 3, no. 3, pp. 366–369, 2012.

[42] K. Matsumoto and H. Nakagaki, "Intramedullary subependymoma occupying the right half of the thoracic spinal cord—case report," *Neurologia Medico-Chirurgica*, vol. 42, no. 8, pp. 349–353, 2002.

[43] B. Orakcioglu, P. Schramm, P. Kohlhof, A. Aschoff, A. Unterberg, and M.-E. Halatsch, "Characteristics of thoracolumbar intramedullary subependymomas: clinical article," *Journal of Neurosurgery: Spine*, vol. 10, no. 1, pp. 54–59, 2009.

[44] C. Sarkar, S. Mukhopadhyay, A. M. Ralte et al., "Intramedullary subependymoma of the spinal cord: a case report and review of literature," *Clinical Neurology and Neurosurgery*, vol. 106, no. 1, pp. 63–68, 2003.

[45] S. Shimada, K. Ishizawa, H. Horiguchi, T. Shimada, and T. Hirose, "Subependymoma of the spinal cord and review of the literature," *Pathology International*, vol. 53, no. 3, pp. 169–173, 2003.

[46] R. K. Yadav, S. Agarwal, J. Saini, and N. K. Sharma, "Imaging appearance of subependymoma: a rare tumor of the cord," *Indian Journal of Cancer*, vol. 45, no. 1, pp. 33–35, 2008.

[47] S. Yamamoto, "Characteristics of intramedullary subependymoma," *Spinal Surgery*, vol. 24, pp. 100–102, 2010.

[48] M. Zenmyo, Y. Ishido, M. Terahara et al., "Intramedullary subependymoma of the cervical spinal cord: a case report with immunohistochemical study," *International Journal of Neuroscience*, vol. 120, no. 10, pp. 676–679, 2010.

36

EEG-Triggered Functional Electrical Stimulation Therapy for Restoring Upper Limb Function in Chronic Stroke with Severe Hemiplegia

Cesar Marquez-Chin,[1,2] **Aaron Marquis,**[2] **and Milos R. Popovic**[1,3]

[1]Rehabilitation Engineering Laboratory, The Lyndhurst Centre, Toronto Rehabilitation Institute-University Health Network, 520 Sutherland Drive, Toronto, ON, Canada M4G 3V9
[2]Neural Engineering Laboratory, University Centre, Toronto Rehabilitation Institute-University Health Network, 550 University Avenue, Toronto, ON, Canada M5G 2A2
[3]Rehabilitation Engineering Laboratory, Institute of Biomaterials and Biomedical Engineering, University of Toronto, Mining Building, 164 College Street, Room 407, Toronto, ON, Canada M5S 3E3

Correspondence should be addressed to Cesar Marquez-Chin; cesar.marquez@uhn.ca

Academic Editor: Norman S. Litofsky

We report the therapeutic effects of integrating brain-computer interfacing technology and functional electrical stimulation therapy to restore upper limb reaching movements in a 64-year-old man with severe left hemiplegia following a hemorrhagic stroke he sustained six years prior to this study. He completed 40 90-minute sessions of functional electrical stimulation therapy using a custom-made neuroprosthesis that facilitated 5 different reaching movements. During each session, the participant attempted to reach with his paralyzed arm repeatedly. Stimulation for each of the movement phases (e.g., extending and retrieving the arm) was triggered when the power in the 18 Hz–28 Hz range (beta frequency range) of the participant's EEG activity, recorded with a single electrode, decreased below a predefined threshold. The function of the participant's arm showed a clinically significant improvement in the Fugl-Meyer Assessment Upper Extremity (FMA-UE) subscore (6 points) as well as moderate improvement in Functional Independence Measure Self-Care subscore (7 points). The changes in arm's function suggest that the combination of BCI technology and functional electrical stimulation therapy may restore voluntary motor function in individuals with chronic hemiplegia which results in severe upper limb deficit (FMA-UE $\leq$ 15), a population that does not benefit from current best-practice rehabilitation interventions.

1. Introduction

Stroke is one of the most common causes of disability [1, 2]. It can be the result of a rupture or infarction of the blood vessels supplying the brain, respectively, referred to as hemorrhagic or ischemic stroke. These events damage neighboring tissue and may lead to necrosis which can have important negative functional repercussions. The location and extent of the lesion often determine the nature and severity of the sequelae. Stroke often results in hemiplegia, in which one side of the body is paralyzed, when only one cerebral hemisphere is affected. This paralysis can have catastrophic effects on the independence and quality of life of individuals who have

had a stroke. Impairments may range from very subtle (mild hemiplegia), in which individuals are able to continue performing movements to assist them in activities of daily living, to high (severe hemiplegia), in which the ability to move is greatly reduced or lost completely.

Despite the advances in the rehabilitation to restore voluntary movement after stroke, there are still individuals for whom effective intervention options are very limited. In particular, people with severe motor impairments may not be able to benefit from existing conventional therapies [1]. This is the case with stroke patients with severe upper limb deficit, measured by Fugl-Meyer Assessment Upper Extremity (FMA-UE) subscore of values equal to or lesser than 15. This situation is even more difficult for individuals with chronic conditions as recovery often takes place during the first months after having a stroke.

One of the few therapies available for individuals with severe hemiplegia following stroke is functional electrical stimulation therapy (FEST) [3]. Several reports suggest that this intervention is one of the most successful strategies to promote recovery after stroke and spinal cord injury [4–8]. Patients receiving FEST are asked to attempt a battery of specific movements and, after a few moments of unsuccessfully trying to perform the movement (e.g., 3 s–6 s), a therapist triggers a train of highly controlled electrical pulses to the paralyzed limb(s) producing the intended movement artificially. As patients recover voluntary function, the use of electrical stimulation is decreased gradually until it is completely discontinued.

The typical format for FEST is 40 one-hour sessions delivered three to five times per week for several months. In each session, patients engage in repetitive tasks focusing on their specific rehabilitation needs. For impaired upper limb movement after stroke, it is common to first focus on restoring reaching. Patients are asked to, for example, reach forward, sustain the arm extended for a few seconds, and then to retrieve their arm with all of the phases of movement assisted by electrical stimulation (i.e., reach, hold, and retract). Once recovery of reaching function is evident, grasping movements are practiced in subsequent therapeutic sessions, sometimes together with reaching movements and sometimes in isolation.

Brain-computer interfaces use brain signals to control electronic devices. Their operation does not require any voluntary movement, making this technology very promising to assist individuals with little or no ability to move. Populations that may benefit directly from this technology include individuals with amyotrophic lateral sclerosis, severe cases of cerebral palsy, and stroke resulting in total loss of motor function (e.g., brain stem stroke) [9]. Originally intended as an assistive device, this technology has been used to facilitate communication [10] and control computer cursors [11, 12], orthotic devices [13], and neuroprostheses [14–16], among other applications.

In the last decade, there has been an increased interest in the potential use of BCI technology to promote recovery of voluntary function after an insult to the nervous system, including stroke and spinal cord injury. One approach to use BCIs as part of a rehabilitation intervention to restore movement consists of training individuals to operate a BCI through motor imagery. Specifically, patients learn how to produce changes in the amplitude of the alpha (8 Hz–12 Hz) and/or beta (13 Hz–30 Hz) frequency ranges of their EEG by imagining voluntary movements [17–19]. These decreases in power, frequently referred to as event related desynchronization (ERD), can typically be observed during preparation, execution, and imagination of voluntary movement and have been used extensively for implementing BCI systems.

The main rationale behind training patients to produce ERD stems from observations in other forms of therapy, not including BCI technology, in which the EEG undergoes changes as functional improvement takes place; the brain

activity can transform from a lack of response at the beginning of therapy to normalized ERD during movement at the time of discharge. The driving hypothesis of this intervention is that teaching patients how to produce normal motor-related EEG activity will result in improvements in voluntary motor function [20].

A recent report described an intervention consisting of motor-imagery-based BCI sessions held immediately before regular physical therapy sessions [21]. Participants in the intervention group were trained to produce voluntary power decreases in sensorimotor rhythms, recorded from their ipsilesional motor cortex, to control hand and arm orthosis. The participants in the control group did not use BCI system to control the hand and arm orthosis; instead it was activated randomly. Both the intervention and control groups received physiotherapy immediately after using the BCI. The "BCI therapy" produced a higher and significant increase in upper limb function at the end of the intervention compared to the control group.

More recently, a randomized control trial conducted by Pichiorri and colleagues [22] explored the use of BCI technology to monitor motor imagery during sessions conducted in addition to regular rehabilitation. In that study, 28 patients who had sustained a stroke a maximum of six weeks before the study underwent an intervention in which they were required to perform kinesthetic imagery of grasping and finger extension with their affected hands. The changes in power in the EEG activity resulting from the imagined movements by the participants in the intervention group ($n = 14$) controlled the movements of a life-size virtual hand projected on a screen placed over their hands. The individuals in the control group had a similar setup but excluded online control of the virtual hand. Their results showed greater functional outcomes for the intervention group, which also had an increased probability of achieving clinically significant changes.

A second method for incorporating a BCI into a rehabilitation intervention, and the one followed in this report, consists of activating an external device designed to facilitate movement of a paralyzed limb upon detecting the intention to move through analysis of brain activities during the rehabilitation sessions. The main hypothesis supporting this approach is that the paring of a motor command (produced when patients attempt to move) and relevant and correct sensory information (resulting from the artificially produced movement) will produce neuroplastic changes that in turn will result in improved voluntary motor function [20].

Control of orthotic and neuroprosthetic devices using BCI technology has been demonstrated several times [13–16], but exploration of the therapeutic effects of the combined technologies has only started recently with efforts focused primarily on the control of robotic rehabilitation systems. A recent randomized control trial conducted by Ang et al. tested the effects of a BCI-controlled robotic system to restore two-dimensional upper limb function [23]. Participants of that study attempted to reach to eight different targets with the assistance of the robotic device. The robot was triggered automatically or with mechanical cues for the control group and with a motor imagery-based BCI for the experimental group. Both groups experienced an improvement of arm's function after four weeks of treatment, with the intervention group requiring lower intensity therapy to experience the improvements (136 versus 1,040 repetitions for the intervention and control groups, resp.).

Daly and colleagues conducted an important study in which they used a BCI-controlled FEST for restoring voluntary finger's function [24]. The participant of that study had lost the ability to move her fingers individually as a result of a stroke she had sustained 10 months prior to the study. During the intervention, she was asked to attempt moving her fingers individually, and a BCI detected her intention to move, identified as a power reduction in the 13 Hz–30 Hz frequency range. The BCI, in turn, triggered a neuroprosthesis that produced the intended movement. The participant's ability to perform isolated finger movements increased after nine sessions.

We present here a proof of concept use of a BCI-triggered FEST for restoring upper limb's function. This combination of technologies was created as an enhancement to FEST in which activation of the stimulation was achieved by identifying changes in the EEG oscillatory activity indicating the attempt to move. The system was tested with a person with chronic hemiplegia (6 years after stoke) with severe upper limb deficit (FMA-UE ≤ 15), for whom all other forms of therapy had failed to produce any functional improvements in his ability to reach and for whom the expectations for recovery were low. This report describes our findings as well as some of the experiences that we had during this practical application of BCI technology.

2. Materials and Methods

2.1. Participant. The participant was a 64-year-old man who had sustained a right hemorrhagic stroke 72 months (six years) prior to his participation in this research study. Tomographic images confirmed an intraparenchymal hemorrhage deep in the right brain involving the subinsular and general capsule extending upward to the corona radiate. He had severe left hemiplegia with no residual movement. Prior to the stroke, he was left-handed. His arm and hand were at stage 1 on the Chedoke-McMaster Stages of Movement Recovery [25] and his FMA-UE subscore was 13. Prior to receiving BCI+FET, every other therapeutic intervention, including FET (without EEG activation) completed six months before this study, had failed to produce any clinically meaningful changes in his upper limb's function. He provided written informed consent to participate in this study, which was approved by the Toronto Rehabilitation Institute-University Health Network Research Ethics Board.

2.2. Experimental Setup

2.2.1. Neuroprosthesis for Reaching. The neuroprosthesis for reaching was implemented with a four-channel programmable stimulator (Compex, Switzerland) [26], which was configured to produce the following reaching movements.

Forward Reaching and Retrieving. It was produced by delivering stimulation to the *anterior deltoid* and the *triceps brachii* muscles (forward reaching) and posterior deltoid and biceps brachii (retrieve).

Reaching to the Mouth. It was achieved by stimulating to the *anterior deltoid* and the *biceps brachii muscles* (forward reaching) and *posterior deltoid* and *triceps brachii* (retrieve).

Lateral Reaching. Lateral reaching included stimulating *biceps brachii* followed by *anterior* and *posterior deltoid* and finally by the *triceps brachii* (lateral reaching); retrieving was produced with stimulation of the *biceps brachii* muscle, interrupting stimulation to the deltoid muscle, and stimulating *triceps brachii* again to produce extension of the arm.

In addition to these movements, the stimulation sequence for forward reaching and retrieving was used to produce *reaching to the right knee and retrieving*, and the stimulation synergy for reaching to the mouth was also used to facilitate *reaching to the right shoulder and retrieving*.

The neuroprosthesis was designed to perform agonist and antagonist movements, each triggered in response to a command signal (e.g., external switch or BCI activation). For example, one BCI activation would facilitate a forward reaching motion of the arm and a second activation would trigger retrieval of the arm and its return to the starting (relaxed) position. Stimulation sequences for all of the facilitated movements can be found in Figure 1.

2.2.2. Brain-Computer Interface. The participant first completed a calibration session in which he was asked to attempt a series of six different hand movements with his left (affected) hand following a READY-GO-STOP cue (details provided in Figure 2). The movements included precision pinch, lateral and palmar grasps, and hand opening. Hand movements were chosen due to their common use in the configuration of motor-imagery-based BCIs. The numbers of repetitions for each movement are displayed in Table 1. At the same time, we recorded EEG from six different locations (F3, Fz, F4, C3, Cz, and C4 of the 10–20-electrode placement system) over premotor and motor cortical areas using the linked ears as a reference and the right mastoid as ground. No additional preprocessing was performed, as we wanted to create a BCI using a single electrode. The signals were digitized at 1,000 samples per second and band-limited between 0.05 Hz and 40 Hz. The EEG and the experimental cues were recorded using a SynAmps RT EEG amplifier (Compumedics, USA).

We segmented the EEG data into each one of the repetitions, which were aligned with respect to the GO cue. We then inspected each one of the repetitions for all movements visually and discarded any that was affected by interference, in which an incorrect movement was performed or in which the movement was not performed within the allotted time. All of the remaining repetitions for each movement were pooled together for further processing. After this, a spectrogram was generated for each one of the segments. To perform a quick inspection, we averaged all of the

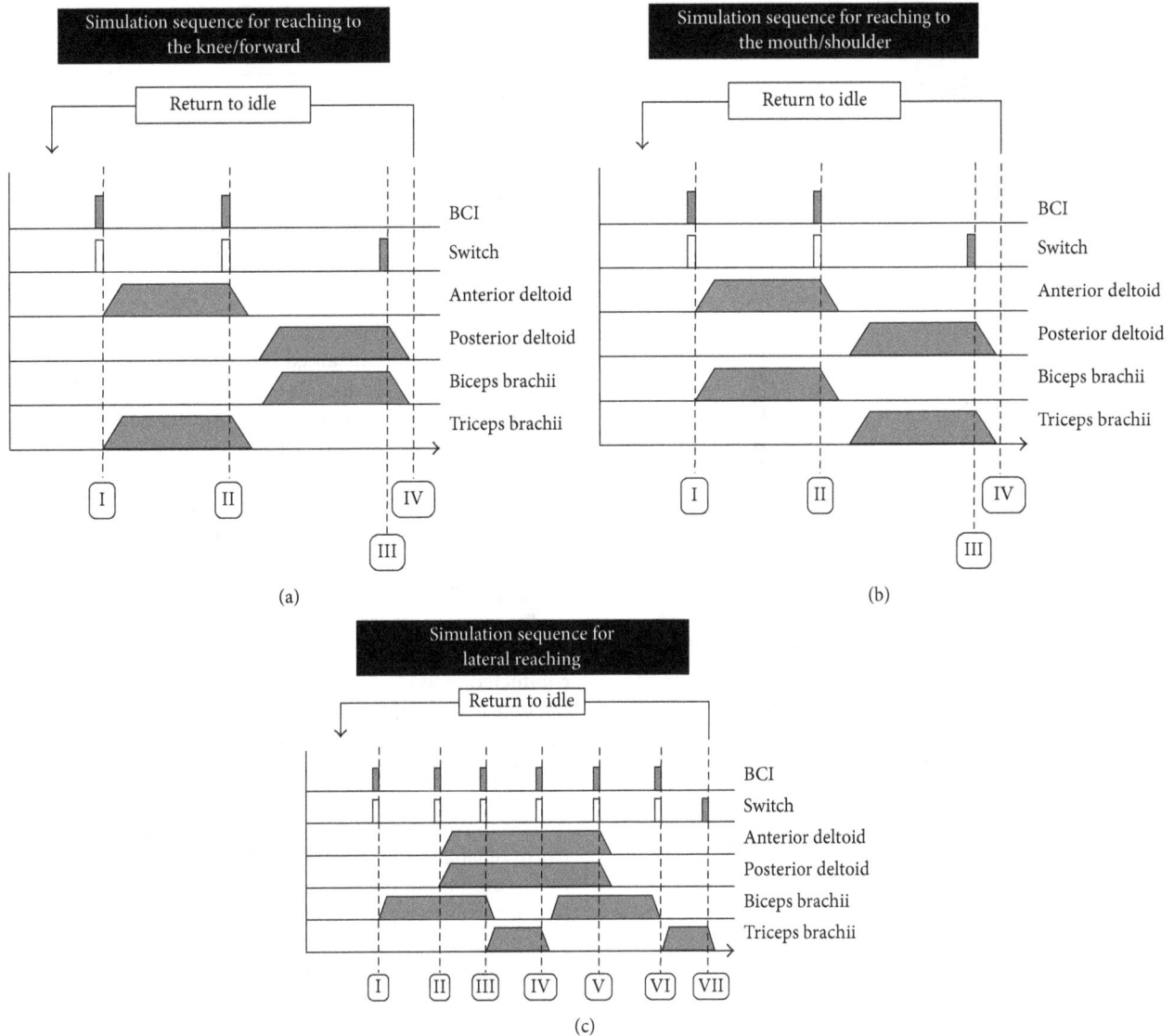

FIGURE 1: Stimulation sequences to facilitate (a) reaching to the right knee/forward, (b) reaching to the mouth/right shoulder, and (c) lateral reaching. For all sequences, activation of the BCI or switch would produce transition into the next phase of the movement. Empty rectangles in the "switch" component indicate optional activation.

spectrograms from all of the electrodes, which revealed the potential locations and frequency bands displaying ERD. This preliminary step helped us in the process of generating ERD maps.

We generated ERD maps following the procedure described in [27]. Briefly, we applied a bank of band pass filters from 4 Hz to 30 Hz with overlapping bandwidths; the filters' center frequencies were separated by 1 Hz and had a bandwidth of 2 Hz. We squared every sample of every trial and applied a moving average filter (1 second) to smooth the resulting power signals, which we then averaged. The two seconds prior to the Go signal were averaged over time to obtain an estimate of baseline power for every sample and every spectral component. The remaining samples of the average power signal were expressed as relative changes (percentage) of the baseline power. We used t-statistic ($t =$

0.05) bootstrapping (500 bootstraps) to perform statistical validation of the observed changes in power. The process revealed Fz to be the site with the strongest ERD within the beta frequency band (18 Hz–28 Hz). This electrode and frequency band were used for the implementation of the BCI.

Once the suitable electrode placement and frequency range were determined, we created the BCI using a single EEG channel (Fz) recorded using a desktop biopotential amplifier (QP511, Grass-Telefunken, Germany) and a data acquisition system (USB-6363, National Instruments, USA) at a rate of 200 Hz prior to its acquisition. The EEG activity was band-limited between 10 Hz and 100 Hz and amplification gain of 20,000.

The BCI was implemented as a "brain-switch" that produced a monostable binary (on/off) control signal. This design supported the immediate integration of the BCI into

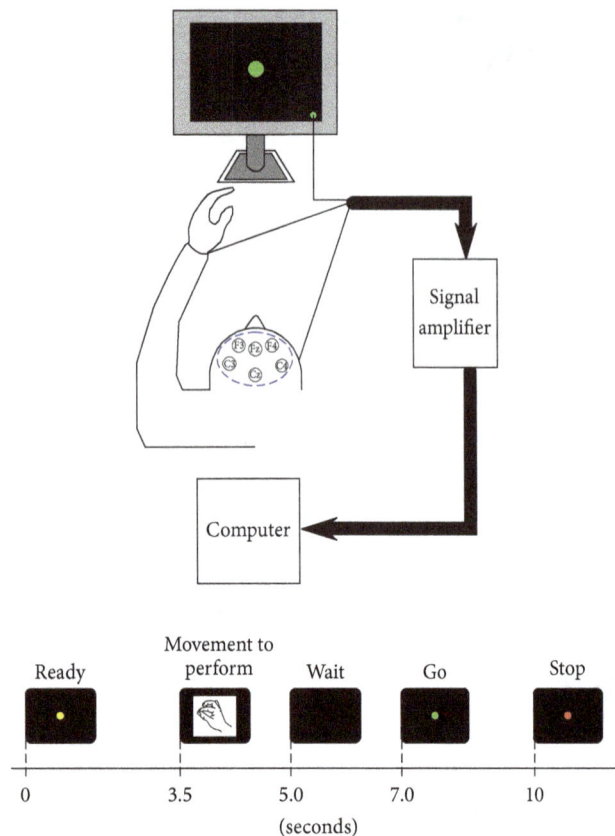

TABLE 1: Movements performed for BCI configuration.

Movement	Number of repetitions
Precision pinch	20
Hand closing (fist)	26
Lateral pinch	34
Hand opening	24
Total	104

FIGURE 2: Experimental sequence used during calibration of the brain-computer interface. The participant sat comfortably in front of a computer monitor that provided cues indicating when to attempt specific movements with his paralyzed hand. These movements included precision pinch, hand closing (fist), lateral pinch, and hand opening and were presented at random.

The brain-switch was activated whenever the power in the resulting signal was sustained below an activation threshold for a prespecified duration. As with the parameters for the line equation used to constrain the range of the moving average, the activation threshold and latency values were also set manually by the second experimenter using the online display of the corrected RMS moving average. Adjustment of these two parameters changed the responsiveness of the BCI. Figure 3 describes the implementation of the BCI used in this work, which was developed originally for creating BCI systems in environments with severe temporal and equipment restrictions (e.g., a limited number of electrodes), common in work conducted with electrocorticographic recordings [28]. Once the switch was activated, it was not possible to trigger it until the second experimenter "armed" it again. This made it possible for the participant to perform the motor tasks without a temporal restriction.

It is important to mention that while continuous BCI control of rehabilitation technologies provides a unique opportunity to monitor online the cerebral activity as related to motor attempt or imagery, a triggering approach does not imply that patients only attempt a motor task prior to the activation of the rehabilitation device (whether this is accomplished with a manual switch, electromyographic signal, mechanical cue, or BCI) but they rather continue with this attempt throughout the duration of each movement. In the context of FES therapy, the continued attempt to perform a voluntary movement is accomplished by asking patients to perform complete functional tasks (e.g., reach, grasp, retrieve, and release an object). In addition, there are several important factors that make FES unsuitable for online control. First, the movements produced by FES do not have the precision of other rehabilitation devices (such as a mechanized orthosis or a rehabilitation robotic system), which requires the intervention of an external agent (e.g., a therapist) to guide the limb in motion. Second, the dynamical behaviour of FES as it acts on the neuromuscular system has not been characterized successfully, severely restricting close-loop control FES applications.

FES therapy in which a switch is typically used to activate the electrical stimulation. The efficacy of "manually triggered" FEST has been demonstrated by several studies [4–8] and it is a current standard of practice within our clinical services. To do this, the root mean square (RMS) value of the EEG activity in the beta frequency range (18 Hz–30 Hz) was estimated every 125 ms. This value was then used to calculate a moving average that included the RMS values over the previous 500 ms (i.e., four estimates). This moving average was then processed with a simple line equation (i.e., $y = mx + b$) and the resulting modified moving average was displayed continuously on a computer screen in both graphical and numerical forms. This information was available to both experimenters constantly and it allowed for selecting the activation parameters for the BCI (all of them available through a graphical user interface). The same information also made it possible to monitor the BCI performance. The parameters m and b of the equation were adjusted heuristically by the second experimenter throughout each experimental session and allowed him to constrain the range of the signal (moving average). This range could be chosen arbitrarily at the preference of the experimenter.

2.2.3. Integrated BCI and FEST System. Integration of the BCI and FEST system was achieved with a single pulse (Transistor-Transistor-Logic (TTL) levels) that could produce a change in the state of the electrical stimulation sequence (Figure 1). In addition to the BCI, the stimulation sequence could also be triggered/controlled using an external switch. This was done to allow for bypassing the BCI in cases

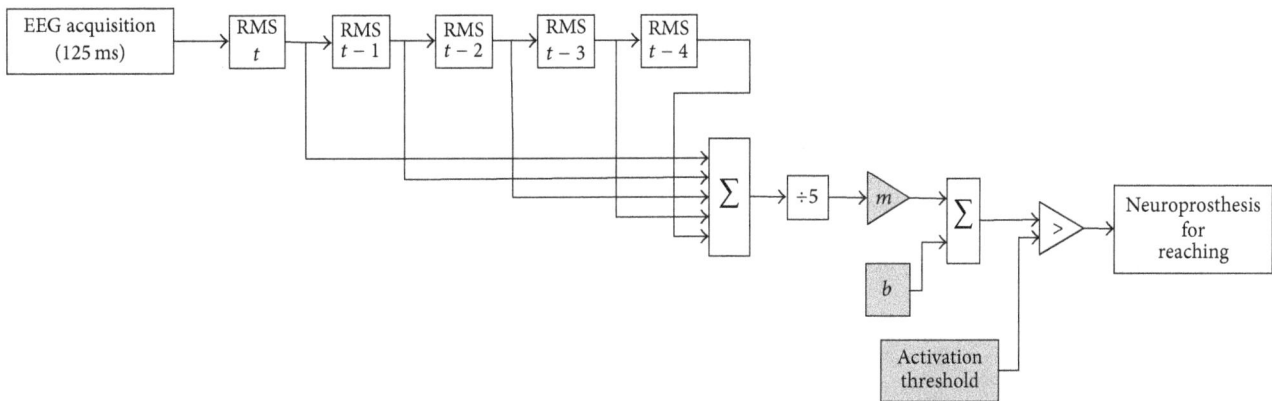

FIGURE 3: Implementation of the BCI. The BCI was implemented as "brain-switch" by comparing a moving average of the RMS values calculated over 625 ms decreased below an activation threshold. Elements in grey (m, b, and the activation threshold) were set heuristically by one of the experimenters throughout the experimental sessions using an online display of the RMS moving average as reference. The external switch is not shown in the figure.

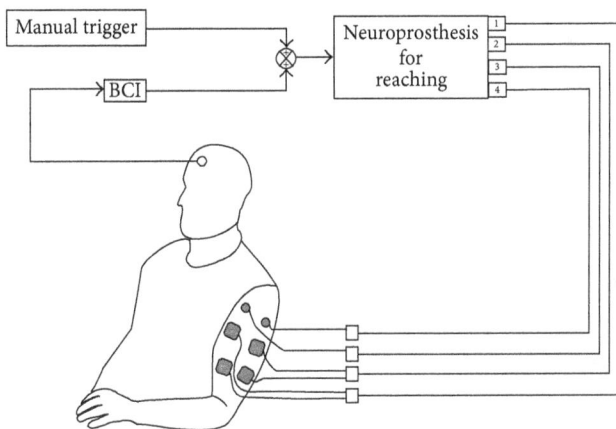

FIGURE 4: Illustration of the integrated BCI and FEST system. The electrical stimulation was delivered with a four-channel neuroprosthesis for reaching which could be triggered with a BCI or a manual switch. The BCI used the signal from a single electrode (positioned at location Fz of the 10–20 EEG electrode placement system), and the manual switch allowed for activating the stimulator whenever the BCI failed to identify the intention to move (note that ground channels for the anterior and posterior deltoid stimulation channels are not shown).

in which it failed to detect the intention to move. Operation with the manual switch was identical to that normally used in standard FEST (without integration with BCI). Figure 4 displays the BCI+FEST system.

2.2.4. Intervention.
Two researchers delivered the EEG-triggered FEST. The first experimenter guided the movement of the arm, facilitated by the neuroprosthesis, while the participant actively attempted the movement. The researcher could also trigger the stimulation using a switch, bypassing the BCI system altogether. This was done to ensure that the stimulation was delivered when required (i.e., when the participant was attempting the movement) even if the BCI

failed to identify the participant's intention to move. Manual activation of the stimulation is used commonly in FEST.

The second experimenter was responsible for making any necessary adjustments to the BCI throughout the duration of each session. These included increasing or decreasing the BCI activation thresholds and enabling or disabling EEG control of the neuroprosthesis for reaching. In addition, he also demonstrated the movements to perform.

The intervention consisted of 40 sessions, each lasting 90 minutes, delivered three times a week. The first 30 minutes of each session were used to prepare all the instrumentation required including placement of the EEG recording electrodes as well as donning and verifying the neuroprosthesis for reaching. The remaining 60 minutes were used to deliver the EEG-triggered FEST.

During the first week of the intervention, the participant received an explanation prior to the beginning of each trained movement including the trajectory to be followed, the starting and final positions of the hand, and the cue indicating the moment in which the movement was to be attempted. He was given the opportunity to practice several times the entire sequence of events until he indicated he was ready to start. It soon became evident that the participant had great difficulty remembering the sequence of actions to follow, which interfered with the intervention. For this reason, starting on the second week, one of the experimenters demonstrated the movement by performing it together with the patient at every repetition during the treatment.

2.2.5. Sequence of Events.
In each session, the participant attempted multiple repetitions of reaching to the mouth and right (opposite) shoulder and reaching forward and to the right (opposite) knee, as well as lateral reaching. All the movements started with the participant's left arm on his side and him sitting with good posture with both feet firmly planted on the ground. One of the experimenters cued the participant as to which specific movement to perform as well as when to attempt the movement. This was done by physically demonstrating the movement to perform, which the

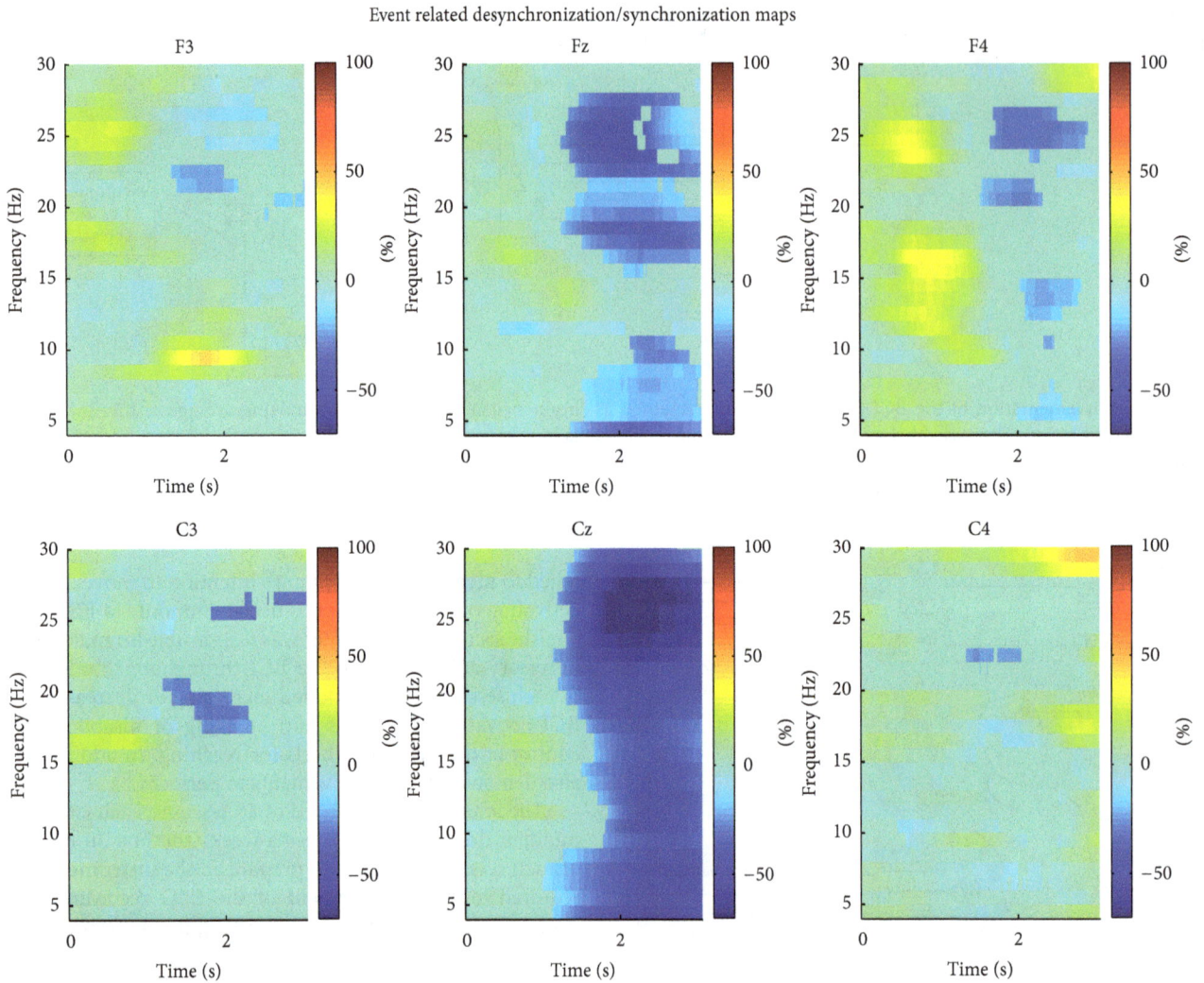

FIGURE 5: Event related desynchronization maps. We decided to use channel Fz for implementation of the BCI as it displayed behaviour resembling typical ERD (i.e., decreases in the alpha and beta ranges), compared to channel Cz, which showed a decrease of power across the entire spectrum. The plots display significant changes in power as a percentage of a two-second baseline period immediately before the Go cue ($t = 0$). Short increases in power were associated with ocular artifacts.

participant followed simultaneously. The movements were performed in phases with a brief pause between them. For example, in the case of reaching to the mouth, the participant would first attempt to touch his mouth with this left (affected) hand, he would then hold the hand in contact with his mouth for 2-3 seconds, and finally he would actively lower his arm back to the starting position. Once the arm was in the starting position, he was allowed to relax for a few moments (in which no electrical stimulation was applied), after which another cycle would start. Each movement was repeated between 20 and 30 times, and the participant was allowed to rest after completing all of the repetitions for each movement.

2.3. Outcomes Measures. We performed five assessments during the baseline, midpoint, and end of the intervention. These included Toronto Rehabilitation Institute-Hand Function Test (TRI-HFT) [29], Action Research Arm Test (ARAT) [30], Functional Independence Measure (FIM) [31], Self-Care Component of the Functional Independence Measure [31], and Fugl-Meyer Assessment Upper Extremity (FMA-UE) subscore [32]. The measured values are shown in Table 4. The Toronto Rehabilitation Institute-Hand Function Test was designed specifically to measure the changes produced during upper limb's rehabilitation using FEST, while the ARAT is an assessment of activity limitations of the upper limb. The FIM and FMA are two of the most widely accepted scales to measure changes during stroke rehabilitation.

3. Results and Discussion

3.1. BCI Configuration. The most reactive electrode was found to be Fz, with decreases in power of 49.4% between the rest and the attempt to move (spectral differences and ERD maps are shown in Figure 5).

TABLE 2: Performance for movements with two phases (reach and retrieve).

| | Movement target | | | | Total |
	Mouth	Shoulder	Forward	Knee	
Number of repetitions	150	123	158	93	524
	Performance figures during reaching				
Expected BCI activation	150	123	158	93	524
Recorded BCI activation	122	100	118	74	414
Successful BCI activation	81.3%	81.3%	74.7%	79.6%	79.0%
	Performance figures during retrieving				
Expected BCI activation	150	123	158	93	524
Recorded BCI activation	87	72	118	58	335
Successful BCI activation	58.0%	58.5%	74.7%	62.4%	63.9%

3.2. BCI Performance.

Transition within each movement phase could be achieved by the BCI so movements with two phases (reaching to the mouth, shoulder, knee, and forward) required two instances of BCI activation, while lateral reaching required six instances of activation. A sample of 6 sessions was chosen to estimate the performance of the BCI. In total, 573 reaching tasks were included in the analysis of which 524 consisted of movements with two phases (i.e., reach and retrieve) and 49 were lateral reaching movements consisting of six different phases. Of the 1048 instances of BCI activation required for two-phase movements, 79% (414/524) and 63.9% (335/524) were successful for reaching and retrieving phases, respectively. Inspection of individual motor tasks revealed 81.3% as the highest BCI performance figure, which was achieved for movements targeting the mouth and shoulder during the reaching phase. In comparison, the lowest performance was recorded during the retrieve phase while reaching to the mouth with a value of 58%. Table 2 provides details of the movements used to generate these results.

With respect to lateral reaching, 63.9% (188/294) of movement phase transitions were achieved with the BCI. Closer inspection showed that the highest accuracy was recorded during the first phase of the movement (performing elbow flexion starting with the arm relaxed on the side of the body) with a value of 93.9% (46/49). The poorest performance was recorded while extending the elbow with the arm abducted (phase III) with a success rate of 36.7% (18/49). Table 3 shows BCI performance figures during lateral reaching.

The BCI responded well to the patient's attempted movements. This was evident by its activation almost exclusively during active periods in which he was instructed to reach with his arm (i.e., not during rest periods).

3.3. Changes in Arm Function.

The Fugl-Meyer Assessment Upper Extremity subscore had a value of 13 points at baseline and of 19 at the end of the intervention. The FIM assessment had a baseline value of 104 points and 118 when the study was completed with the FIM Self-Care subscores registering 28 at baseline and 35 at the time of discharge. The Toronto Rehabilitation Institute-Hand Function Test Object Manipulation subscore and the Action Research Arm Test had a

TABLE 3: Performance for lateral reaching.

Number of repetitions	49
Total expected BCI activation	294
Phase I	Arm relaxed to elbow flexion
Expected BCI activation	49
Recorded BCI activation	46
Successful BCI activation	93.9%
Phase II	Shoulder abduction with elbow flexion
Expected BCI activation	49
Recorded BCI activation	40
Successful BCI activation	81.6%
Phase III	Elbow extension with shoulder abduction
Expected BCI activation	49
Recorded BCI activation	18
Successful BCI activation	36.7%
Phase IV	Shoulder abduction with elbow flexion
Expected BCI activation	49
Recorded BCI activation	22
Successful BCI activation	44.9%
Phase V	Shoulder adduction with elbow flexion
Expected BCI activation	49
Recorded BCI activation	24
Successful BCI activation	49.0%
Phase VI	Elbow flexion to arm relaxed
Expected BCI activation	49
Recorded BCI activation	38
Successful BCI activation	77.6%

TABLE 4: Performed assessments.

	Baseline	Midpoint	Discharge
TRI Hand Function Test Object Manipulation subscore	0	0	0
Action Research Arm Test	0	0	0
FIM Self-Care subscore	28	35	35
FIM total	104	118	118
Fugl-Meyer Assessment Upper Extremity subscore	13	18	19

baseline value of zero and displayed no change at the end of the intervention.

3.4. Unique Aspects of the Integration of BCI and FEST Technologies. In addition to exploring the efficacy of a BCI-controlled FEST for restoration of upper limb's movements, this work also allowed us to identify elements that may be important for future integration of BCI and FEST technologies. There were unique technical challenges evident throughout the process of using BCI and FEST simultaneously. In addition, operation of a BCI by an individual with chronic severe hemiplegia resulting from stroke, with considerable cortical damage, presented a new set of challenges not commonly observed when BCI systems are tested on able-bodied individuals.

3.4.1. Interference due to Voluntary Movement. One of the most obvious elements for the integration of BCI and FEST, as described here, was that the person using the BCI was actively attempting to move. This is different from one of the fundamental motivations of BCI development in which the technology was envisioned as a method to compensate for a severely limited or nonexisting ability to move voluntarily. We observed frequently muscle contractions unrelated to the required reaching motion, when the person was attempting/struggling to perform a movement. These movements often included pronounced facial gestures and bilateral shoulder contractions and were likely a manifestation of the physical and mental effort that the person was making while trying to move his affected arm. Although we did not measure EMG as part of our intervention, it was evident that the BCI failed to recognize the intention to move in these cases. The severity of this problem was reduced by asking the participant to keep his face and shoulders relaxed.

3.4.2. Interference due to Electrical Stimulation. The electrical stimulation used by the neuroprosthesis to produce the movement may also produce electrical interference affecting the quality of the EEG recordings and subsequent operation of the BCI. The operation of our system did not appear to be affected by the electrical stimulation likely due to the fact that the stimulation pulses were delivered at 40 Hz, while the EEG frequency band used by the BCI was restricted to the beta activity (18 Hz–28 Hz). However, it should be noted that it is not uncommon to use asymmetric pulses, sometimes with discontinuities, which may still affect the spectral content of the EEG activity.

3.4.3. Unobtrusive BCI. Another important feature of the presented work was that the operation of the BCI took a secondary role behind the delivery of FEST. In other words, we considered the delivery of FEST, and not the operation of the BCI, as the most important aspect of the intervention. One potential consequence that should not be overlooked is the level of motivation that the participant had, even at the end of the intervention, which is often not the case for regular FEST (i.e., not integrated with a BCI). This, in combination with the ease by which he could generate (FES assisted) reaching movements, allowed us to complete a much larger number of repetitions per session (approximately 35) than those typically practiced during standard FEST (approximately 10 per movement).

3.5. Potential Impact for Patients. The results observed in this case report suggest that triggering functional electrical stimulation therapy with the intention to move, using EEG indicators signaling motor intent, may produce restoration of reaching movements even 6 years (72 months) after having a stroke. It is also important to mention that the therapeutic effects may apply to individuals with severe hemiplegia (such as the case presented here), a population for which the options for therapy are very limited.

3.6. Weaknesses of the Study. The results show that, with the exception of three intermediate movement phases during lateral reaching, the BCI produced most of the transitions in the state of the electrical stimulation. We were pleasantly surprised by this finding along with the observed significant change in FMA-UE scores as well as the small increment in FIM Self-Care subscores. However, it is important to acknowledge the external manual switch as a confounding factor. The switch was included in our design as we were trying to create an enhanced version of FEST and we wanted to avoid a situation in which the operation of the BCI interfered with the actual FEST intervention. Future investigations of BCI-triggered FEST targeting multiple movements excluding the use of an external switch are warranted.

With respect to the manual selection of range-limiting and activation parameters, all values could be adjusted automatically in future versions of the system presented here. This could be accomplished using an online recursive calibration approach allowing us to obtain a measure of power at rest (baseline) and during attempting to perform a movement. However, it is important to point out that in the work described here activation of the BCI triggered a transition between different phases of the movement (e.g., forward reach and retract) which may require different processing including, for example, movement-phase-specific activation thresholds.

Another important potential weakness of the work presented is the demonstration performed by one of the experimenters to the participant. This, while it allowed the intervention to proceed without interruptions by the patient to clarify the type of movement to perform and the moment to execute it (both constant problems during the initial sessions), may have diverted the patient's attention towards the experimenter and away from the execution of the motor task. However, it should be mentioned that a fundamental therapeutic component of FEST is the use of functional tasks during the therapeutic intervention, which requires that patients be fully engaged in the motor task. In addition, verbal, visual, and tactile cues are commonly used in rehabilitation to facilitate the initiation of movement.

Also important is to discuss the use of different movements for creating the BCI (i.e., grasping movements) and those facilitated by the FES (i.e., reaching movements). Hand movements were selected due to their common use for the development of ERD-based BCI system. Although suitable for this initial proof-of-concept work, the next versions of our work will try to ensure that configuration of the BCI is performed using the same movements targeted during rehabilitation.

4. Conclusions

A 64-year-old man with chronic severe left hemiplegia resulting from stroke received 40 90-minute sessions of BCI+FEST (brain-computer interface triggered functional electrical stimulation therapy) to restore reaching function (forward, mouth, knee, opposite shoulder, and lateral). Every other intervention that the patient received since having the stroke had failed to produce improvements in his upper limb's function. The BCI used a single EEG channel and triggered individual phases of each of the reaching tasks, when it detected the individual's intention to move.

Competing Interests

Milos R. Popovic is the cofounder, Director, and Chief Technology Officer of the Canadian company MyndTec Inc., which develops and distributes equipment and therapies for the rehabilitation after stroke and spinal cord injuries. All other authors have no competing interests.

Acknowledgments

The authors wish to thank Ms. Kathryn Atwell for her help in the preparation of the illustrations included in this document. Funding for this project was provided by the Natural Sciences and Engineering Research Council (Discovery Grant no. 249669) and Toronto Rehab Foundation.

References

[1] B. H. Dobkin, "Strategies for stroke rehabilitation," *The Lancet Neurology*, vol. 3, no. 9, pp. 528–536, 2004.

[2] B. Cheeran, L. Cohen, B. Dobkin et al., "The future of restorative neurosciences in stroke: driving the translational research pipeline from basic science to rehabilitation of people after stroke," *Neurorehabilitation and Neural Repair*, vol. 23, no. 2, pp. 97–107, 2009.

[3] M. B. Popovic, D. B. Popovic, T. Sinkjær, A. Stefanovic, and L. Schwirtlich, "Restitution of reaching and grasping promoted by functional electrical therapy," *Artificial Organs*, vol. 26, no. 3, pp. 271–275, 2002.

[4] M. R. Popovic, T. A. Thrasher, V. Zivanovic, J. Takaki, and V. Hajek, "Neuroprosthesis for retraining reaching and grasping functions in severe hemiplegic patients," *Neuromodulation*, vol. 8, no. 1, pp. 58–72, 2005.

[5] M. R. Popovic, T. A. Thrasher, M. E. Adams, V. Takes, V. Zivanovic, and M. I. Tonack, "Functional electrical therapy: retraining grasping in spinal cord injury," *Spinal Cord*, vol. 44, no. 3, pp. 143–151, 2006.

[6] T. A. Thrasher, V. Zivanovic, W. McIlroy, and M. R. Popovic, "Rehabilitation of reaching and grasping function in severe hemiplegic patients using functional electrical stimulation therapy," *Neurorehabilitation and Neural Repair*, vol. 22, no. 6, pp. 706–714, 2008.

[7] N. Kapadia, K. Masani, B. Catharine Craven et al., "A randomized trial of functional electrical stimulation for walking in incomplete spinal cord injury: effects on walking competency," *Journal of Spinal Cord Medicine*, vol. 37, no. 5, pp. 511–524, 2014.

[8] N. M. Kapadia, M. K. Nagai, V. Zivanovic et al., "Functional electrical stimulation therapy for recovery of reaching and grasping in severe chronic pediatric stroke patients," *Journal of Child Neurology*, vol. 29, no. 4, pp. 493–499, 2014.

[9] J. R. Wolpaw, N. Birbaumer, W. J. Heetderks et al., "Brain-computer interface technology: a review of the first international meeting," *IEEE Transactions on Rehabilitation Engineering*, vol. 8, no. 2, pp. 164–173, 2000.

[10] N. Birbaumer, N. Ghanayim, T. Hinterberger et al., "A spelling device for the paralysed," *Nature*, vol. 398, no. 6725, pp. 297–298, 1999.

[11] J. R. Wolpaw and D. J. McFarland, "Control of a two-dimensional movement signal by a noninvasive brain-computer interface in humans," *Proceedings of the National Academy of Sciences of the United States of America*, vol. 101, no. 51, pp. 17849–17854, 2004.

[12] G. Schalk, K. J. Miller, N. R. Anderson et al., "Two-dimensional movement control using electrocorticographic signals in humans," *Journal of Neural Engineering*, vol. 5, no. 1, pp. 75–84, 2008.

[13] G. Pfurtscheller, C. Guger, G. Müller, G. Krausz, and C. Neuper, "Brain oscillations control hand orthosis in a tetraplegic," *Neuroscience Letters*, vol. 292, no. 3, pp. 211–214, 2000.

[14] C. Márquez-Chin, M. R. Popovic, T. Cameron, A. M. Lozano, and R. Chen, "Control of a neuroprosthesis for grasping using off-line classification of electrocorticographic signals: case study," *Spinal Cord*, vol. 47, no. 11, pp. 802–808, 2009.

[15] G. Pfurtscheller, G. R. Müller, J. Pfurtscheller, H. J. Gerner, and R. Rupp, "'Thought'—control of functional electrical stimulation to restore hand grasp in a patient with tetraplegia," *Neuroscience Letters*, vol. 351, no. 1, pp. 33–36, 2003.

[16] G. R. Müller-Putz, R. Scherer, G. Pfurtscheller, and R. Rupp, "EEG-based neuroprosthesis control: a step towards clinical practice," *Neuroscience Letters*, vol. 382, no. 1-2, pp. 169–174, 2005.

[17] G. Pfurtscheller, D. Flotzinger, and J. Kalcher, "Brain-computer interface—a new communication device for handicapped persons," *Journal of Microcomputer Applications*, vol. 16, no. 3, pp. 293–299, 1993.

[18] G. Pfurtscheller and A. Aranibar, "Evaluation of event-related desynchronization (ERD) preceding and following voluntary self-paced movement," *Electroencephalography and Clinical Neurophysiology*, vol. 46, no. 2, pp. 138–146, 1979.

[19] G. Pfurtscheller, C. Neuper, D. Flotzinger, and M. Pregenzer, "EEG-based discrimination between imagination of right and left hand movement," *Electroencephalography and Clinical Neurophysiology*, vol. 103, no. 6, pp. 642–651, 1997.

[20] J. J. Daly and J. R. Wolpaw, "Brain-computer interfaces in neurological rehabilitation," *The Lancet Neurology*, vol. 7, no. 11, pp. 1032–1043, 2008.

[21] A. Ramos-Murguialday, D. Broetz, M. Rea et al., "Brain-machine interface in chronic stroke rehabilitation: a controlled study," *Annals of Neurology*, vol. 74, no. 1, pp. 100–108, 2013.

[22] F. Pichiorri, G. Morone, M. Petti et al., "Brain-computer interface boosts motor imagery practice during stroke recovery," *Annals of Neurology*, vol. 77, no. 5, pp. 851–865, 2015.

[23] K. K. Ang, K. S. G. Chua, K. S. Phua et al., "A randomized controlled trial of EEG-based motor imagery brain-computer interface robotic rehabilitation for stroke," *Clinical EEG and Neuroscience*, vol. 46, no. 4, pp. 310–320, 2015.

[24] J. J. Daly, R. Cheng, J. Rogers, K. Litinas, K. Hrovat, and M. Dohring, "Feasibility of a new application of noninvasive brain computer interface (BCI): a case study of training for recovery of volitional motor control after stroke," *Journal of Neurologic Physical Therapy*, vol. 33, no. 4, pp. 203–211, 2009.

[25] C. Gowland, P. Stratford, M. Ward et al., "Measuring physical impairment and disability with the chedoke-mcmaster stroke assessment," *Stroke*, vol. 24, no. 1, pp. 58–63, 1993.

[26] M. R. Popovic and T. Keller, "Modular transcutaneous functional electrical stimulation system," *Medical Engineering and Physics*, vol. 27, no. 1, pp. 81–92, 2005.

[27] B. Graimann, J. E. Huggins, S. P. Levine, and G. Pfurtscheller, "Visualization of significant ERD/ERS patterns in multichannel EEG and ECoG data," *Clinical Neurophysiology*, vol. 113, no. 1, pp. 43–47, 2002.

[28] C. Márquez-Chin, M. R. Popovic, E. Sanin, R. Chen, and A. M. Lozano, "Real-time two-dimensional asynchronous control of a computer cursor with a single subdural electrode," *Journal of Spinal Cord Medicine*, vol. 35, no. 5, pp. 382–391, 2012.

[29] N. Kapadia, V. Zivanovic, M. Verrier, and M. R. Popovic, "Toronto rehabilitation institute-hand function test: assessment of gross motor function in individuals with spinal cord injury," *Topics in Spinal Cord Injury Rehabilitation*, vol. 18, no. 2, pp. 167–186, 2012.

[30] R. C. Lyle, "A performance test for assessment of upper limb function in physical rehabilitation treatment and research," *International Journal of Rehabilitation Research*, vol. 4, no. 4, pp. 483–492, 1981.

[31] T. A. Dodds, D. P. Martin, W. C. Stolov, and R. A. Deyo, "A validation of the functional independence measurement and its performance among rehabilitation inpatients," *Archives of Physical Medicine and Rehabilitation*, vol. 74, no. 5, pp. 531–536, 1993.

[32] A. R. Fugl-Meyer, L. Jääskö, I. Leyman, S. Olsson, and S. Steglind, "The post-stroke hemiplegic patient. 1. A method for evaluation of physical performance," *Scandinavian Journal of Rehabilitation Medicine*, vol. 7, no. 1, pp. 13–31, 1975.

Permissions

The contributors of this book come from diverse backgrounds, making this book a truly international effort. This book will bring forth new frontiers with its revolutionizing research information and detailed analysis of the nascent developments around the world.

We would like to thank all the contributing authors for lending their expertise to make the book truly unique. They have played a crucial role in the development of this book. Without their invaluable contributions this book wouldn't have been possible. They have made vital efforts to compile up to date information on the varied aspects of this subject to make this book a valuable addition to the collection of many professionals and students.

This book was conceptualized with the vision of imparting up-to-date information and advanced data in this field. To ensure the same, a matchless editorial board was set up. Every individual on the board went through rigorous rounds of assessment to prove their worth. After which they invested a large part of their time researching and compiling the most relevant data for our readers.

The editorial board has been involved in producing this book since its inception. They have spent rigorous hours researching and exploring the diverse topics which have resulted in the successful publishing of this book. They have passed on their knowledge of decades through this book. To expedite this challenging task, the publisher supported the team at every step. A small team of assistant editors was also appointed to further simplify the editing procedure and attain best results for the readers.

Apart from the editorial board, the designing team has also invested a significant amount of their time in understanding the subject and creating the most relevant covers. They scrutinized every image to scout for the most suitable representation of the subject and create an appropriate cover for the book.

The publishing team has been an ardent support to the editorial, designing and production team. Their endless efforts to recruit the best for this project, has resulted in the accomplishment of this book. They are a veteran in the field of academics and their pool of knowledge is as vast as their experience in printing. Their expertise and guidance has proved useful at every step. Their uncompromising quality standards have made this book an exceptional effort. Their encouragement from time to time has been an inspiration for everyone.

The publisher and the editorial board hope that this book will prove to be a valuable piece of knowledge for researchers, students, practitioners and scholars across the globe.

List of Contributors

Michiko Arima, Atsuko Ogata, Kazumi Kawahira and Megumi Shimodozono
Department of Rehabilitation and Physical Medicine, Kagoshima University Graduate School of Medical and Dental Sciences, Kagoshima, Japan

Valentina Arnao, Marianna Riolo, Giovanni Savettieri and Paolo Aridon
Dipartimento di Biomedicina Sperimentale e Neuroscienze Cliniche, Universit`a degli Studi di Palermo, Palermo, Italy

Firas Ido, Reina Badran, Brandon Dmytruk and Zain Kulairi
Wayne State University School of Medicine, 1101W. University Drive, 2 South, Rochester, MI 48307, USA

Jung koo Lee, Hak-cheol Ko and Jin-gyu Choi
Department of Neurosurgery, Seoul St. Mary's Hospital, College of Medicine, The Catholic University of Korea, Seoul, Republic of Korea

Byung-chul Son
Department of Neurosurgery, Seoul St. Mary's Hospital, College of Medicine, The Catholic University of Korea, Seoul, Republic of Korea
Catholic Neuroscience Institute, College of Medicine, The Catholic University of Korea, Seoul, Republic of Korea

Youn Soo Lee
Department of Hospital Pathology, Seoul St. Mary's Hospital, College of Medicine, The Catholic University of Korea, Seoul, Republic of Korea

Chiaki Takahashi
Department of Neurosurgery, Takaoka City Hospital, 4-1, Takara-machi, Takaoka, Toyama, Japan

Christopher Payne, Kristen Stabingas, Dunbar Alcindor, Khaled Abdel Aziz and Alexander Yu
Department of Neurosurgery, Allegheny General Hospital, Pittsburgh, PA, USA

Ali Batouli and Robert Williams
Department of Radiology, Allegheny General Hospital, Pittsburgh, PA, USA

Cunfeng Pu
Department of Pathology, Allegheny General Hospital, Pittsburgh, PA, USA

Elizabeth Tyler-Kabara
Department of Neurological Surgery, Children's Hospital of Pittsburgh, University of Pittsburgh, Pittsburgh, PA, USA

Ahmed Mustafa Ibrahim, Tarek Talaat ElSefi, Maha Ghanem, Akram Muhammad Fayed and Nesreen Adel Shaban
Faculty of Medicine, Alexandria University, Alexandria, Egypt

James Fowler, Brian Fiani, Vladimir Cortez and Javed Siddiqi
Department of Neurosurgery, Desert Regional Medical Center, Palm Springs, CA, USA

Syed A. Quadri
Department of Neurosurgery, Desert Regional Medical Center, Palm Springs, CA, USA
Department of Neurology, University of New Mexico, Albuquerque, NM, USA

Mudassir Frooqui, Atif Zafar and Asad Ikram
Department of Neurology, University of New Mexico, Albuquerque, NM, USA

Fahad Shabbir Ahmed
Department of Pathology, Yale School of Medicine, New Haven, CT, USA

Anirudh Ramachandran
College of Osteopathic Medicine of the Pacific, Western University of Health Sciences, Pomona, CA, USA

Ryota Tamura, Yoshiaki Kuroshima and Yoshiki Nakamura
Department of Neurosurgery, Tokyo Medical Center, 2-5-1 Higashigaoka, Meguro-ku, Tokyo 152-8902, Japan

Jin-gyu Choi and Hak-cheol Ko
Department of Neurosurgery, Seoul St. Mary's Hospital, College of Medicine, The Catholic University of Korea, Seoul, Republic of Korea

Byung-chul Son
Department of Neurosurgery, Seoul St. Mary's Hospital, College of Medicine, The Catholic University of Korea, Seoul, Republic of Korea
Catholic Neuroscience Institute, College of Medicine, The Catholic University of Korea, Seoul, Republic of Korea

Suma Shah, Anastasie Dunn-Pirio, Matthew Luedke, Mark Skeen and Christopher Eckstein
Duke University Department of Neurology, USA

Joel Morgenlander
Duke University Departments of Neurology and Orthopedic Surgery, USA

Sara Khodor
University of South Florida, Tampa, FL, USA

Scott Blumenthal
South Florida Neurology Associates, Boca Raton, FL, USA

Francesco Berti and Zeeshan Arif
Division of Clinical Neuroscience, University of Nottingham School of Medicine, Nottingham, UK

Cris Constantinescu
Division of Clinical Neuroscience, University of Nottingham School of Medicine, Nottingham, UK
Department of Neurology, Nottingham University Hospitals NHS Trust, Nottingham, UK

Bruno Gran
Department of Neurology, Nottingham University Hospitals NHS Trust, Nottingham, UK

Yiolanda-Panayiota Christou, Elena Kkolou, Annita Ormiston and Kleopas A. Kleopa
Neurology Clinics, The Cyprus Institute of Neurology and Genetics, Nicosia, Cyprus

George A. Tanteles
Clinical Genetics Clinic, The Cyprus Institute of Neurology and Genetics, Nicosia, Cyprus

Kostas Konstantopoulos
European University Cyprus, Nicosia, Cyprus

Maria Beconi, Randall D. Marshall and Horacio Plotkin
Retrophin Inc., New York, NY, USA

Hussein Algahtani
King Abdulaziz Medical City/King Saud bin Abdulaziz University for Health Sciences, Jeddah 21483, Saudi Arabia

Ahmad Subahi
King Saud bin AbdulazizUniversity for Health Sciences, Jeddah 21483, Saudi Arabia

Bader Shirah
King Abdullah International Medical Research Center/ King Saud bin Abdulaziz University for Health Sciences, Jeddah 21483, Saudi Arabia

Jin-gyu Choi
Department of Neurosurgery, Seoul St.Mary'sHospital College ofMedicine, The Catholic University of Korea, Seoul, Republic of Korea

Byung-chul Son
Department of Neurosurgery, Seoul St.Mary'sHospital College ofMedicine, The Catholic University of Korea, Seoul, Republic of Korea
Catholic Neuroscience Institute, College of Medicine, The Catholic University of Korea, Seoul, Republic of Korea

Elizabeth O'Keefe
Department of Neurology, Division of Physical Medicine and Rehabilitation, Washington University School of Medicine, Campus 4444 Forest Park Blvd., St. Louis, MO 63108, USA

Katherine E. Schwetye
Department of Pathology and Immunology, Division of Neuropathology, Saint Louis University School of Medicine, 1402 South Grand Blvd., Saint Louis, MO 63104, USA

John Nazarian
Department of Radiology, Wake Radiology, 3949 Browning Place, Raleigh, NC 2760, USA

Richard Perrin and Robert E. Schmidt
Department of Pathology and Immunology, Division of Neuropathology, Washington University School ofMedicine, Campus 660 S. Euclid Ave., St. Louis, MO 63110, USA

Robert Bucelli
Department of Neurology, Divisions of Neuromuscular and General Neurology, Washington University School of Medicine, Campus 660 S. Euclid Ave., St. Louis, MO 63110, USA

E. Frezza, C. Terracciano, M. Giacanelli, E. Rastelli, G. Greco and R.Massa
Neuromuscular Diseases Unit, Department of Systems Medicine, University of Rome Tor Vergata, Rome, Italy

Semiha Kurt, Betul Cevik and Durdane Aksoy
Department of Neurology, Gaziosmanpasa University Faculty of Medicine, 60100 Tokat, Turkey

E. Irmak Sahbaz, Aslı Gundogdu Eken and A. Nazli Basak
Suna and Inan Kırac¸ Foundation Neurodegeneration Research Laboratory, Molecular Biology and Genetics Department, Bogazici University, 34342 Istanbul, Turkey

Shinji Shimato, Toshihisa Nishizawa, Takashi Yamanouchi, Takashi Mamiya, Kojiro Ishikawa and Kyozo Kato
Department of Neurosurgery, Kariya Toyota General Hospital, 5-15 Sumiyoshi-cho, Kariya City, Aichi 448-8505, Japan

Jun Takei, Toshihide Tanaka, Yohei Yamamoto, Akihiko Teshigawara, Satoru Tochigi and Yuzuru Hasegawa
Department of Neurosurgery, Jikei University School of Medicine Kashiwa Hospital, 163-1 Kashiwa-shita, Kashiwa, Chiba 277-8567, Japan

Yuichi Murayama
Department of Neurosurgery, Jikei University School of Medicine, 3-25-8 Nishi-Shinbashi, Minato-ku, Tokyo 105-8461, Japan

François-Xavier Sibille, Philippe Hantson and Simone Giglioli
Department of Intensive Care, Université Catholique de Louvain, Cliniques St-Luc, 1200 Brussels, Belgium

Thierry Duprez
Department of Neuroradiology, Université Catholique de Louvain, Cliniques St-Luc, 1200 Brussels, Belgium

Vincent van Pesch
Laboratory of Neurophysiology, Université Catholique de Louvain, Cliniques St-Luc, 1200 Brussels, Belgium

Matthew Herrmann, Prissilla Xu and Antonio Liu
White Memorial Medical Center Department of Internal Medicine, Los Angeles, CA, USA

L. M. Conners, P. H. Janda and Z. Mudasir
Department of Neurology, Valley Hospital Medical Center, Las Vegas, NV, USA

R. Ahad
Pediatric Neurology, University of Las Vegas School of Medicine, Las Vegas, NV, USA

Ritsuo Hashimoto, Tomoko Ogawa, Asako Tagawa and Hiroyuki Kato
Department ofNeurology, International University of Health andWelfare Hospital, Tochigi, Japan

Lauren Surdyke, Jennifer Fernandez, Hannah Foster and Pamela Spigel
Brooks Rehabilitation Hospital, 3599 University Blvd S, Jacksonville, FL 32216, USA

Waqar Waheed, Christopher Trevino and W. Pendlebury
Department of Neurological Sciences, University of Vermont College of Medicine, Burlington, VT 05401, USA

Anjali L. Varigonda
Department of Psychiatry, University of Vermont College of Medicine, Burlington, VT 05401, USA

Chris E. Holmes
Hematology/Oncology Division, Department of Medicine, University of Vermont College of Medicine, Burlington, VT 05401, USA

Neil M. Bordenfv
Department of Radiology, University of Vermont College of Medicine, Burlington, VT 05401, USA

Robert Gross
Department of Neurology, Icahn School of Medicine at Mount Sinai, New York, NY 10029, USA

Jennifer Davis
Department of Psychiatry, Rhode Island Hospital, Brown University School of Medicine, Providence, RI 02903, USA

Julie Roth and Henry Querfurth
Department of Neurology, Rhode Island Hospital, Brown University School of Medicine, Providence, RI 02903, USA

Sonal Saran, Rengarajan Rajagopal, Pushpinder S. Khera and Neeraj Mehta
Department of Radiology, AIIMS Jodhpur, Jodhpur 342005, India

Kaylan M. Brady
Department of Pediatrics, Staten Island University Hospital-Northwell Health, Staten Island, NY, USA

Jonathan A. Blau
Division of Neonatology, Department of Pediatrics, Staten Island University Hospital-Northwell Health, Staten Island, NY, USA

Spencer J. Serras
Division of Neuroradiology, Department of Radiology, Staten Island University Hospital-Northwell Health, Staten Island, NY, USA

Jeremy T. Neuman
Division of Pediatric Radiology, Department of Radiology, Staten Island University Hospital-Northwell Health, Staten Island, NY, USA

Richard Sidlow
Division of Pediatric Hospitalist Medicine, Department of Pediatrics, Staten Island University Hospital-Northwell Health, Staten Island, NY, USA

A. G. T. A. Kariyawasam
Registrar in Medicine, University Medical Unit, Teaching Hospital Karapitiya, Sri Lanka

C. L. Fonseka and H. M. M. Herath
Consultant Physician, Department of Internal Medicine, Faculty of Medicine, University of Ruhuna, Sri Lanka
Consultant Physician, University Medical Unit, Teaching Hospital, Karapitiya, Galle, Sri Lanka

S. D. A. L. Singhapura and J. S. Hewavithana
Consultant Physician, University Medical Unit, Teaching Hospital, Karapitiya, Galle, Sri Lanka

K. D. Pathirana
Professor in Neurology, Department of Internal Medicine, Faculty of Medicine, University of Ruhuna, Sri Lanka

Yi Zhang and Abhay Kumar
Department of Neurology, Saint Louis University, Saint Louis, MO 63110, USA

John B. Tezel and Yihua Zhou
Department of Radiology, Saint Louis University, Saint Louis, MO 63110, USA

Ha Son Nguyen
Neurosurgery, Medical College of Wisconsin, Milwaukee, WI 53226, USA

Peter Pahapill
Neurosurgery, Medical College of Wisconsin, Milwaukee, WI 53226, USA
Neurosurgery, Clement J. Zablocki VA Medical Center, Milwaukee, WI 53295, USA

Harvey Woehlck
Anesthesiology, Medical College of Wisconsin, Milwaukee, WI 53226, USA

Hiroyuki Toi, Yukari Ogawa, Keita Kinoshita, Satoshi Hirai, Hiroki Takai, Keijiro Hara, Nobuhisa Matsushita, Shunji Matsubara and Masaaki Uno
Department of Neurosurgery, Kawasaki Medical School, Kurashiki, Okayama, Japan

Aaron Marquis
Neural Engineering Laboratory, University Centre, Toronto Rehabilitation Institute-University Health Network, 550 University Avenue, Toronto, ON, Canada M5G 2A2

Philippe Hantson
Department of Intensive Care, Cliniques St-Luc, Université Catholique de Louvain, Brussels, Belgium

Thierry Duprez
Department of Neuroradiology, Cliniques St-Luc, Université Catholique de Louvain, Brussels, Belgium

Cesar Marquez-Chin
Rehabilitation Engineering Laboratory, The Lyndhurst Centre, Toronto Rehabilitation Institute-University Health Network, 520 Sutherland Drive, Toronto, ON, Canada M4G 3V9
Neural Engineering Laboratory, University Centre, Toronto Rehabilitation Institute-University Health Network, 550 University Avenue, Toronto, ON, Canada M5G 2A2

Milos R. Popovic
Rehabilitation Engineering Laboratory, The Lyndhurst Centre, Toronto Rehabilitation Institute-University Health Network, 520 Sutherland Drive, Toronto, ON, Canada M4G 3V9
Rehabilitation Engineering Laboratory, Institute of Biomaterials and Biomedical Engineering, University of Toronto, Mining Building, 164 College Street, Room407, Toronto, ON, Canada M5S 3E3

Index

www.ingramcontent.com/pod-product-compliance
Lightning Source LLC
Chambersburg PA
CBHW070153240326

41458CB00126B/4509